A Practical Guide to
First Trimester of Pregnancy

A Practical Guide to
First Trimester of Pregnancy

Editors

Mala Arora FRCOG (UK) FICOG FICMCH
Director, Noble IVF Centre, Faridabad, Haryana, India
Consultant, Fortis La Femme, Greater Kailash, New Delhi, India

Alok Sharma MD DHA MICOG
Consultant, Obstetrics and Gynecology
Deen Dayal Upadhyaya Hospital
Shimla, Himachal Pradesh, India

Foreword

Hema Divakar

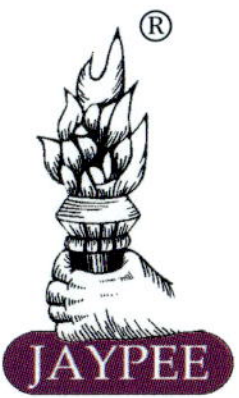

JAYPEE BROTHERS MEDICAL PUBLISHERS (P) LTD.

New Delhi • London • Philadelphia • Panama

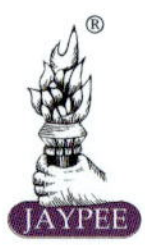

Jaypee Brothers Medical Publishers (P) Ltd

Headquarters

Jaypee Brothers Medical Publishers (P) Ltd
4838/24, Ansari Road, Daryaganj
New Delhi 110 002, India
Phone: +91-11-43574357
Fax: +91-11-43574314
Email: jaypee@jaypeebrothers.com

Overseas Offices

J.P. Medical Ltd
83 Victoria Street, London
SW1H 0HW (UK)
Phone: +44-2031708910
Fax: +02-03-0086180
Email: info@jpmedpub.com

Jaypee Medical Inc
The Bourse
111 South Independence Mall East
Suite 835, Philadelphia, PA 19106, USA
Phone: +1 267-519-9789
Email: joe.rusko@jaypeebrothers.com

Jaypee Brothers Medical Publishers (P) Ltd
Bhotahity, Kathmandu, Nepal
Phone: +977-9741283608
Email: kathmandu@jaypeebrothers.com

Jaypee-Highlights Medical Publishers Inc
City of Knowledge, Bld. 237, Clayton
Panama City, Panama
Phone: +1 507-301-0496
Fax: +1 507-301-0499
Email: cservice@jphmedical.com

Jaypee Brothers Medical Publishers (P) Ltd
17/1-B Babar Road, Block-B, Shaymali
Mohammadpur, Dhaka-1207
Bangladesh
Mobile: +08801912003485
Email: jaypeedhaka@gmail.com

Website: www.jaypeebrothers.com
Website: www.jaypeedigital.com

A Practical Guide to First Trimester of Pregnancy / Eds. Mala Arora and Alok Sharma

First Edition: **2014**

ISBN 978-93-5152-178-5

Printed at: Samrat Offset Pvt. Ltd.

Dedications

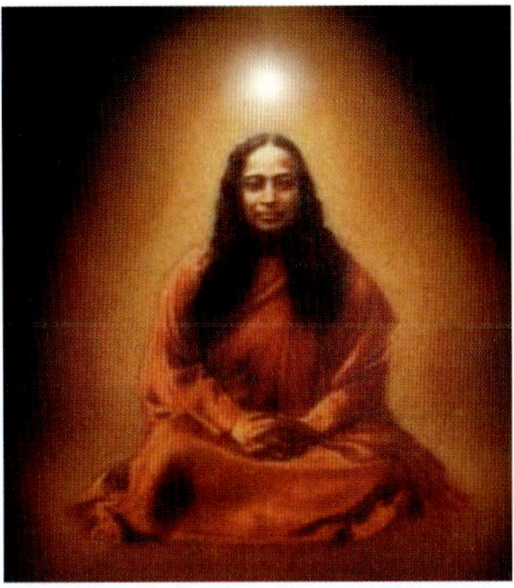

This book is dedicated to my eternal guru Sri Paramhansa Yogananda, founder of Self Realization fellowship (USA) and Yogoda Satsanga Society (India). His invisible guidance was vital for the completion of this manuscript.

My parents who have laid the foundation stone of literacy in me.

My husband Dr Narinder Pal who has not only allowed me to concentrate on my writing but has guided me at every step.

My children who have made me proud by out shining me in every aspect.

Mala Arora

My parents, Smt Dhanwanti Sharma and Shri Hansraj Sharma for shaping my character in my formative years.

My wife, Dr Pratibha Sharma for her immense patience and guidance.

My lovely daughter, Hiranya Sharma.

Alok Sharma

Contents

Contributors

Editors

Mala Arora FRCOG (UK) FICOG FICMCH
Director, Noble IVF Centre, Faridabad
Haryana, India
Consultant, Fortis La Femme, Greater Kailash
New Delhi, India

Alok Sharma MD DHA MICOG
Consultant, Obstetrics and Gynecology
Deen Dayal Upadhyaya Hospital
Shimla, Himachal Pradesh, India

Contributing Authors

Prashant Acharya MD FICOG
Consultant, Fetal Medicine and High Risk Obstetric care
Paras Advanced Centre for Fetal Medicine
Ahmedabad, Gujarat, India

Ashini Acharya MD
Consultant, Fetal Medicine and High Risk Obstetric Care
Paras Advanced Centre for Fetal Medicine
Ahmedabad, Gujarat, India

Sarita Agarwal MD FICOG FIAMS FCGP
Professor and Head, Department of Obstetrics and Gynecology
All India Institute of Medical Sciences
Raipur, Chhattisgarh, India

Maninder Ahuja DGO FICOG
Director, Ahuja Hospital and Infertility Centre
Visiting Consultant, Asian Institute of Medical Sciences
Faridabad, Haryana, India

Ananya Banerjee MD
Senior Resident, Department of Obstetrics and Gynecology
Vardhman Mahavir Medical College and Safdarjung Hospital
New Delhi, India

Kanthi Bansal MD DGO FICOG
Director, Safal Fertility Foundation
Ahmedabad, Gujarat, India

Punita Bhardawaj MD
Senior Consultant, Division of Minimally Invasive Gynecology
Institute of Minimal Access, Metabolic Surgery
Max Hospital, Saket
New Delhi, India

Subhash C Biswas MD FICOG FIMSA
Professor and Head, Department of Obstetrics and Gynecology
Burdwan Medical College
Kolkata, West Bengal, India

Rahul Chauhan MD
Senior Resident, N Wadia Maternity Hospital
Mumbai, Maharashtra, India

Sagnika Dash MBBS
Junior Resident
CSS College of Obstetrics, Gynecology and Childhealth
Kolkata, West Bengal, India

Deepali Dhingra MD
Senior Resident, Department of Obstetrics and Gynecology
Vardhman Mahavir Medical College and Safdarjung Hospital
New Delhi, India

Bharati Dhorepatil DNB DGO Diploma Endoscopy (Germany) FICS PGDCR
Director and Chief IVF Consultant
Pune Fertility Centre
Pune, Maharashtra, India

Yogita Dogra MD
Registrar, Kamla Nehru State Hospital for Mother and Child
IGMC, Shimla, Himachal Pradesh, India

Kusum G Kapoor MD FICOG FICS
Consultant, Obstetrics and Gynecology
Ex Professor and Head, Department of Obstetrics and Gynecology
Nalanda Medical College Hospital
Patna, Bihar, India

Anupam Gupta MS FICMU FICMCH
Consultant, Aakanksha Test Tube Baby Centre
Agra, Uttar Pradesh, India

Sadhana Gupta MS MNAMS FICOG FICMU FICMCH
Senior Consultant, Jeevan Jyoti Hospital and Medical Research Centre
Gorakhpur, Uttar Pradesh, India

Ritu Joshi MS
Honorary Consultant, Obstetrics and Gynecology
Monilek Hospital and Research Centre
Consultant, Fortis Escorts Hospital
Jaipur, Rajasthan, India

Ashis K Mukhopadhyay MD
Professor and Unit-in-Charge, Obstetrics and Gynecology
Medical Superintendent-cum-Vice Principal
CSS College of Obstetrics, Gynecology and Childhealth, Kolkata, West Bengal, India

Anita Kaul MD
Senior Consultant, Apollo Centre for Fetal Medicine
Indraprastha Apollo Hospitals
New Delhi, India

Krishna Kavita Ramavath MD FICOG
Physician Observer Fellow, Gynec-Oncology, Doctors Hospital, Baptist Hospital
South Florida, Miami, USA

Pratap Kumar MD DGO FICS FIGOG
Professor, Department of Obstetrics and Gynecology
Kasturba Medical College, Manipal University
Manipal, Karnataka, India

S Shantha Kumari MD
Professor, Obstetrics and Gynecology
Deccan College of Medical Sciences
Hyderabad, Andhra Pradesh, India

Kiran Kurtkoti DGO DNB
Kurtkoti Nursing Home
Pune, Maharashtra, India

Pooja Lodha DNB Fellow, Fetal Medicine and Fetal Therapy
Lead Consultant
Deparment of Fetal Medicine and Fetal Therapy
Ruby Hall Clinic, Pune, Maharashtra, India

Pragya M Choudhary DFFP MRCOG (London) PhD MICOG
Consultant, Obstetrics and Gynecology
NuLife Test Tube Baby Centre
MGM Hospital and Research Centre
Patna, Bihar, India

Asmita M Rathore MD MRCOG
Director, Professor, Department of Obstetrics and Gynecology, Maulana Azad Medical College and LNJP Hospital, New Delhi, India

Nalini Mahajan MD MMedSci (ART FICOG)
Director, Mother and Child Hospital
New Delhi, India

Sujata Misra MD FICOG
Associate Professor, Department of Obstetrics and Gynecology
SCB Medical College
Cuttack, Odisha, India

Bhavana Mittal FNB, MNAMS, Post Doctoral Fellow in Reproductive Medicine ART
Consultant, Shivam Surgical and Maternity Centre
Delhi
Pushpanjali Institute of IVF and Infertility
Ghaziabad, Uttar Pradesh, India

Neela Mukhopadhaya MBBS DGO (India) MRCOG (UK) FIGOG (India) DRMCH (UK)
Consultant, Obstetrics and Gynecology
Luton and Dunstable Teaching Hospital
Lewsey Road, Luton, United Kingdom

Sudhanshu Nanda MD
Consultant, Obstetrics and Gynecology
Cuttack, Odisha, India

Roza Olyai MS MICOG FICMCH FICOG
Director, Olyai Hospital
Gwalior, Madhya Pradesh, India

Ram P Dey MD DCH MICOG
Assistant Professor, Department of Obstetrics and Gynecology
IPGMER and SSKM Hospital
Kolkata, West Bengal, India

Deepali P Kale DNBE FCPS DGO (MUHS) DGO (CPS)
Assistant Proffessor, Nowrosjee Wadia Maternity Hospital and Seth GS Medical College
Parel, Mumbai, Maharashtra, India

Bhaskar Pal DGO MD DNB FICOG FRCOG
Senior Consultant, Obstetrics and Gynecology
Apollo Gleneagles Hospital
Kolkata, West Bengal, India

Seetha Ramamurthy Pal DGO MD MRCOG RCOG/RCR Diploma in Advanced Obstetric Ultrasound
Consultant, Obstetrics and Gynecology
Apollo Gleneagles Hospital
Kolkata, West Bengal, India

Suchitra N Pandit MD DNBE FRCOG FICOG DFP MNAMS: B Pharm
Consultant, Obstetrics and Gynecology
Kokilaben Dhirubhai Ambani Hospital and Research Centre
Mumbai, Maharashtra, India

Harshad Parasnis MD DNB FCPS DGO FICOG
Consultant Gynecologic Oncologist
Honorary Associate Professor
Bharati Vidyapeeth Medical College
Pune, Maharashtra, India

Madhuri Patel MD DGO FICOG
Honorary Consultant, N Wadia Maternity Hospital
Mumbai, Maharashtra, India

MC Patel MD
Gynecologist and Medicolegal Counsellor
Niru Maternity and Nursing Home
Ahmedabad, Gujarat, India

Deepali Patil MD DGO FCPS
Consultant, Obstetrics and Gynecology
Shri Mahalaxmi Nursing Home
Kolhapur, Maharashtra, India

Ameet Patki MD DNB FCPS FICOG FRCOG (UK)
Medical Director, Fertility Associates, Mumbai
Consultant, Obstetrics and Gynecology
Sir Harkisondas Hospital and Research Centre
Hinduja HealthCare Surgicals
Honorary Associate Professor, Obstetrics and Gynecology
KJ Somaiya Medical College and Hospital
Mumbai, Maharashtra, India

Shashi Prateek MD
Professor and Head, Department of Obstetrics and Gynecology
Vardhman Mahavir Medical College and Safdarjung Hospital
New Delhi, India

Reena Rani MBBS
Postgraduate Student (Obstetrics and Gynecology)
Maulana Azad Medical College
New Delhi, India

Aarti Rapol DNB DGO
Assistant Consultant, Pune Fertility Centre
Pune, Maharashtra, India

Rajat Ray MD
Assistant Professor, Hi-Tech Medical College
Rourkela, Odisha, India

Suvarna S Khadilkar MD DGO FICOG
Consultant, Gyne-Endocrinologist
Bombay Hospital and Medical Research Centre
Mumbai, Maharashtra, India

Jayprakash Shah MD FICOG
Rajni Hospital, Ahmedabad
CIMS Hospital, Science City Road, Ahmedabad
Akar IVF Centre Anand, Ahmedabad
Gujrat, India

Parth Shah MD DGO FIGE
Laproscopist and Fetal Medicine Expert
Rajni Hospital
Ahmedabad, Gujrat, India

Shivani Singh MD DNB FNB (Reproductive Medicine)
Associate Consultant, Mother and Child Hospital
New Delhi, India

Sunita Tandulwadkar MD (OBGY) FICS FICOG Dip in Endoscopy (USA and Germany)
Head of the Department (Obstetrics and Gynecology), Ruby Hall Clinic
Pune, Maharashtra, India

Sangeeta Tejpuria MD
Consultant, Gynecologist and Infertility Specialist
Rajashree Nursing Home
Nagpur, Maharashtra, India

Ajay V Valia MD
Consultant, Isha Hospital, Krishna Hospital
Vadodra, Gujarat, India

D Vidyadhari MD
Professor, Obstetrics and Gynecology
Mediciti Medical College
Hyderabad, Andhra Pradesh, India

Foreword

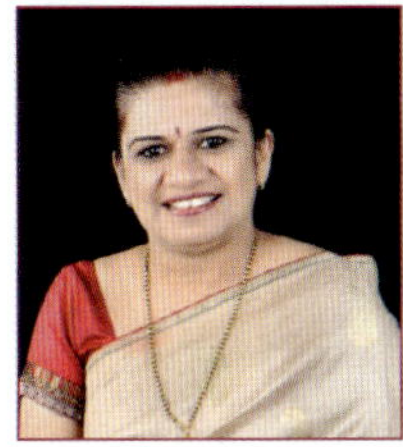

Hema Divakar DGO MD FICMCH FICOG PGDMLE
President, FOGSI 2013
Senior Consultant, Divakar Speciality Hospital
JP Nagar, Bengaluru, India
Director, Mediscan Divakar's Ultrasound Training Program, Bengaluru, India

Eccentricity was once a prized attribute of famous clinicians. However, aberrations in obstetrics such as use of thalidomide resulting in tens and thousands of children with phocomelia have led to widespread reluctance on the part of couples to accept bland reassurances from the doctors. In these days of ready access to internet, one needs to justify one's choice of management.

Fortunately help is at hand. Dr Mala Arora and Dr Alok Sharma have done a superb job in persuading top class clinicians to summarize for us topics related to crucial issues in first trimester of pregnancy. This book is a collection and expansion of the very popular management options, to inform the reader and guide their practice. Our patients deserve it.

This book on "*A Practical Guide to First Trimester of Pregnancy*" is an essential read for all clinicians to help their patients embark on healthy foundations for the journey through a safe pregnancy and successful outcome. I congratulate Dr Mala Arora and Dr Alok Sharma, and all the authors for providing practical and insightful information for best practices in managing routine and complex situations in the first trimester.

Hema Divakar

Preface

"The magical moment of creation of a new life ushers the first trimester"

It gives us immense pleasure to bring forth this '*A Practical Guide to First Trimester of Pregnancy*'. The first trimester is fraught with danger, with a 20% risk of losing the fetus during this time. It requires careful vigilance in patients with assisted conceptions, recurrent miscarriages, advanced maternal age, and preexisting medical disorders. Events of the first trimester lay the foundation, as well as seal the fate of a pregnancy. The booking visit is the most crucial visit for the obstetrician and the triaging of antenatal care is decided in the first trimester. We believe that if the first trimester is handled competently, it can save many adverse pregnancy outcomes for both, the mother and the baby.

In this issue, we have touched on all relevant aspects of the first trimester where the obstetrician may need guidance in decision making. First trimester is the platform on which obstetricians, fetomaternal specialists, endocrinologists, geneticists, sonologists, medical and surgical specialists, dieticians, endoscopists and IVF specialists converge, to ensure a healthy pregnancy.

This book is a practical guide to management of first trimester and its complications and incorporates a blend of accepted guidelines, practical inputs and recent advances. On the journey of pregnancy '*Well Begun is half done!*'

Mala Arora

Alok Sharma

Acknowledgments

We are indebted to all the authors for their contribution to this book, who despite their busy schedule have provided outstanding, up-to-date, and evidence-based chapters on various aspects of first trimester of pregnancy.

We are especially thankful to Dr Surveen Ghumman who has helped us at the conception of the book in elaborating and refining the content list.

We wish to thank Mr JP Vij, CEO Jaypee Brothers Medical Publishers for his encouragement in bringing out this book. The editorial team under the able leadership of Dr Madhu Choudhary has extended excellent support to me and worked untiringly to shape up this manuscript.

Mala Arora

Alok Sharma

Physiological Changes

1

CHAPTER

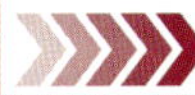

Suvarna S Khadilkar, Deepali Patil

INTRODUCTION

The anatomical, physiological, and hormonal changes in pregnancy are significant and occurr in response to stimuli from the placenta and the fetus. Due to these changes, there are physiological symptoms in first trimester of pregnancy. The understanding of these changes is essential to treat symptomatology of pregnant woman, and also to know the physiological basis for certain conditions of pregnancy. For majority of these complaints, only reassurance may be enough, but for some therapeutic measures may have to be undertaken to ensure good maternal and fetal outcome.

The changes occur in all systems of the body starting from the first trimester and gradually increasing toward the last trimester. Major changes in first trimester occur in the genital system, gastrointestinal system, cardiovascular systems, and central nervous system. Systemic changes, leading to physiological symptoms in first trimester of pregnancy occur from first trimester onward (Box 1). The major factors responsible for the physiological changes in pregnancy are increasing levels of human chorionic gonadotropin (hCG), estrogen, and progesterone.

Box 1: Physiological symptoms of first trimester of pregnancy

- Amenorrhea
- Morning sickness
- Giddiness, weakness, and leg cramps
- Drowsiness or excessive sleepiness
- Anorexia
- Headache and heaviness in the head
- Frequency of micturition
- Leucorrhea or excessive vaginal discharge
- Breast discomfort

GENITAL SYSTEM

Increased level of progesterone is associated with increased vascularity of pelvic organs and decreased vascular resistance. This leads to congestion of genital organs.[1]

Uterus

Uterine size is increased both due to intrauterine growth of the gestational sac (distension), and also due to myohyperplasia and hypertrophy of myometrium under the influence of estrogen. Progesterone excess is associated with increased vascularity.

The shape of the pre-pregnant uterus is pyriform which becomes globular by end of the first trimester and then it again changes to oval, from 12 weeks onward. Due to increasing tension in the growing amniotic sac, there is downward pressure on the cervix.

Uterine Signs

- *Size, shape, and consistency*: The uterus is enlarged to the size of hen's egg at 6th week, size of a cricket ball at 8th week, and size of a fetal head by 12th week. The pyriform shape of the non-pregnant uterus becomes globular by 12 weeks. The uterus becomes acutely anteverted between 6 weeks and 8 weeks. There may be a symmetrical enlargement of the uterus if there is lateral implantation. This is called *Piskacek's sign* where one half is more firm than the other half. As pregnancy advances, symmetry is restored. The pregnant uterus feels soft and elastic
- *Hegar's sign*: It is present in two-thirds of cases. It can be demonstrated between 6 weeks and 10 weeks, a little earlier in multiparae. This sign is based on the fact that: (1) Upper part of the body of the uterus is enlarged by the growing fetus, (2) lower part of the body is empty and extremely soft, and (3) the cervix is comparatively firm. Because of variation in consistency, on bimanual examination (two fingers in the anterior fornix and the abdominal fingers behind the uterus), the abdominal and vaginal fingers seem to appose below the body of the uterus
- *Palmer's sign*: Regular and rhythmic uterine contraction can be elicited during bimanual examination as early as 4–8 weeks. Palmer in 1949, first described it and it is a valuable sign when elicited.

Cervix

Congestion and softening of cervix occurs during early trimester. Non-pregnant cervix has a firm feel on touch but, during pregnancy it is soft. Increased vascularity causes congestion of cervix giving rise to bluish discoloration of cervix and is known as *Goodell's sign.* During the first trimester, isthmus elongates to three times original length and after 12 weeks it unfolds from above downward. Thus, lower segment starts to form from the end of the 12th week. If the circular fibers of the internal os are weak then the abortion takes place due to incompetent cervix.

Vagina

Vaginal mucosa appears bluish and congested due to increased vascularization, this leads to excessive non-purulent vaginal discharge (physiological leucorrhea). There is increased pulsation, felt through the lateral fornices at 8th week called *Osiander's sign*. Similar pulsation is, however, felt in acute pelvic inflammation.

External Genitalia

A dusky view of vestibule and anterior vaginal wall usually seen in multipare is known as *Chadwick's* or *Jacquemier's Sign* and is due to altered vascularity.

Ovaries

Ovulation ceases during pregnancy and the maturation of new follicles is suspended. A single corpus luteum of pregnancy may be found in the ovary of pregnant women and functions maximally during the first 6–7 weeks of pregnancy.

Breast

Breast changes are evident in primigravidas. There is deeper pigmentation of the areola and nipples are larger and erectile. The breast changes are evident between 6 weeks and 8 weeks. There is enlargement with vascular engorgement evidenced by the delicate veins visible under the skin. The nipple and the areola (primary) become more pigmented specially in dark women. Montgomery's tubercles are prominent. Thick yellowish secretion (colostrum) can be expressed as early as 12th week.

GASTROINTESTINAL SYSTEM

Morning sickness is a common complaint in the first trimester and its severity very well correlates with level of hCG. Relaxation of the cardiac sphincter of stomach causes regurgitation of food and leads to recurrent vomiting and retrosternal burning in early trimester. Under the influence of progesterone, there is decreased gastrointestinal motility and a decreased muscle tone of the intestinal tract which is responsible for anorexia, indigestion, and constipation during pregnancy. Liver function is depressed during pregnancy but there are no changes in the liver function test. There is delayed emptying of gall bladder.

URINARY SYSTEM

Enlarged size of the uterus along with its exaggerated anteverted position leads to frequency of urine due to bladder irritability. This may also be due to congestion of the bladder mucosa.

CARDIOVASCULAR SYSTEM

Effect of hormonal changes on the cardiovascular system leads to hyperdynamic circulation. There is relaxation of smooth muscles of vessels leading to decreased vascular resistance in almost all vasculature. This effect is measured as overall fall of diastolic blood pressure and mean arterial blood pressure by 5–10 mm of Hg. The cardiac output starts rising since 5 week of pregnancy.[2] Blood volume starts rising from 10th week onward. All these changes in the cardiovascular system are responsible for complaints like giddiness, weakness, headache, and heaviness in the head.[3]

MUSCULOSKELETAL SYSTEM

During early weeks of pregnancy, there is secretion of relaxin. Under the influence of relaxin, there is relaxation in joint synovial membranes leading to instability of synovial joints like sacroiliac joint and pubic symphysis. Usually, there is no movement in these joints, but because of these changes, there is instability in the pelvis leading to pain in the hips during walking, and turning while in lying down position.[4] Pregnant women commonly complain of cramps in the legs and calf muscle pain, which may be due to decreased availability of energy resources like adenosine triphosphate.

CENTRAL NERVOUS SYSTEM

Increased level of hormones may have effect on central nervous system causing nausea and vomiting.

CUTANEOUS CHANGES

Hyperdynamic circulation in pregnancy leads to increased vascularity of the skin during pregnancy and disturbed thermoregulation of the body, leading to rise in basal body temperature by 1°F. Due to this, pregnant women complain of heat intolerance.

WEIGHT

In the first trimester, a woman may lose weight because of nausea, vomiting, and anorexia

OSMOREGULATION

During pregnancy, there is increased sodium retention due to estrogen, progesterone, aldosterone, and antidiuretic hormone. Increased accumulation of fluid leads to decrease in colloid osmotic pressure due to hemodilution.

METABOLISM

Initially during the first trimester, there is negative protein metabolism and lipolysis. Gradually, as symptoms of early pregnancy subside, protein synthesis and lipogenesis develop due to estrogen effect.

ENDOCRINE SYSTEM

Before the placental function starts corpus luteum acts as a rescue till 6–8 weeks of pregnancy. Syncytiotrophoblasts secrete a number of protein and steroidal hormones that simulate pituitary hormones.[5] Some of the important hormones are:

- *Human chorionic gonadotropin*: is a glycoprotien hormone which simulates luteinizing hormone, plays a major role in maintenance of pregnancy and immunosuppression. It stimulates the adrenal and placental steroidogenesis, and maternal thyroid gland
- *Human placental lactogen:* is lactogenic and functions as growth hormone in pregnancy
- *Human chorionic thyrotropin*
- *Human chorionic corticotropin*
- *Steroidal hormones*: estrogen and progesterone start rising since 9th week of pregnancy.

EMBRYONAL AND FETAL DEVELOPMENT

Normal embryonal and fetal development during first trimester is illustrated in table 1. It is amply clear that any insult during this phase may cause first trimester abortion.

Physiological maternal adaptation in pregnancy starts as soon as conception occurs. These changes are necessary for implantation and healthy growth in early pregnancy. The understanding of these changes and influence of age, parity, race, multiple gestation, and other variables has to be understood to appreciate the adaptations and disease process that occur during pregnancy.

TABLE 1: Carnegie stages of embryonic development

Day post-ovulation	*Carnegie stages*	*Embryonal development*
0	1	Fertilization
1	2	2-cell stage blastomere
2	-	4-cell stage
3	-	12-cell stage
4	-	16-cell stage morula
5	3	Blastocyst
6	4	Interstitial implantation
11	5	Implantation completed
13	6	Primitive streak gastrulation primary villi
16	7	Secondary villi neurulation
17–19	8	Primitive pit, notochordal canal, and neurenteric canals
21	9	Appearance of (mesoderm) tertiary villi somites
22	10	Neural folds/heart folds begin to fuse fetal heart and fetal circulation
23–25	11	Two pharyngeal arches appear
25–27	12	Upper limb buds appear
27–30	13	The first thin surface layer of skin appears covering the embryo
31–35	14	Esophagus formation takes place
35–38	15	Future cerebral hemispheres distinct
38–42	16	Hindbrain begins to develop
42–44	17	A four chambered heart
44–48	18	Lens vesicle, nasal pit, and hand plate begins to develop
48–51	19	Semicircular canals forming in inner ear
51–53	20	Spontaneous movement begins

Contd...

Contd...

Day post-ovulation	*Carnegie stages*	*Embryonal development*
53–54	21	Intestines recede into body cavity
54–56	22	Brain can move muscles, begins to transform into bone cartilage
56–60	23	End of embryonic period (all major structures form recognizably human)
60–68	-	External genitalia develops
70 days	-	Fetus begins to move

REFERENCES

1. Ganong WF. The gonads: development and function of reproductive system. In: Ganong WF, editor. Review of Medical Physiology. 2nd ed. Philadelphia, PA: McGraw-Hill; 2009. p. 142-7.
2. Pandey AK, Banerjee AK, Das A, et al. Evaluation of maternal myocardial performance during normal pregnancy and post partum. Indian Heart J. 2010;62(1):64-7.
3. McFadyn IR. Maternal changes in normal pregnancy. In: Turnbull A, Chamberlin G, editors. Obstetrics. 3rd ed. Edinburgh: Churchill Livingstone; 1994. p. 151-71.
4. Stirrat GM. Physiological changes in pregnancy. In: Stirrat GM, editor. Obstetrics. 2nd ed. Blackwell Oxford, Boston: Scientific Publication; 1986. p. 7-22.
5. Roti E, Gnudi A, Braverman LE. The placental transport, synthesis and metabolism of hormones and drugs which effect thyroid function. Endocrinal review. 1983;4(2):131-49.

Dating and Chorionicity

2

CHAPTER

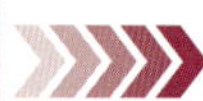

Jayprakash Shah, Parth Shah

INTRODUCTION

Sonography is an indispensable tool for early pregnancy assessment. Its initial use was for gestational age assessment, i.e., dating.[1] Dating during early pregnancy has the advantage that at this time embryo does not reflect biological variations. Factors, such as race, geographical distribution, and nutrition do not affect its size significantly. Early pregnancy scan will also define the number of gestational sacs in multiple pregnancy and their chorionicity and amnionicity. During the 11–14 weeks scan, one can predict dating with almost equal accuracy, at the same time, we can assess fetal structure, chromosomal markers, and rule out major gross malformation. In some cases, we can predict early growth problems. At the same time, one can define chorionicity and amnionicity in multiple pregnancy with almost equal accuracy.

In obstetrics, many decisions require accurate gestational age for:

- Deciding the timing of invasive procedures like chorion villous sampling and amniocentesis
- Biochemical screening like double marker between 9 weeks and 12 weeks and triple marker at 16 weeks
- Deciding about medical termination of pregnancy
- Induction of labor in intrauterine growth restriction and sick fetuses for better outcome of neonate.

TERMINOLOGY

- *Menstrual age*: It is calculated from last menstrual period
- *Conception age*: It is calculated from day of conception
- *Gestational age*: Conception age +14 days. Gestational age is currently used in place of menstrual age.

Early pregnancy scan gives the best chance to date the pregnancy accurately. The best time to date pregnancy is between 6 weeks and 9 weeks by crown-rump length (CRL),[2] and best chorionicity and amnionicity can be defined at 8 weeks of pregnancy.

DATING OF EARLY PREGNANCY

Gestational Sac

Gestational sac is visible earliest from 4 weeks and 3–4 days. It is nothing but the chorionic sac with thick echogenic (>2 mm) border produced by the developing chorionic villi. It is eccentric and embedded completely in decidua—

intradecidual sign (Fig. 1). As it grows, it distorts the endometrial cavity. Toward the side of uterine cavity, it is covered by two layers of decidua, i.e., decidua capsularis and parietalis, separated by endometrial cavity—*double decidual sign* (Fig. 2). Gestational sac grows at a rate of 1.1 mm/day up to 8 weeks of pregnancy. It is filled by slightly echogenic fluid called chorionic fluid. Gestational sac should be measured from inner to inner border, i.e., only the anechoic area, excluding the trophoblast. It is to be measured in three dimensions, two transverse, and one vertical to get the average mean sac diameter (MSD). Many studies have been published using confirmed conception age as in *in vitro* fertilization pregnancies. These studies have confirmed that gestational sac is very accurate in gestational age assessment with variability of ±2 days. MSD when measured, gives the gestational age in days by a simple formula—MSD in mm +30 = gestational age in days. One can tabulate gestational age from gestational sac measurement. All machines are now equipped with these tables.

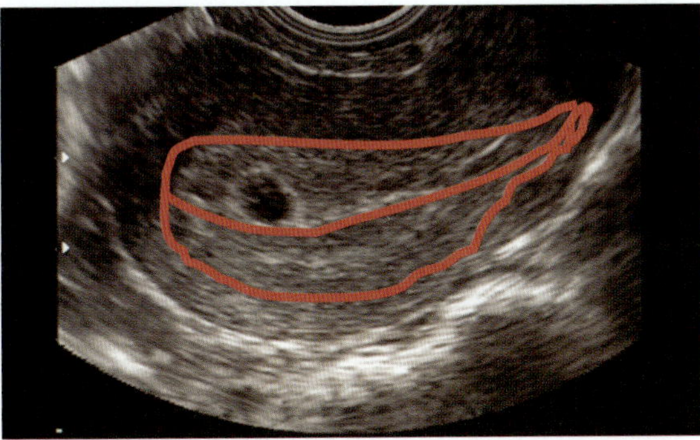

FIGURE 1 Intradecidual sign.

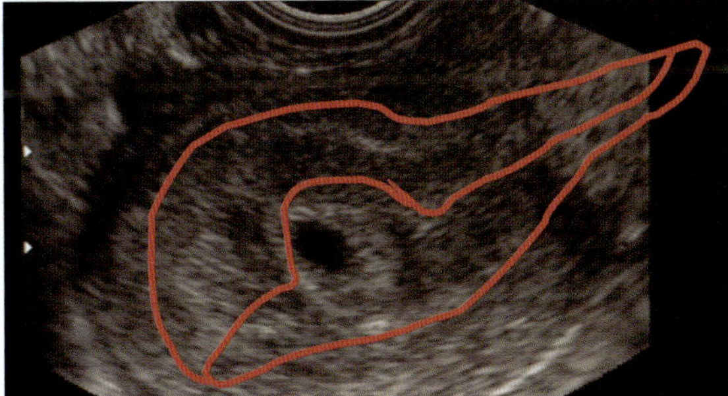

FIGURE 2 Double decidual sign.

Rules for Gestational Sac Measurement

- Largest sac diameter in longitudinal sagittal and transverse planes should be selected (Fig. 3)
- Inner to inner (anechoic area) to be measured excluding trophoblast
- Two transverse and one vertical measurement, and mean of all three is to be taken
- Accuracy is ±2 days
- Once embryo is visible, it loses its accuracy, and now it is time to switch to CRL for gestational age assessment.

Crown-rump Length

Crown-rump length is crown to rump length but in practice it is maximum length measurement of the embryo (Fig. 4). Embryo is visible from 5 weeks 5 days (CRL 2 mm) just at the periphery of the yolk sac, because at this stage there is no yolk stalk. As soon as the embryo is visible, cardiac activity is visible, but it may not appear in few cases till the embryo size is 5 mm. Measurement of CRL gives the most accurate gestational age

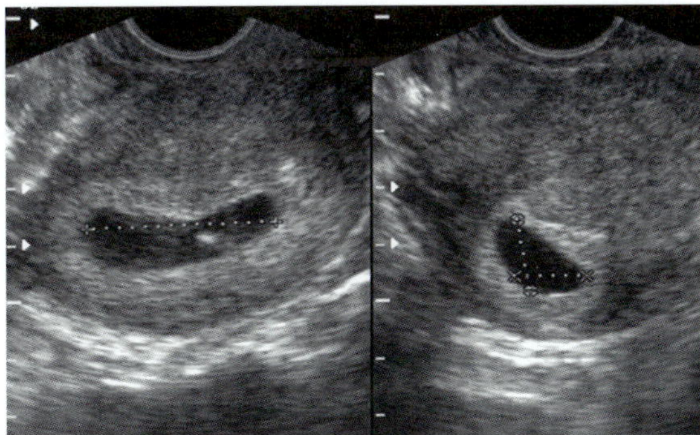

FIGURE 3 Gestational sac measurement in three planes.

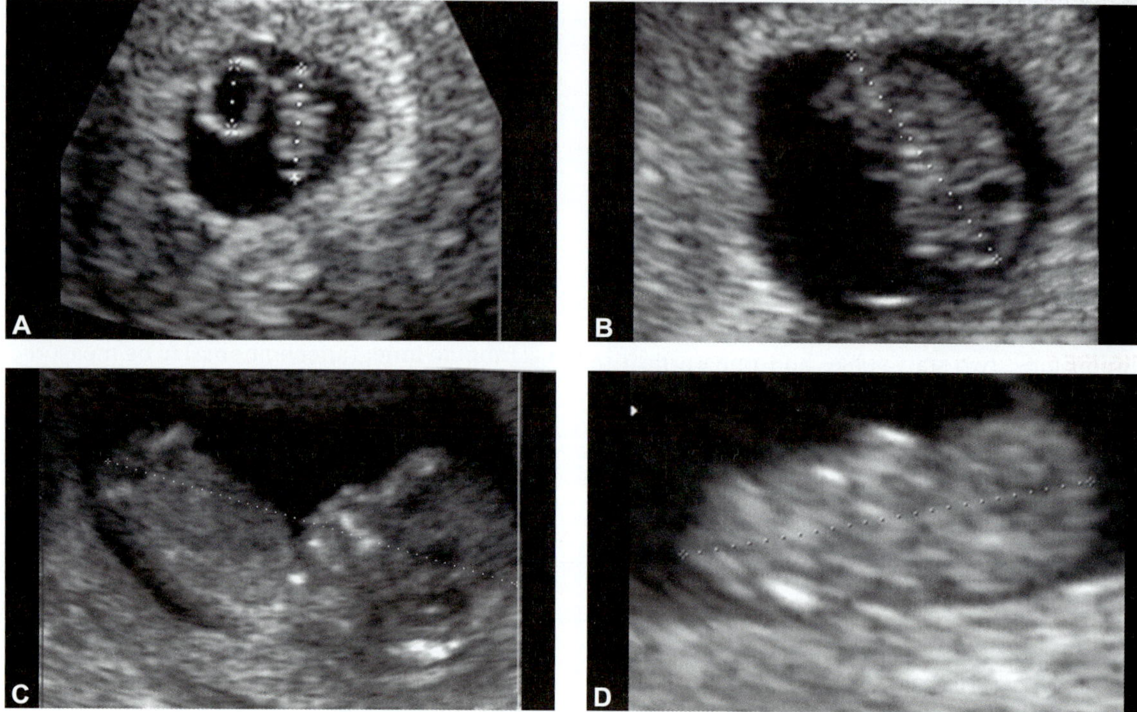

FIGURE 4 Measurement of crown-rump length.

±3–5 days.[3] All the data and studies that have been published unanimously agree upon the accuracy of the CRL for gestational age assessment from 7 weeks to 15 weeks gestation. Transition period of 13–15 weeks is considered best to switch over to other biometry like biparietal diameter.

Rules for Crown-rump Length Measurement

- The embryo shall be with spine towards the probe or away from probe so that the neutral position can be judged accurately. Chin not touching the chest in late early pregnancy. Limbs shall not be visible confirming exact sagittal plane
- Mid sagittal section of embryo—bladder visible and no limb visible in full length
- Maximum length of embryo to be measured.

In a study by MacGregor et al.[4] accuracy of CRL was found to be low with increasing gestational age—toward end of first trimester, probably reflecting the early biological variability. It was observed from various studies that overall accuracy of CRL gestational age has a ±8% variability, i.e., at CRL 11 weeks—gestational age is 11 weeks ±8%, i.e., 11 weeks ±9.5 days.

Biparietal Diameter

With the availability of high resolution machines equipped with transvaginal probe, many studies have been published on assessment of gestational age by other biometric parameters like biparietal diameter (BPD), femur length (FL), and abdominal circumference (AC). Although, BPD, FL, and AC are reasonably accurate, they do not have an upper edge compared to CRL. It is difficult to measure other biometry compared to CRL with accuracy before 13 weeks of pregnancy, although data on BPD are published

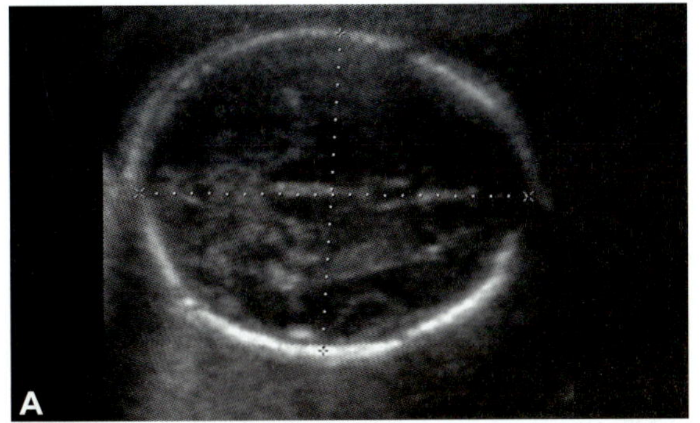

FIGURE 5 Measurement of biparietal diameter (BPD).

from seventh weeks onward. However, after 13 weeks—transition from first trimester to second trimester, it becomes important to switch over to other biometry.[5] Measurement of BPD is most accurate after 14 weeks of pregnancy (Fig. 5).

CHORIONICITY

All multifetal pregnancies are at high risk. It's risk depends on the chorionicity. Chorion is nothing but the developing placenta and when the fetuses in a multifetal pregnancy share the placenta, it means that they share their circulation as well. When circulation is shared among fetuses, one of them may get more blood supply at the cost of other due to arterio-arterial (A-A), arterio-venous (A-V), or veno-venous (V-V) connections. Both fetuses are be at risk. Complications associated with of monochorionicity include twin-to-twin transfusion syndrome (TTTS), acardiac twin, cord entanglement, conjoined twins, parasitic twins, and fetus *in fetu*, which has a direct impact on the outcome of pregnancy. Table 1 shows the outcome of pregnancy based on chorionicity.

Chorionicity and amnionicity are depicted in figure 6. The frequency and perinatal mortality rates are shown in table 1. Figure 7 graphically depicts the higher mortality rate in monochorionic twins.

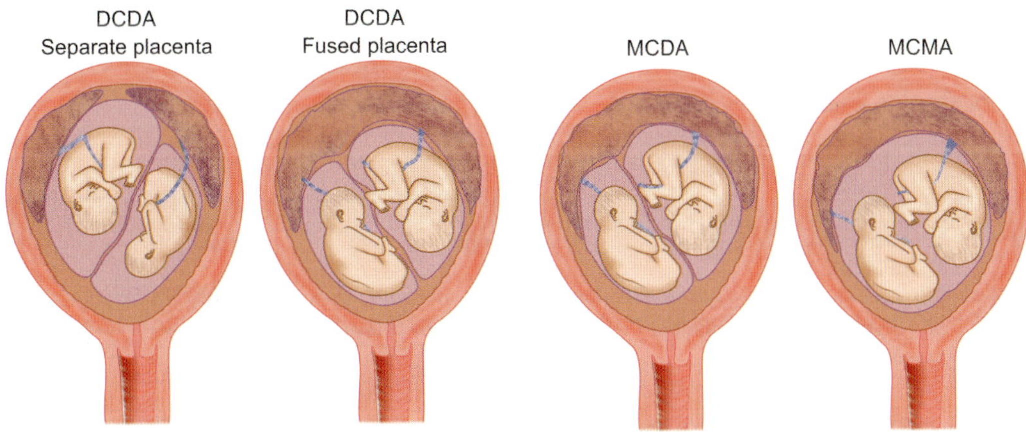

DCDA, dichorionic- diamniotic; MCDA, monochorionic- diamniotic, MCMA, monochorionic-monoamniotic.

FIGURE 6 Chorionicity and amnionicity.

TABLE 1: Frequency and perinatal mortality with different chorionicity

	Dichorionic- diamniotic separate placenta (%)	*Dichorionic- diamniotic fused placenta (%)*	*Monochorionic-diamniotic (%)*	*Monochorionic-monoamniotic (%)*
Frequency	35	27	36	2
Mortality	13	11	32	44

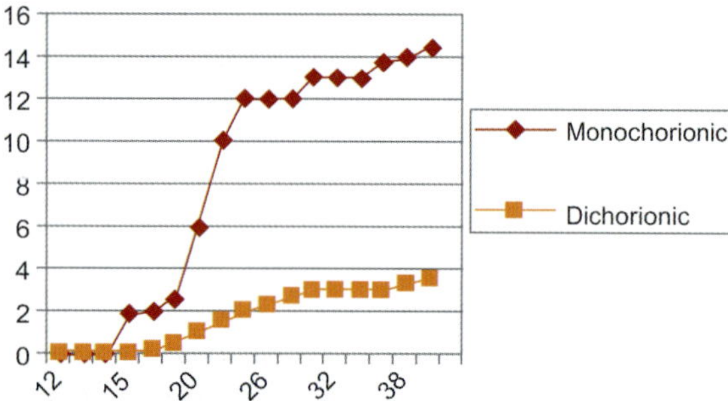

FIGURE 7 Higher perinatal mortality in monochorionic twins.

Chroionicity and amnionicity are prognostic markers in multifetal pregnancy. It is important to define chorionicity by an early scan for better management of these pregnancies.[6] High perinatal morbidity and mortality is associated with monochorionic twins. Selective fetal reduction and invasive testing for chromosomal analysis also require defining chorionicity, as in monochorionic twins, fetal reduction using potassium chloride injection will lead to death of other fetus also. In dichorionic twins, sampling of both fetuses is mandatory.

Assessment of chorionicity using the twin peak lambda sign has a very high sensitivity and specificity.[7] Although chorionicity and amnionicity can be predicted with more than 91% sensitivity by ultrasound, zygosity may not be predicted in all cases.[8] Chorionicity can be assessed as early as 5 weeks gestation but amnionicity cannot be confirmed before the eighth week of gestation.[9] If there has been no earlier scan then the ideal time to check for chorionicity will be the 11–14 weeks nuchal scan. The lambda sign and membrane thickness seem to be superior to other markers listed in table 2.[10] Monochorionic and dichorionic pregnancies are easily identified in early scans (Fig. 8).

In order to understand chorionicity and amnionicity we need to understand the embryology of early pregnancy events. Type of twinning depends upon:

- Two fertilized ova (dizygotic twins)
- Single zygote division (monozygotic twins).

TABLE 2: Defining chorionicity

Step 1	Define number of placentas (Fig. 9)	Separate placenta	Dichorionic
		Placenta together	Chorionicity undetermined
Step 2	Define lambda sign/T sign (Fig. 10)	Lambda sign	Dichorionic
		"T"Sign	Monochorionic
Step 3	Thickness of membrane (Fig. 11)	Thick membrane (4 layers)	Dichorionic
		Thin membrane (2 layers)	Monochorionic
Step 4	Sex of fetus	Different sex	Dichorionic
		Same sex	Chorionicity undetermined

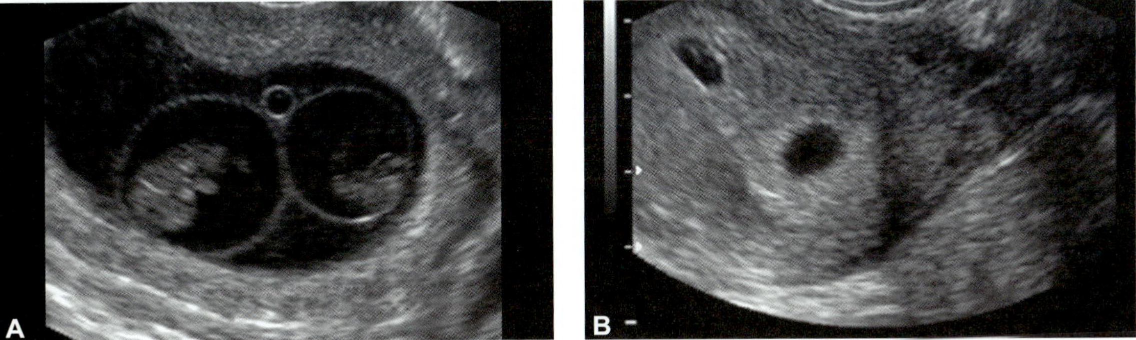

FIGURE 8 Early scan for chorionicity and amnionicity. **A,** Monochorionic-diamniotic twins; **B,** Dichorionic-diamniotic twins.

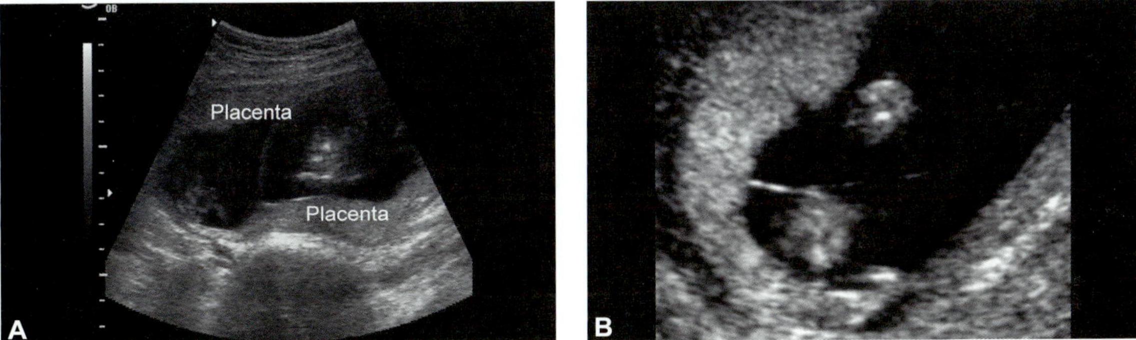

FIGURE 9 Number of placenta. **A,** Two placenta; **B,** Single placenta.

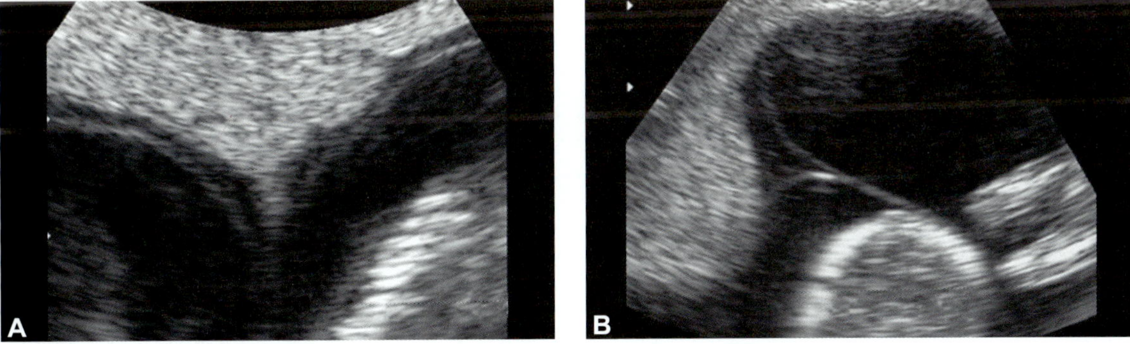

FIGURE 10 **A,** Lambda sign; **B,** "T" sign.

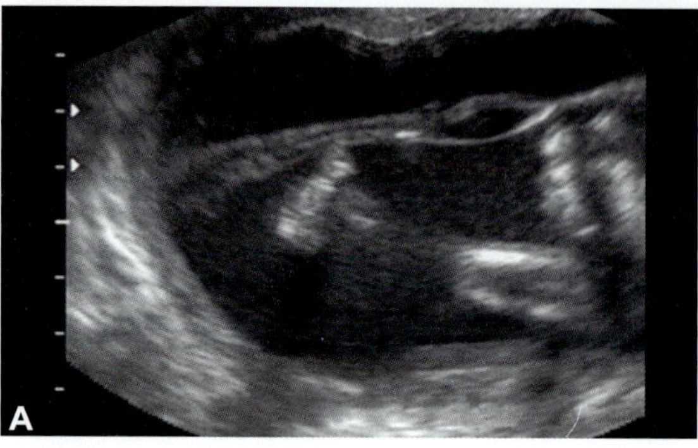

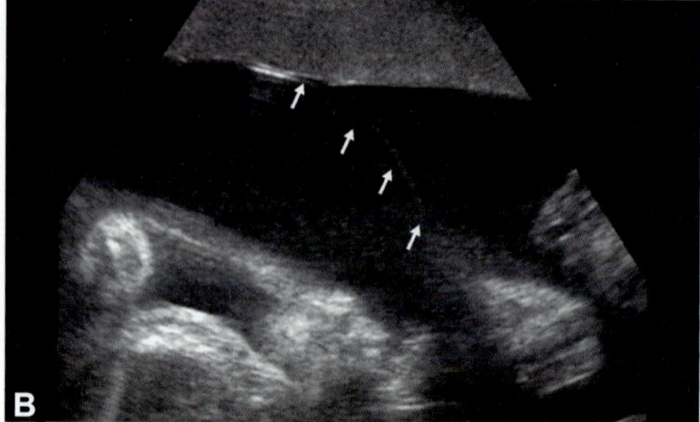

FIGURE 11 Thickness of membrane. **A,** Thick membrane; **B,** Thin membrane.

ZYGOSITY (FIG. 12)

- Can only be determined by DNA fingerprinting
- Prenatally, such testing would require an invasive procedure:
  - Amniotic fluid (amniocentesis)
  - Placental tissue (chorionic villous sampling
  - Fetal blood (cordocentesis).

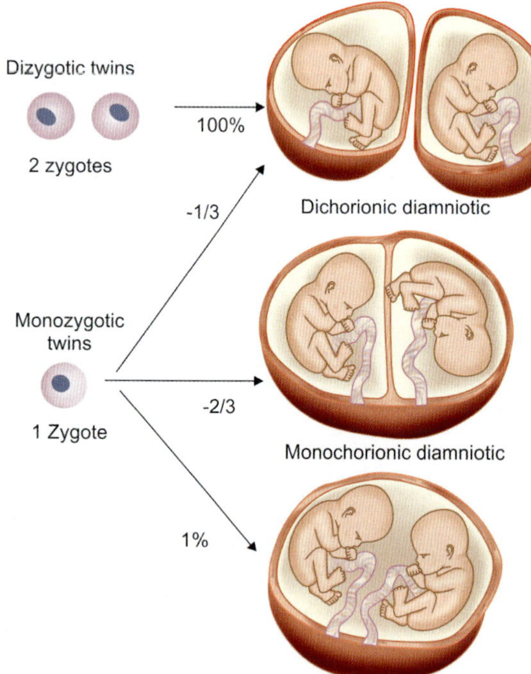

FIGURE 12 Zygosity and chorionicity.

Dizygotic Twins

- All dizygotic twins are dichorionic.

Monozygotic Twins (Fig. 13)

- Dichorionic-diamniotic
- Dichorionic-monoamniotic
- Monochorionic-monoamniotic.

It is believed that a single blastocyst splits the inner cell mass in half, and each half develops into a fetus.

In monozygotic twins all monochorionic twins are:

- Diamniotic
- Monoamniotic
  - Normal fetuses
  - Acardiac twins
  - Parasitic twins
  - Fetus *in fetu*.

Complications in Monochorionic Twins

- Twin-to-twin transfusion syndrome is also known as the *twin oligohydramnios polyhydramnios sequence*. It results in one twin being under perfused and oligoamniotic while the other twin is over perfused and develops polyhydramnios. It carries a mortality of more than 60%. Fetoscopic laser ablation of placental vessels will improve survival rates
- Acardiac twin or twin reversed arterial perfusion syndrome. Also known as the

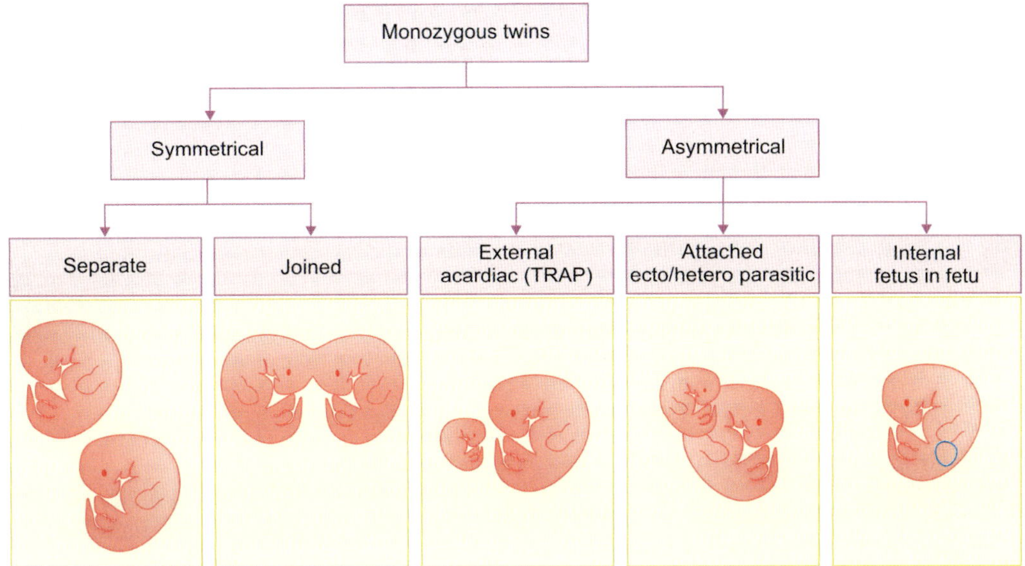

TRAP, twin reverse arterial perfusion.

FIGURE 13 Monozygotic twins.

parasitic twin, or asymmetrical twin, where one embryo maintains dominant development at the expense of the other

- Conjoined twins may be joined at the head or torso and require surgical separation after birth
- Cord entanglement
- Fetus in fetu where a rudimentary fetus is found inside the live fetus.

Ultrasound is hence of immense value in dating a pregnancy accurately. This ensures that we perform prenatal screening procedures at the right time and the decision to intervene and induce labor is also taken at the correct time. Determining the chorionicity and amnionicity in multifetal pregnancy is extremely important. It allows us to follow monochorionic pregnancies more carefully to identify cases of TTTS and take corrective measures.

REFERENCES

1. Reece EA, Gabrieli S, Degennaro N, et al. Dating through pregnancy: a measure of growing up. Obstet Gynecol Surv. 1989;44(7):544-55.
2. Callen PW. Ultrasonography in Obstetrics and Gynecology. 5th ed. Philadelphia, PA: Saunders; 2007.
3. Pederson JF. Fetal crown-rump length in measurement by ultrasound normal pregnancy. Br J Obstet Gynaecol. 1982;89(11):926-30.
4. MacGregor SN, Tamura RK, Sabbagha RE, et al. Underestimation of gestational age by conventional crown-rump length dating curves. Obstet Gynecol. 1987;70(3 pt 1):344-8.
5. Hadlock FP, Shah YP, Kanon DJ, et al. Fetal crown-rump length: reevaluation of relation to menstrual age (5-18 weeks) with high-resolution real time US. Radiology. 1992;182(2):501-5.
6. Weisz B, Pandya P, Dave R, et al. Scanning for chorionicity: comparison between sonographers and perinatologists. Prenat Diagn. 2005;25(9):835-8.
7. Wood SL, St Onge R, Connors G, et al. Evaluatiolon of twin peak or lambda sign in determining chorionicity in multiple pregnancy. Obstet Gynecol. 1996;88(1):6-9.
8. Scardo JA, Ellings JM, Newman RB. Prospective determination of chorionicity, amnionicity, and zygosity in twin gestations. Am J Obstet Gynecol. 1995;173(5):1376-80.
9. Monteagudo A. Sonographic assessment of chorionicity and amnionicity in twin pregnancies: how, when and why? Croat Med J. 1998;39(2):191-6.
10. D'Alton ME, Dudley DK. The ultrasonographic prediction of chorionicity in twin gestation. Am J Obstet Gynecol. 1989;160(3):557-61.

The Booking Visit

3

CHAPTER

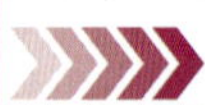

Bhaskar Pal, Seetha Ramamurthy (Pal)

INTRODUCTION

A positive pregnancy test opens a Pandora's box throwing more questions than answers. The first antenatal visit or the booking visit is the most important visit, both for the patient and for the doctor as it has a major bearing on further course of the pregnancy. Ideally, preconception counseling is better, especially for patients with potential problems in pregnancy. The aim is to identify pregnancies with maternal or fetal conditions associated with maternal or perinatal morbidity/mortality and provide interventions to prevent such complications.[1]

Preferably, the first appointment should be early in pregnancy (prior to 12 weeks).This is something we need to educate our patients on, as the first trimester offers a large volume of information. There may be need in early pregnancy for two appointments. However, in women with recurrent miscarriages and assisted reproductive technologies or high risk pregnancies several first trimester visits may be required to ensure fetal well-being and growth.

ORGANIZATIONAL ISSUES

There is no evidence that physicians need to be involved in the prenatal care of every woman experiencing an uncomplicated pregnancy, and some problems in particular those involving social issues, may be better handled by midwives or general practitioners.[2] Involvement of an obstetrician is usually recommended when complications are present or anticipated. However, a recent Cochrane review (2010) reported that where the standard number of visits is low, visits should not be reduced without close monitoring of fetal and neonatal outcome, as it was seen that reduced visits program of antenatal care is associated with an increase in perinatal mortality compared to standard care.[3]

The booking visit does not necessarily have to be in a hospital. It should be in a place that is readily and easily accessible to all women and should be sensitive to the needs of individual women and the local community. If any potential problem is identified, then further visits can be scheduled at the nearest referral center.

FOCUSED ANTENATAL CARE

- Focused antenatal care (ANC) emphasizes quality of visits over quantity
- Is based on the premise that every pregnant woman is at risk for complications
- Relies on evidence-based, goal-directed interventions appropriate to gestational age of pregnancy

- Targets most prevalent health issues affecting pregnant women
- Is given by skilled healthcare provider (midwife, doctor, nurse) with basic midwifery and life-saving skills.

Goals of Antenatal Care

- *Promotion of health and prevention of disease*:
  - Nutrition
  - Prevention of anemia and tetanus
  - Counseling and testing for human immunodeficiency virus (HIV)
  - Care for common discomforts
  - Use of potentially harmless substances
  - Prevention of infection
  - Maintenance of hygiene
  - Adequate rest and activity
  - Sexual relations and safer sex
  - Early and exclusive breast feeding
  - Family planning

  In disease or deficiency endemic areas:
  - Insecticide treated bed nets for malaria
  - Presumptive treatment for hookworm infection
  - Vitamin supplementation
  - Iodine supplementation
- *Detection of existing diseases and treatment*:
  If not treated, existing diseases can complicate or be complicated by pregnancy. Examples include anemia, syphilis and sexually transmitted infections, HIV/AIDS (acquired immunodeficiency syndrome), hepatitis, diabetes, malnutrition, malaria, tuberculosis, heart disease, etc
- *Early detection and management of complications*:
  Management of following complications can affect survival/death of women and, or new born. These are hemorrhage, sepsis, and pre-eclampsia/eclampsia
- *Birth preparedness and complication readiness*:
  As part of focused ANC, skilled provider assists women and her family in developing a birth plan
- *Help and ensure arrangements for clean and safe birth with skilled provider*: These arrangements include:
  - Skilled provider to attend birth
  - Appropriate place of birth
  - Transportation of/to skilled provider
  - Funds for normal birth
  - Blood donor
  - Identification of danger signs

  Help family to prepare for possible emergency as every woman is at risk for complications and most complications cannot be predicted.

Core Components of Basic Antenatal Care Visit

- *Quick check*:
  Screen for danger signs. This helps to quickly identify woman who need immediate medical attention, stabilize (if necessary), and to treat or refer as quickly as possible.
  These *danger signs* include:
  - Severe headache/blurred vision
  - Convulsions/loss of consciousness
  - Difficulty in breathing
  - Fever
  - Foul smelling vaginal discharge
  - Vaginal bleeding
  - Leaking of fluid from vagina
  - Severe abdominal pain
- *Basic assessment and care provision*:
  - Ensures maternal and fetal well-being
  - Helps identify common discomforts and special needs
  - Screens for conditions beyond the scope of basic care, including life threatening complications
- *During every visit*
  - Consider each finding in context of other findings to target assessment and make more accurate diagnosis
  - If abnormal signs and symptoms are observed, one should conduct additional assessment

- *During return visits*
  - Ensure continued normal progress
  - Identify changes whether positive or negative
  - Determine whether care plan has been effective or requires modification.

Irrespective of the place or person providing care, it should be systematic, evidence-based, and provide both medical and psychological support, as well as risk assessment. It should result in informed decision making between the patient and the provider.

At the first visit, women should receive written/pictorial information regarding their pregnancy care services, lifestyle issues, such as nutrition and exercise and sufficient information to enable informed decision-making about screening tests. All information should be made available in local languages and in pictorial formats for easy understanding and acceptance. Addressing women's choices should be recognized as being integral to the decision making process. The main aim is to identify women who may need additional care (Box 1) and plan their pattern of care for the pregnancy. Major parts of the visit include history, physical examination, laboratory testing, and counseling (Box 2).

Box 1: Women requiring additional care

- Underweight (BMI <18) or obese (BMI >30)
- Extremes of age
- History of medical disorders like cardiac, renal, and hypertension
- Psychiatric disorders
- Previous history of recurrent pregnancy loss, preterm birth, stillbirth, preeclampsia, previous uterine surgery including LSCS, and baby with a congenital anomaly.

BMI, body mass index; LSCS, lower segment caesarean section.

Box 2: The booking visit at a glance

- Comprehensive history—Calculate EDD
- Directed physical examination—includes weight, BMI, BP, and urine dipstick
- First trimester ultrasound
- Laboratory screening: Hb, blood group, Rh type, blood sugar, HBSAg, HIV, VDRL, and urine routine
- Offer aneuploidy screening (first trimester or sequential)
- Screening and counseling for lifestyle/workplace issues
- Genetic screening
- Identify women who may need additional care
- Additional laboratory screening as needed
- Management of symptoms—nausea, vomiting, heartburn, constipation, and vaginal discharge

EDD, expected delivery date; BMI, body mass index; BP, blood pressure; Hb, hemoglobin; HBSAg, hepatitis B surface antigen; HIV, human immunodeficiency virus; VDRL, venereal disease research laboratory test; Rh, Rhesus factor.

HISTORY

A comprehensive history should be taken preferably using structured and standardized record forms. Maternity services should have a system in place whereby women preferably carry a copy of their own case notes. History should include present pregnancy, past obstetric history, past medical and surgical history, family history, and history of social habits and allergies. This would primarily classify the patient as low risk or high risk.

PHYSICAL EXAMINATION

The physical examination should be not only general, but also directed to any risks identified in the history.

Weight and Height

Weight and height should be determined at the first visit, so as to determine the body mass index. Women who are obese or underweight are at increased risk of pregnancy complications and need counseling accordingly.

Blood Pressure

Initial blood pressure evaluation may help in identifying women with chronic hypertension. Pressure should be taken in the sitting position using an appropriately sized cuff and correct technique.

Pelvic Examination

A routine pelvic examination is not accurate for assessment of gestational age and is not a reliable predictive test of preterm birth or cephalopelvic disproportion. It is not recommended for the above. However, abdominal and pelvic examination to confirm suspected gynecologic pathology can be included.

LABORATORY SCREENING

Universal Tests

These tests are done in all pregnant women.

Hemoglobin/Hematocrit

Anemia screening should be offered early in pregnancy and repeated later. This gives a baseline value and also allows enough time for treatment and further investigations if required.

Platelet Count

Initial determination of platelet count may help in later diagnosis of gestational thrombocytopenia, HELLP syndrome (hemolysis, elevated liver enzymes and low platelet count), and other conditions.

Hemoglobin Electrophoresis

Due to the high prevalence of hemoglobinopathies in our population, hemoglobin electrophoresis should ideally be done for all pregnant women at the booking visit, if not done earlier (as part of pre-marriage or pre-conception testing or in previous pregnancy). If the woman is identified as a carrier for hemoglobinopathy, partner has to be tested and evaluation of fetus should be offered if partner is also a carrier. However, this is not universally implemented. Hence women with microcytic anemia and raised values of red cell distribution width should be screened as they are more likely to be carriers of hemoglobinopathies.

ABO/Rh (D) Type and Antibody Screen

Testing for blood group, rhesus factor (Rh) status and atypical red cell antibodies at the initial visit is recommended to determine which patients would need anti-D immunoglobulin.

Blood Sugar

Fasting blood sugar or a glucose load test should be routinely done to detect prediabetes, gestational diabetes mellitus, and pre-existing diabetes mellitus, so that effective intervention can be started early.

Syphilis Screening

Screening for syphilis should be offered to all pregnant women at an early stage, because the condition can be treated timely, thereby avoiding detrimental effects of the disease on the mother and fetus.

Hepatitis B Virus

Serological screening for hepatitis B virus (hepatitis B surface antigen) should be offered to all pregnant women so that effective postnatal intervention can be offered to infected women to decrease the risk of vertical transmission.

HIV Serology

Screening for HIV should be offered as a routine for all women and decliners should be encouraged to sign "opt out" consent. Providers should emphasize to women who decline screening that testing not only provides opportunity to maintain maternal health but also dramatically reduces the risk of vertical transmission to the fetus through effective interventions.

Thyroid Status

In our country, thyroid deficiency is endemic in many areas and thyroid screening should be done at least once, preferably at the booking visit.

Urine for Asymptomatic Bacteriuria

A midstream routine urine examination should be done to screen for asymptomatic bacteriuria.

Rubella IgG

Rubella IgG test identifies women who are non-immune to rubella. A positive report indicates immunity to rubella infection while women who test negative, i.e., non-immune, can be vaccinated against rubella immediately after delivery. Ideally, rubella IgG testing should be part of routine booking antenatal investigations in women who are not known to be immune to rubella; however, the cost-effectiveness of testing should be determined locally before it is adopted as routine in resource-poor settings.

Selective Tests

These tests are done only in women with risk factors.

Infectious Diseases

Hepatitis C serology, screening for bacterial vaginosis, chlamydia, gonorrhea, and TORCH (Toxoplasmosis, rubella, cytomegalovirus, and herpes simplex) serology should not be offered as a routine, as there is no benefit in routine screening. Only patients with positive risk factors should be considered for the same.

PAP Screening

A Papanicolaou (PAP) test may be offered at the first visit if none has been documented previously.

ULTRASOUND SCREENING

Women should be offered an early ultrasound scan to determine gestational age and to detect multiple pregnancies for all cases. This will ensure consistency of gestational age assessments, improve the performance of serum screening for Down's syndrome, and reduce the need for induction of labor after 41 weeks.

SCREENING FOR ANEUPLOIDY

With increasing patient awareness and improved sensitivity of the first trimester screening for Down's syndrome, prenatal screening (both first and second trimester screening) methods should be discussed and offered. These tests are recommended wherever possible, and not mandatory as there may be financial and logistic problems in these tests being made available everywhere.

COUNSELING ABOUT LIFESTYLE ISSUES

Nutrition and Nutritional Supplements

Diet is one of the major concerns of the patient and her family. However, diet and weight gain in general have been insufficiently studied in pregnancy, not allowing for strong recommendations. (*See* Chapter 4: Diet Counseling) It is generally preferable to have small frequent meals especially in the first trimester to avoid hyperacidity. There is no specific food restriction, however, certain food safety issues need to be discussed (Table 1).

TABLE 1: Food safety in pregnancy

Foodborne illness to avoid	*Preventive strategy*
Listeriosis	Cook all foods (especially meats), avoid raw meats and unpasteurized cheese
Toxoplasmosis	Avoid litter of outdoor cats
Salmonella	Avoid uncooked seafood/ shellfish and eggs

Folic acid supplementation is strongly recommended and the patient should be informed of the importance of folic acid and its role in reducing neural tube defects. The recommended dose is 400 µg/day.[4] Iron and calcium should not be ideally started at the first visit as it may aggravate the nausea and constipation present at this time.

There is insufficient evidence at present to recommend routine supplementation with other vitamins like vitamin A, C, and E, and minerals like magnesium and zinc, or other micronutrients or anti-oxidants including docosahexaenoic acid (DHA). The issue about vitamin D supplementation is emerging but lacks consensus yet.

Working and Travel During Pregnancy

Pregnant women should be informed of their rights and benefits. Majority can be reassured that it is safe to continue working during pregnancy provided there are no medical or obstetric complications. Travel is safe and patient should be counseled regarding risks of long distance travel, especially venous thromboembolism (*See* Chapter 13: Travel Guidelines).

Alcohol and Smoking

Pregnant women should be informed of the risks of smoking and alcohol, and strongly advised to quit smoking at the earliest. Dangers of passive smoking at home and workplace should be explained.

Sex and Sexuality

Intercourse has not been associated with adverse outcomes in pregnancy. Most women desire more communication regarding sex in pregnancy by their care providers. Healthcare provider counseling should be reassuring in the absence of pregnancy complications (*See* Chapter 29: Sexual Behavior).

Exercise in Pregnancy

Regular exercise during low-risk pregnancy is beneficial to overall maternal fitness and sense of well-being with insufficient data to assess impact on maternal or fetal outcomes in high risk pregnancies.[5] Twenty minutes of light exercise about three times a week has not been associated with detrimental effects. For further information refer to chapter 14: Role of Exercise and Bed Rest.

Prescribed Medicines

Prescribing medicines should be limited to circumstances where benefits outweigh the risks (*See* Chapter 11: Prescription Writing).

MANAGEMENT OF SYMPTOMS AT THE FIRST VISIT

Most of the women complain of common symptoms at their first visit as disscussed below.

Nausea and Vomiting

Majority need reassurance that these symptoms will resolve spontaneously and most of the antiemetics can be safely prescribed at this stage (*See* Chapter 5: Nausea and Vomiting).

Heartburn

Apart from diet and lifestyle modification, antacids and proton pump inhibitors may be offered, for details *see* chapter 11: Prescription Writing.

Constipation

Increasing fiber in the diet and if necessary, mild laxatives can help this very distressing complaint.

Vaginal Discharge

Increase in vaginal discharge is a common physiological change in pregnancy and patients should be reassured regarding this.

At the end of the visit, proper documentation should be done and plans made for care during the pregnancy, arranging follow up appointments and/or testing. Adequate quality time spent during the booking visit is very important in establishing a good doctor patient relation which itself can have a very positive impact on the rest of the pregnancy.

REFERENCES

1. American Academy of Paediatrics, American College of Obstetricians and Gynecologists. Guidelines for Perinatal care 5th ed. 2002 (review).
2. Villar J, Carroli G, Khan-Neelofur, et al. Patterns of routine antenatal care for low-risk pregnancy. Cochrane Database Syst Rev. 2001;(4):CD000934.
3. Dowswell T, Carroli G, Duley L, et al.Alternative versus standard packages of antenatal care for low-risk pregnancy. Cochrane Database Syst Rev. 2010;6(10):CD000934.
4. Lumley L, Watson L, Watson M, et al. Periconceptional supplementation with folate and/or multivitamins for preventing neural tube defects. Cochrane Database Sys Rev. 2001;(3): CD001056.
5. Kramer MS, Mc Donald SW. Aerobic exercise for women during pregnancy. Cochrane Database Sys Rev. 2006;19(3): CD000180.

FURTHER READING

1. NICE Guidelines on Antenatal Care. Routine Care for the Healthy Pregnant Woman.
2. FOGSI and ICOG Recommendations for Good Clinical Practice.
3. RCOG Guidelines for Care of a Healthy Pregnant Patient.
4. WHO book on EmOC and Basic Obstetric Care for Pregnant Patients.
5. UNFPA Manual in Obstetric Care.

Diet Counseling

4

CHAPTER

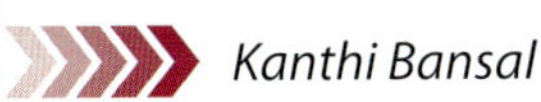

Kanthi Bansal

INTRODUCTION

Nutrition has always played a pivotal role during pregnancy since ancient times. Pregnancy has held a special importance for the family and with it are linked many customs and traditions that mainly aim for the well-being of the mother and child. Proper nutrition of the pregnant lady is important for both maternal well-being and the critical role it plays in development of the fetus. Adequate nutrition before and during pregnancy has a greater potential for long-term health impact than it does at any other time. The diet of a pregnant woman has been the subject of many a discussion. The opinions are varied ranging from rigid calorie control to liberal protein and calcium consumption. This is mainly because it is difficult to do a methodological study in nutrition during pregnancy due to ethical reasons. Nutrition in pregnancy refers to the nutrient intake and dietary planning that is undertaken before, during, and after pregnancy. It is important for the intrauterine growth of the fetus and the future well-being of the baby as it plays a significant role in childhood morbidity and mortality. Mothers taking inadequate food give birth to low birth weight babies, small for date babies, and premature babies.[1]

Pregnancy is a period where nutrition should be optimized in the mother as she is nurturing a growing fetus in her body. Fetal development is accompanied by many physiological, biochemical, and hormonal changes occurring in the maternal body which influence the need for nutrients and the efficiency with which the body uses them. These changes include:

- Increased basal metabolic rate
- Gastrointestinal changes
- Hormonal changes
- Changes in the body fluid.

The three trimesters during pregnancy have different emotional and physical demands that make them unique. Dietary counseling is important before and throughout pregnancy and the postpartum period. In 2005, the United States Department of Agriculture released a new version of the food guide pyramid, also known as "My Pyramid" (Fig.1). The newer pyramid has color, vertical stripes of varying widths with an outline of a person climbing stairs alongside the pyramid.

NUTRITIONAL STATUS

Nutritional requirements during pregnancy are dictated by maternal and fetal growth needs.

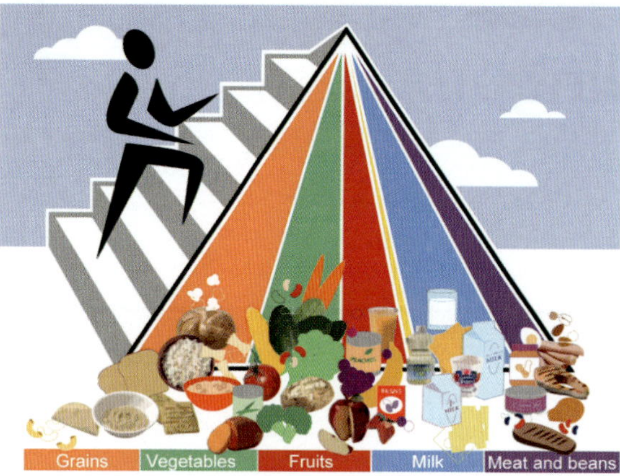

FIGURE 1 Food guide pyramid.

Of the 11–16 kg that a woman of normal weight optimally gains during pregnancy,[2] approximately 40% consists of fetus, placenta, and amniotic fluid, whereas the remainder represents an increase in maternal tissues, including the uterus, breasts, blood, tissue fluid, and body fat.[3] Fetal survival strongly correlates with the birth weight, up to an optimal weight of 3,000–4,000 g.[4] Low birth weight increases the risk of neonatal complications.[5] Low birth weight infants (< 2500 g) have a 40 times greater risk of mortality than normal weight infants.[6] Birth weight, in turn, depends largely on adequate maternal nutrition, as evidenced by prepregnancy weight and by weight gain during pregnancy.[6,7]

Weight Gain in Pregnancy

Maternal weight gain has traditionally been used to evaluate the state of pregnancy. Hytten[8] observed that total weight gain through pregnancy in healthy primigravida females eating without any restrictions is approximately 27.5 lb (12.5 kg). The rate of weight gain is about 1 lb (0.45 kg)/week from 20th week of gestation to delivery. The same results were obtained by Petitti and co-workers.[9]

The National Academy of Science recommends that pregnancy weight gain be based on a woman's prepregnancy body mass index (BMI). A woman with prepregnancy BMI between 19.8 and 26 (normal) should gain 11.6 kg and those with BMI 26–29 (high) should gain 7–11 kg. In case the prepregnancy BMI is over 29 (obese women), the obstetrician should closely monitor the patient to detect and manage the disease resulting from excess weight like gestational diabetes and hypertension.

However, dieting during pregnancy is never recommended, even for patients who are morbidly obese. Severe restriction of energy (caloric) intake is associated with a 250 g decrease in average birth weight. Because of the expansion of maternal blood volume and construction of fetal and placental tissues, some weight gain is essential for a healthy pregnancy.

Assessment of Nutritional Status

The best way to assess nutritional status is to refer to standard height and weight tables using prepregnancy maternal height and weight. BMI (weight in kg, height in m^2) also known as quetelet's index is commonly used. Naeye classified pregnant women into 4 categories based on arbitrary BMI values, namely:

1. Thin: BMI less than 20
2. Normal: BMI 20–24
3. Overweight: BMI 25–30
4. Obese: BMI more than 30.

This study considered both under nutrition and obesity as abnormalities of nutrition.[10] The classical anthropometric indicators of nutrition include prepregnancy weight and height, arm circumference, weight gain in pregnancy, and BMI. However, arm circumference is seldom used in practice. Another measure to assess nutritional status is to determine the fetal growth which can be assessed by ultrasound imaging of the fetus.

Preconceptional Counseling

Preconceptional counseling is an essential part of modern management of pregnancy.

Nutritional counseling by an expert dietician can be incorporated as a part of the preconceptional consultation. Foods to be avoided during pregnancy include alcohol and excessive amounts of liver or liver products, caffeine, salt and junk food.

DIET AND FEEDING PATTERN

While planning meals for pregnant women, the basic meal planning principles remain the same as for normal adults (Box 1). Pregnant women should avoid fasting (>13 hours) and should

Box 1: Suggested dietary guidelines for pregnant women

Prior to Pregnancy:

- Eat iron-rich or iron-fortified foods (meat or meat alternatives, breads, and cereals)
- Include vitamin C-rich foods (e.g., orange juice, broccoli, or strawberries) to enhance iron absorption
- Take folic acid supplements (400 µg) daily
- Eat a well-balanced diet, including 3–3.5 cups of fruits and vegetables per day, with a focus on a variety of different colors of these foods
- Eat/drink 3 cups of milk or calcium-rich foods per day, with a focus on low-fat or skimmed milk products
- Do not consume alcoholic beverages
- Vitamin D deficiency causes impaired fetal growth. All women should be informed about the importance of maintaining adequate vitamin D stores before pregnancy to avoid complications during pregnancy and breastfeeding

During Pregnancy:

- Continue to follow the recommendations listed above
- Eat enough food to gain weight at the rate recommended by health-care provider
- No need exists to increase food intake in the first trimester; however, continue to eat well-balanced meals. Increase food intake by only 340 calories per day during the second trimester and 450 calories per day during the third trimester
  - In healthy women on a normal diet, advice on eating 5 portions of fruit and vegetables per day and consuming dairy products to raise stores of vitamins, iron, and calcium is reasonable
- Do not skip meals. Eat three small to moderate-sized meals at regular intervals and two to three nutritious snacks (fruits/vegetables) per day
- If no medical or obstetrical complications exist, exercise 30 minutes or more, employing a moderate intensity of physical activity, on most, if not all, days of the week. Examples include walking briskly (about 3.5 miles per hour); swimming, gardening, dancing, golf, bicycling (<10 miles per hour); and general light workout
- Because of the dangers of toxoplasmosis/listeriosis/amebiasis, women should avoid:
  - Street food
  - Uncooked meat, fish, and eggs
  - Unpasteurized milk
  - Soft cheeses
  - Unwashed fruit and vegetables

Breastfeeding:

- Losing weight after giving birth does not affect the nursing newborn's weight gain
- Exercise does not affect the ability to successfully breastfeed

never skip breakfast to avoid the increased risk of ketosis, which can increase the risk of preterm delivery. Most nutrition experts caution that it is never healthy to diet during pregnancy.[11] The body is bombarded with hormonal changes in early pregnancy and, at least 70% of women experience nausea, vomiting, fatigue, stress, and/or other discomforts in the first trimester.[12]

Healthy Diet during Pregnancy

A healthy diet during pregnancy contains much the same balance of vitamins, minerals, and nutrients as a healthy diet in general (Table 1).

Calories

It is recommended that pregnant women consume an additional 300 calories over their normal requirement. Avoid dieting and the urge to binge eating during pregnancy. The key is moderation.

Complex Carbohydrates

Whenever possible, it is recommended to take complex carbohydrates (like whole-grain breads and pastas, vegetables, beans, and legumes) rather than nutritionally deficient simple carbohydrates (white bread, cookies, pretzels, chips, sugar, and sweeteners).

Protein

Four servings of protein daily (60–75 g daily) should be included. If the pregnancy is a high-risk one, higher amount is recommended.

Fat

High-fat foods should be limited to four servings daily. However, eliminating all fat is dangerous; essential fatty acids are important, including omega-3 fatty acids.

Note: No more than 30% of total calories should be from fat.

Fiber

Twenty to thirty-five grams of fiber a day is needed to help prevent constipation and hemorrhoids. Whole grains have to be taken.

TABLE 1: Recommended dietary allowance for select nutrients (Institute of Medicine, 2006)[13]

Recommended dietary allowance	*Women 19–50 years*		
	Nonpregnant	*Pregnant*	*Breastfeeding*
Folate (μg/day)	400	600	500
Iron (mg/day)	18	27	9
Vitamin A (μg/day)	700	770	1,300
Vitamin C (mg/day)	75	85	120
Vitamin D (mcg/day)	5	5	5
Calcium (mg/day)	1,000	1,000	1,000
Zinc (mg/day)	8	11	12
Vitamin B6 (mg/day)	1.3	1.9	2.0
Magnesium (mg/day)	310 (19–30 years) 320 (31–50 years)	350 (19–30 years) 360 (31–50 years)	310 (19–30 years) 320 (31–50 years)
Vitamin B12 (μg/day)	2.4	2.6	2.8

Iron

Iron-rich foods should be consumed daily. Since many women don't get enough iron in their diet, iron is an important part of prenatal supplements.

Salt

Salty foods should be consumed in moderation.

Fluids

Fluids are an important part of a healthy diet. At least 64 ounces (8 glasses) should be consumed per day, and more is better, preferably 80 ounces.

Importance of fluids:
- Water reduces the chance of constipation and subsequent hemorrhoids
- It increases flow of urine thus reducing the risk of developing urinary tract infection.

Vegetables

Three or more servings daily of green and yellow vegetables, which contain significant amounts of vitamin A, β-carotene, fiber, vitamin E, riboflavin, folic acid, vitamin B6, calcium, and trace minerals is recommended. Four additional servings per day should come from fruits and other (non-green/ yellow) vegetables. These provide fiber, vitamins, potassium, and magnesium.

Grains and Legumes

Whole grains and legumes (dried peas and beans) should comprise nine or more servings a day; they provide B vitamins (B1, B2, and B3) and trace minerals (zinc selenium, magnesium). These foods supply energy. Refined grains like white bread and instant white rice have fewer vitamins and fiber.

Essential Minerals and Vitamins for Pregnant Women

There are many important minerals and vitamins needed for a healthy pregnancy.

Minerals

Calcium: Calcium is an important nutrient throughout pregnancy. The fetus demands a huge supply of calcium during development and is thought to have a total body store of 25 g of calcium at birth, all of which is received from the mother. Pregnant women need 1,000 mg of calcium daily. Adequate calcium intake may also help prevent pregnancy induced high blood pressure and pre-eclampsia.[14] Adequate vitamin D intake is also important, as it aids in calcium absorption.

Source: Milk and dairy products are great sources of calcium, as is calcium-fortified orange juice and bread.

Iron: Iron is a crucial element in many of the body's processes. It is present in every molecule of hemoglobin. Iron supplements are important for most women, as few women get enough iron through their diet. The Center for Disease Control and Prevention recommends that all pregnant women take a daily supplement containing 30 mg of iron, since many women have difficulty maintaining iron stores during pregnancy.[15] Iron is often poorly absorbed from foods, which is why it is difficult for many people to reach the proper requirement. For example, while many vegetables have significant iron content, only 3–8% of the iron in these foods is absorbed, as compared to 20% of the iron in meat and fish.

Source:
- Green leafy vegetables, like spinach, turnip greens, and beet root
- Fruits, such as apple
- Seeds, such as pumpkin seeds
- Nuts like cashew, pine, peanut, and almond
- Beans especially soy beans, kidney beans, and chickpeas
- Whole grains like barley, quinoa, and oatmeal
- Jaggery, molasses, dark chocolate, and cocoa powder
- Red meat, liver, and fortified breakfast cereals. The best dietary sources of iron are oysters, clams, and mussels followed by liver chicken lamb pork and beef.

Magnesium: Magnesium is a major mineral important for bone building and essential to keep the body functioning properly. Mother needs 350–400 mg of magnesium for building and repairing of body tissues. A deficiency of magnesium during pregnancy may lead to nausea and vomiting, preeclampsia, eclampsia, and hamper fetal development. It has also been linked to preterm labor. Taking magnesium during pregnancy is important as it aids in functioning of enzymes, supports bones, regulates insulin, and blood sugar levels. Expectant woman can also control her cholesterol and palpitations, if she is maintaining proper magnesium levels.

Source: Seeds, whole grains, fish, leafy green vegetables, banana's, figs, and some legumes, but excellent sources are dairy products, dark chocolate, coffee, and water.

Iodine: Iodine is critical for the development and functioning of the thyroid gland and regulation of metabolism. The Recommended Dietary Allowance (RDA) for pregnant women is 200 μg per day.

Source: Iodine is obtained from fluoridated drinking water, iodized salt (table salt), eggs, milk, and brewer's yeast.

Potassium: Potassium is a mineral that affects cellular function, fluid balance, and blood pressure regulation, as well as proper nerve and muscle function. While there is no RDA for any pregnant adults, it is assumed that pregnant women require at least 2,000 mg per day.

Source: Prenatal vitamins can provide potassium, but potassium is present in high levels in foods, such as bananas, cantaloupe, oranges, watermelon, meats, milk, grains, potatoes, sweet potatoes, and legumes.

Phosphorus: Along with calcium, phosphorus is required for bone formation. Maternal serum inorganic phosphorus level remains constant during pregnancy because of maternal adaptations. Well-balanced diets easily provide the RDA for phosphorus in nonpregnant, pregnant, and lactating women; hence supplementation is not recommended.

Zinc: Zinc is involved in nucleic acid and protein metabolism and is, therefore, important in early gestation. Low plasma zinc concentrations during pregnancy have been associated with congenital abnormalities, abortions, intrauterine growth restriction, premature births, and preeclampsia. Zinc deficiency can also affect the immune response because it results in reductions in T cell development, thymic hormone release, and T cell functions. Well-balanced diets provide the RDA for zinc in women who are pregnant and lactating, and supplementation is not recommended. However, both iron and copper compete with zinc at absorption sites. Therefore, zinc supplementation is recommended when elemental iron supplementation exceeds 60 mg/day. Likewise, whenever zinc supplements are used, copper should also be supplemented.

Copper: Copper deficiency affects many cupro-enzymes leading to defects in adenosine triphosphate production, hormone activation, and angiogenesis, which can cause abnormalities of the vasculature, skeleton, and lungs. Although maternal copper level rises during pregnancy, its validity is questionable. There is an association between low copper levels and premature rupture of membranes.

Selenium: Selenium participates in antioxidant cellular protection and energy metabolism. However, there is very little evidence of detrimental effects of selenium deficiency on the fetus other than in conjunction with iodine deficiency.

Sodium: Sodium is present in large quantities in the average diet and its importance has often been overstated. Whether pregnant or not, sodium should neither be restricted nor used excessively. Well-balanced diets "salted to taste" satisfy sodium requirements and obviate any need for supplementation. Pregnant women should remember that most processed and prepreprepared foods are high in sodium, and hence the consumption of such products should be within limits.

Vitamins

Prenatal vitamins provide an abundance of other vitamins and minerals important in early pregnancy. However, vitamins should act more as insurance than as the primary source of nutrition.

Note: Large intake of some vitamins may be harmful, for instance, consumption of more than 10,000 International Units of vitamin A in early pregnancy can actually cause birth defects.[16]

Vitamin A: Vitamin A is critical for proper cell growth and the development of eyes, skin, blood, and immunity and resistance to infection.

Thiamine (B1): Thiamine is important for metabolism and development of the brain, nervous system, and heart. During pregnancy, the requirement of vitamin B1 is increased. The RDA for pregnant women is about 1.3 mg. Thiamine is present in many foods, with highest amounts in brewer's yeast, pork and ham, wheat germ, and peas.

Riboflavin (B2): This vitamin is important for fetal development and growth. The RDA for pregnant women is 1.6 mg and 1.8 mg for nursing women. A prenatal vitamin may be the best consistent source, but B2 can be found in liver, with smaller amounts present in soybeans, yogurt, and mushrooms.

Folic acid: Folic acid is another important vitamin that stimulates red blood cell formation and the production of important chemical signals in the nervous system. It has been identified as a critical vitamin to prevent neural tube defects in the baby and supplementation is initiated in the first several weeks of pregnancy, since the neural tube closes about 3–4 weeks after conception. It is taken in a dose of 400 μg daily.

Vitamin B6 (pyridoxine): Vitamin B6 is important for body's metabolism and for the development of the fetal brain and nervous systems. The RDA for pregnant women is 2.2 mg. There are a number of good food sources of vitamin B6, including bananas, chickpeas, potatoes, and chicken.

Vitamin B12: Vitamin B12 is important for hematopoiesis. It is found mainly in meats and dairy products, it can be low in vegans or strict vegetarians, resulting in macrocytic anemia during pregnancy. It will then require to be supplemented during pregnancy.

Vitamin C (ascorbic acid): Vitamin C is essential for wound healing and production of body's connective tissue. Vitamin C also helps the body absorb iron. The RDA for pregnant women is 80 mg per day. The best sources of vitamin C include fresh oranges and orange juice, strawberries, grapefruit and grapefruit juice, broccoli, tomatoes, and cabbage.

Vitamin D: Humans produce vitamin D in their skin in response to sunlight. Vitamin D itself is found naturally only in some fish liver oils. Since exposure to sunlight is variable and this vitamin is important for pregnant women and growing children. Low vitamin D levels are seen in many pregnant women and require supplementation during pregnancy.

Choline: Choline is a vital nutrient related to the vitamin B family and it is present in eggs, spinach, bacon, milk, cauliflower, kidney, soybean, salmon, white fish, bananas, lentils, and wheat germ. Discovered in 1862, it remained unrecognized as an essential nutrient till 1998. Although it can be produced within the body, the amount is not adequate to meet human needs; therefore, it must be obtained from the diet. The majority of body's choline is found in phospholipids, the most common being lecithin, the structural component of cell membrane. Choline is the key metabolic precursor of two physiological compounds—phosphatidylcholine and acetylcholine. Choline is essential for the structural integrity and signaling functions of cell membranes. It directly affects cholinergic neurotransmission and lipid transport from liver, and it is the major source of methyl groups in the diet. Betaine, one of the choline's metabolites, participates in the methylation of homocysteine to form methionine.

The demand for choline is especially high during pregnancy and lactation because of transport of choline from mother to fetus.[17] Choline plays an important role in fetal development as it influences stem cell proliferation and apoptosis as well as brain and spinal cord structure and function.[18]

Because of the insufficient scientific evidence which is needed to assign a RDA for choline, Food and Nutrition Board of the Institute of Medicine had recommended an adequate intake of choline in 1998. According to that recommendation, adult men need 550 mg of choline; whereas, adult women need 425 mg of the nutrient daily. For pregnant women, the amount is 450 mg.

Choline deficiency may lead to elevated levels of the amino acid homocysteine in the body which may in turn cause reduced cognitive functioning and increased risk of cardiovascular diseases. Adequate choline intake during pregnancy and lactation has been seen to improve attentiveness in the infant. Choline deficient diets during pregnancy had two times greater the risk of giving birth to babies who has neural tube defects and could cause the baby to have insufficient blood vessels in the brain that could lead to learning and memory difficulties later in life.

Maintaining a Vegetarian Diet

A woman can maintain a vegetarian diet and have a healthy pregnancy and a healthy baby. The body requires 15% more protein during pregnancy than usual, so consumption of 60 mg/day of protein is advised.

It is important for pregnant women to get adequate protein. For women who are lacto-ovo vegetarian (meaning they include dairy products and eggs in their diet), this is usually not a problem because eggs, cheese, milk, and yogurt provide plenty of protein.[19] Pregnant women should also focus on other protein sources, such as tofu and other soy proteins, beans and rice, legumes, and some nuts. Ideal menu plan is given in table 2.

TABLE 2: Ideal menu plan

Meal	*Menu*
Early morning	Tea/biscuits/nuts
Breakfast	Tea
	Spinach/besan/parathas/egg-toast
	Curd/milk
	Fruits – Apple guava
Mid-morning	Sprouts/chana chat
	Lemon water
Lunch	Channa curry/dal
	Stuffed vegetables/paneer
	Mint raita
	Salad
	Rice/chapattis
Evening tea	Banana shake in milk/soup
	Poha
Dinner	Pea paneer curry
	Mixed vegetable
	Chapattis/rice
	Fruit custard
Post dinner	Nuts/raisins/dates

Many vegetables and other foods provide calcium, such as nuts, dark leafy greens like kale and collard greens, broccoli, and dried fruit.

ENERGY NEEDS OF PREGNANCY— JUST A LITTLE MORE FOOD

Pregnant women's energy needs increase during their second and third trimesters according to Institute of Medicine, 2002 (Table 3).

TABLE 3: Estimated energy requirements by life stage group (Institute of Medicine, 2006)[20]

Age group	*Nonpregnant (kcal/day)*	*Pregnant*	*Breastfeeding*
Women 19–30 years	1,900	First trimester: 1,900 + 0 Second trimester: 1,900 + 340 Third trimester: 1,900 + 452	0–6 months postpartum: 1,900 + 330 7–12 months postpartum: 1,900 + 400
Women 31–50 years	1,800	First trimester: 1,800 + 0 Second trimester: 1,800 + 340 Third trimester: 1,800 + 452	0–6 months postpartum: 1,800 + 330 7–12 months postpartum: 1,800 + 400

Women who have a normal body weight at the start of their pregnancy need about 350 extra calories a day in their second trimester and 450 extra calories a day in their third trimester. These extra calories help them gain the amount of weight needed to support the baby's growth and development.

FOODS TO AVOID DURING PREGNANCY

- Canned food—can cause food poisoning
- Uncooked meats
- Coffee and tea
- Alcohol
- Greasy or heavily spiced foods
- Junk food with lots of calories and too few nutrients
- Cut down on salt as this can cause water retention and high blood pressure complications especially in the last trimester.

COMMON AILMENTS IN PREGNANCY AFFECTING NUTRITION

Common ailments in pregnancy are frequent and affect nutritional intake. The objectives of giving advice should be clear. Ailments during pregnancy include nausea and vomiting, which are most common in the first 3 months of pregnancy; heartburn and indigestion; and constipation.

Morning Sickness

- Avoid being hungry
- Eat some biscuits or toast in the morning
- Avoid strong food odors by eating food cold or at room temperature and using good ventilation while cooking
- Avoid fragrances that might trigger nausea, such as perfume, household cleaners, and air fresheners
- Drink a cup of ginger tea.

Heartburn and Indigestion

- Eat small, low-fat meals and snacks, such as fruits, pretzels, crackers, and low-fat yogurt, slowly and frequently
- Drink fluids between meals
- Avoid foods that may irritate the stomach, such as caffeine, spearmint, peppermint, citrus fruits, spicy foods, high-fat foods, and tomato products
- Take a walk after meals
- Avoid eating or drinking for 1–2 hours before lying down
- Slowly eating a bland snack, such as milk with cereal or low-fat yogurt can help ease heartburn. Yogurt is also a good source of calcium.

Medications

Laxatives, diuretics, and other medications taken may be harmful to the developing baby. These substances take away nutrients and fluids before they are able to feed and nourish the baby. It is possible that they may lead to fetal abnormalities as well, particularly if they are used on a regular basis.

NUTRITIONAL RISK FACTORS IN PREGNANCY

There are many nutritional risk factors associated with pregnancy and one should look out for them (Table 4).

Maintaining optimal nutrition through healthful food choices, such as fruits, vegetables, dairy products, whole grains, and lean protein is a must during pregnancy. Supplements of iron, calcium, folic acid and vitamin B_{12} may be required in pregnancy. Teenage pregnancy requires special attention to nutrition. Adequate amount of dietary fiber and fluid intake is also essential to prevent constipation.

TABLE 4: Nutritional risk factors in pregnancy

Risk factors present at onset of pregnancy	*Risk factors occurring during pregnancy*

• Age less than 15 years or greater than 35 years
• Frequent pregnancies—3 or more during approximately 2 years
• Poor obstetric history or poor fetal performance
• Poverty
• Bizarre food habits
• Abuse of caffeine, nicotine, alcohol, or drugs
• Therapeutic diet required for chronic disorders
• Inadequate weight
  ○ Less than 85% of standard
  ○ Greater than 120% of standard
	• Low hemoglobin—less than 12 g/mL
	• Inadequate weight gain
	  ○ Any weight loss
	  ○ Weight gain less than 1 kg per month after first trimester
	  ○ Excessive weight gain after first trimester 1 kg per week

REFERENCES

1. Kramer MS, Seguin L, Lydon J, et al. Socio-economic disparities in pregnancy outcome: why do the poor fare so poorly? Paediatr Perinat Epidemiol. 2000;14(3):194-210.
2. Committee on Nutritional Status During Pregnancy and Lactation, Institute of Medicine. Nutrition During Pregnancy Part I: Weight Gain, Part II: Nutrient Supplements. Washington DC: National Academy Press; 1990.
3. Hurley LS. Developmental Nutrition Englewood Cliffs (NJ): Prentice Hall; 1980.
4. Mac Burney M, Wilmore DW. Parenteral nutrition in pregnancy. In: Rombeau JL, Caldwell MD, editors. Clinical Nutrition: Parenteral Nutrition 2nd edition. Philadelphia: WB Sauders; 1993. pp. 696-715.
5. Osrin D, de L Costello AM. Maternal nutrition and fetal growth: practical issues in international health. Semin Neonatal. 2000;5(3):209-19.
6. Stone Neuhouser ML. Nutrition during pregnancy and lactation. In: Mahan LK, Escott-Stump S, editors. Food, Nutrition and Diet 9th ex. Philadelphia: WB Saunders; 1996. pp. 181-212.
7. Fawzi WW, Forman MR, Levy A, et al. Maternal anthropometry and infant feeding practices in Israel in relation to growth in infancy: the North African Infant Feeding Study. Am J Clin Nutr. 1997;65(6):1731-7.
8. Hytten FE. Weight gain in pregnancy. In: Hytten Fe, Chamberlain G, editors. Clinical Physiology in Obstetrics 2nd edition. Oxford: Blackwell Scientific Publication; 1991. p. 173.
9. Petitti DB, Croughan-Minihane MS, Hiatt RA. Weight gain by gestational age in both black and white women delivered of normal-birth-weight and low birth weight infants. Am J Obstet Gynecol. 1991;164(3):801-5.
10. Naeye RL. Maternal body weight and pregnancy outcome. Am J Clinical Nutr. 1990;52(2):273-9.
11. Hacker N, Moore JG, Gambone JC, editors. Essentials of Obstetrics and Gynecology, 4th edition. Philadelphia: Saunders; 2004. pp. 87-91.
12. ACOG Committee on Practice Bulletin—Obstetrics. ACOG Practice Bulletin: Clinical management guidelines for obstetrician-gynecologists number 92, April 2008 (replaces practice bulletin number 87, November 2007). Use of psychiatric medications during pregnancy and lactation. Obstet Gynecol. 2008;111(4):1001-20.
13. Institute of Medicine. 2006 Dietary Reference Intakes, the Essential Guide to Nutrient Requirements (Washington DC: National Academies Press).
14. Ritchie LD, King, JC. Dietary calcium and pregnancy-induced hypertension: Is there a relation? Am J Clin Nutr. 2000;71(5 Suppl):1371S-74S.

15. Recommendations to prevent and control iron deficiency in the United States. Centers for Disease Control and Prevention. Morbidity and Mortality Weekly Report (MMWR). 1998;47(RR-3):1-29.
16. Rothman KJ, Moore LL, Singer MR, et al. Teratogenicity of high vitamin A intake. New Engl J Med. 1995;333(21):1369-73.
17. Molloy AM, Mills JL, Cox C, et al. Choline and homocysteine interrelations in umbilical cord and maternal plasma at delivery. Am J clin Nutr. 2005;82(4):836-42.
18. Sweiry JH, Yudilevich DL. Characterization of choline transport at maternal and fetal interfaces of the perfused guinea-pig placenta. J Physiol. 1985;366:251-66.
19. Drake R, Reddy S, Davies J. Nutrient intake during pregnancy and pregnancy outcome of lacto-ovo-vegetarians, fish-eaters and non-vegetarians. Veg Nutr. 1998; 2:45-52.
20. Institute of Medicine. 2002. Dietary Reference Intakes for Energy, Carbohydrate, Fiber, Fat, Fatty Acids, Cholesterol, Protein, and Amino Acids (Washington DC: National Academies Press).

Nausea and Vomiting

5

CHAPTER

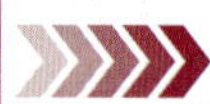

Anupam Gupta

INTRODUCTION

Nausea and vomiting of pregnancy, also known as "morning sickness" is a frequently encountered self-limiting problem, especially during the first trimester of pregnancy. It usually begins between the 4th and the 7th week in 80% of pregnant women and resolves by the 20th week of gestation. It affects more than 70% of pregnant women and is seen more in urban than in rural population. It is more common in housewives than in working women. A small percentage of pregnant women may have a more profound course, with the most severe form being hyperemesis gravidarum where women present with persistent vomiting, dehydration, ketosis, electrolyte disturbances, and weight loss. Multiple gestation, gestational trophoblastic disease, triploidy, trisomy 21 (Down syndrome), and hydrops fetalis have been associated with an increased incidence.

CAUSES

The etiology of nausea and vomiting of pregnancy remains unknown, but a number of possible causes have been investigated.[1]

Psychological

Although many believe that psychological factors are responsible for nausea and vomiting, few data support this theory.

Gastrointestinal Tract Dysfunction

Gastrointestinal tract dysfunction has also been suggested as a cause. *Helicobacter pylori* has been postulated as a possible cause in some.

Hormonal

It has been suggested that elevated levels of human chorionic gonadotropin (hCG) may be the cause. Some studies have also demonstrated elevated estrogen levels in women with this condition while others have not. Therefore, the role of hCG and estrogen remain controversial.[2] Many pregnant women with hyperemesis have shown suppressed TSH (thyroid-stimulating hormone) levels.[3]

DIFFERENTIAL DIAGNOSIS AND EVALUATION

Nausea and vomiting in early pregnancy is usually a self-limiting condition. When the condition is more severe, potentially serious causes need to be ruled out. A thorough history and a complete physical examination are important in the evaluation of pregnant women who present with persistent vomiting. If the findings of the history and physical examination suggest a specific cause, testing is directed toward confirming that cause. Ultrasonography may be helpful in ruling out gallbladder, liver, and kidney disorders. In addition to hyperemesis gravidarum, pregnancy related causes of persistent vomiting include acute fatty liver and preeclampsia.

Nonpregnancy related causes are listed in table 1.

TABLE 1: Nonpregnancy related causes of vomiting

Gastrointestinal	Gastroenteritis
	Hepatitis
	Biliary tract disease/gall stones
	Pancreatitis
	Appendicitis
	Peptic ulcer
	Intestinal obstruction
Genitourinary	Pyelonephritis
	Chronic renal disease
	Renal stones
	Degenerating leiomyoma
	Adnexal torsion
Metabolic	Diabetic ketoacidosis
	Addison's disease
	Hyperthyroidism
	Porphyria
Neurological	Migraine
	Pseudotumor cerebri
	Vestibular lesions
	Central nervous system tumors
Drug toxicity	

Investigations may be directed to them.

Recommendation: If symptoms are very severe and do not subside with treatment, or they appear after 9-weeks of gestation, other causes must be evaluated.

Laboratory Tests

- A chemistry panel is needed to detect and correct any electrolyte imbalances. The potassium concentration is especially important to note
- Thyroid function tests (free T3, free T4, and TSH) are obtained to exclude any thyroid disease
- A hepatitis panel is needed to rule out liver disease, which many times present with vomiting
- hCG is ordered to screen for possibility of molar pregnancy
- Ultrasound is ordered to determine whether a molar or partial molar pregnancy exists.

Maternal and Fetal Outcomes

Women with uncomplicated nausea and vomiting of pregnancy ("morning sickness") have been noted to have improved pregnancy outcomes, including fewer miscarriages, preterm deliveries, and stillbirths. The incidence of low birth weight, growth retardation, and mortality is less in these women. In contrast, hyperemesis gravidarum has been associated with increase in maternal adverse effects, including splenic avulsion, esophageal rupture, Mallory-Weiss tears, pneumothorax, peripheral neuropathy, pre-eclampsia, fetal growth restriction, and mortality.

TREATMENT

The management depends on the severity of the symptoms. Treatment measures range from dietary changes to more aggressive approaches involving antiemetic medications, hospitalization, or even total parenteral nutrition (TPN).

Principle of Management: It is preferable to start with dietary changes, and add medications if necessary. Medications started with milder and going on to stronger preparations, if needed.

Nonpharmacological Therapy

Dietary Modification

Initial treatment of women with mild nausea and vomiting of pregnancy should include diet modification. Affected pregnant women should be instructed to eat frequent small meals as volume overload in the stomach can trigger the vomiting reflex. They should avoid smells and food textures that cause nausea. Solid foods should be bland tasting, high in carbohydrates, and low in fat. Salty foods usually can be tolerated early in the morning. Sour liquids (e.g., lemonade) are often tolerated better than water. Family members should be informed that pregnant women with nausea and vomiting of pregnancy may need to alter meal times and other home routines.

Emotional Support

Although nausea and vomiting of pregnancy are not strongly associated with psychological illness, some women may become depressed or exhibit other mood affective disorders. It is important that these women receive appropriate support and tender loving care from family members and medical and nursing staff.

Ginger

A popular alternative treatment for morning sickness, ginger has been used in teas, preserves, ginger ale, and capsule form. One study demonstrated that ginger powder (1 g per day) was more effective than placebo in reducing the symptoms of hyperemesis gravidarum.[4]

Acupressure

Stimulation of the pericardium (PC) 6 site (called nei guan in Chinese) on the inner aspect of the wrist joint is the most famous and well researched points in acupressure. It is supposed to influence the flow of qi in the digestive tract and make it flow downward. However, large studies have failed to confirm the efficacy of acupressure.

Transcutaneous Nerve Stimulation

Transcutaneous nerve stimulation of PC 6 on the wrist has been effective.[5]

Pharmacologic Therapy

Pyridoxine (Vitamin B_6) and Doxylamine

Pyridoxine can be used as a single agent or in conjunction with doxylamine. A study demonstrated that vitamin B6 in a dosage of 25 mg taken orally every 8 hours (75 mg per day) was more effective than placebo for controlling nausea and vomiting in pregnant women. In pharmacologic doses, vitamin B6 has not been found to be teratogenic. A single 25 mg doxylamine tablet taken at night can be used alone or in combination with pyridoxine (25 mg three times daily).[6,7]

Antiemetics

If the previously discussed therapies are unsuccessful, a trial of antiemetics is warranted. Phenothiazine, prochlorperazine, and chlorpromazine have been shown to reduce nausea and vomiting of pregnancy compared with placebo. A reasonable regimen is prochlorperazine administered rectally in a dosage of 25 mg every 12 hours (50 mg per day) or promethazine (Phenergan) given orally or rectally in a dosage of 25 mg every 4 hours (150 mg per day).

If treatment with prochlorperazine or promethazine is unsuccessful, other antiemetics, such as trimethobenzamide or ondansetron can be tried. Studies have shown no increased benefit of ondansetron over promethazine.[8]

Antihistamines and Anticholinergic

Meclizine, dimenhydrinate, and diphenhydramine have been used to control nausea and vomiting during pregnancy. All have been shown to be more effective than placebo. Although meclizine was previously thought to be teratogenic, studies have demonstrated its safety during pregnancy.

Women with severe nausea and vomiting of pregnancy or hyperemesis gravidarum may benefit from droperidol and diphenhydramine (Benadryl). One study found that continuous intravenous administration of both droperidol and diphenhydramine resulted in significantly shorter hospitalizations and fewer readmissions compared with a variety of other in patient antiemetic therapies.[9,10]

Motility Drugs

Metoclopramide acts by increasing pressure at the lower esophageal sphincter, as well as speeding transit through the stomach. This drug has been shown to be more effective than placebo in the treatment of hyperemesis gravidarum.

Metoclopramide has not been associated with an increased incidence of congenital malformations.

Corticosteroids

Methylprednisolone, in a dosage of 16 mg three times daily (48 mg per day) followed by tapering of dose over 2 weeks, is an important treatment option for women with refractory hyperemesis gravidarum. However, a recent meta-analysis demonstrated a marginally increased risk of major malformation and a 3- to 4-fold increased risk of oral cleft in infants exposed to corticosteroids in the first trimester.[11]

Supportive Treatment

Intravenous Fluids

Women who are not controlled with the above treatment, require intravenous fluids. Normal saline or lactated Ringer's solution is the mainstay of intravenous fluid therapy. Many physicians use solutions that contain dextrose; however, it may be advisable to give thiamine (vitamin B1) first, because of the theoretic risk of Wernicke's encephalopathy. Intravenous fluid may provide relief from nausea and vomiting, but many pregnant women also require an antiemetic administered orally, rectally, or by infusion with the fluid. Depending on the severity of the symptoms, intravenous fluid therapy may be given in the hospital or at home by a visiting nurse.

Enteral or Parenteral Nutrition

Enteral tube feeding and TPN are last resort treatments for pregnant women who continue to vomit and lose weight despite aggressive treatment with any or all of the previously discussed modalities. TPN is administered through a central venous catheter. Its content is determined by the pregnant woman's daily caloric requirements and any existing electrolyte abnormalities. Consultation with a perinatologist experienced in parenteral nutrition, as well as a gastroenterologist or inpatient parenteral nutrition service, may be prudent. Both TPN and central venous access can result in significant complications including sepsis.

An algorithm for the suggested evaluation and management of women with nausea and vomiting of pregnancy is provided in figure 1.

Nausea and vomiting of pregnancy is usually a mild, self-limiting condition which is often controlled with conservative measures. Although several theories have been proposed,

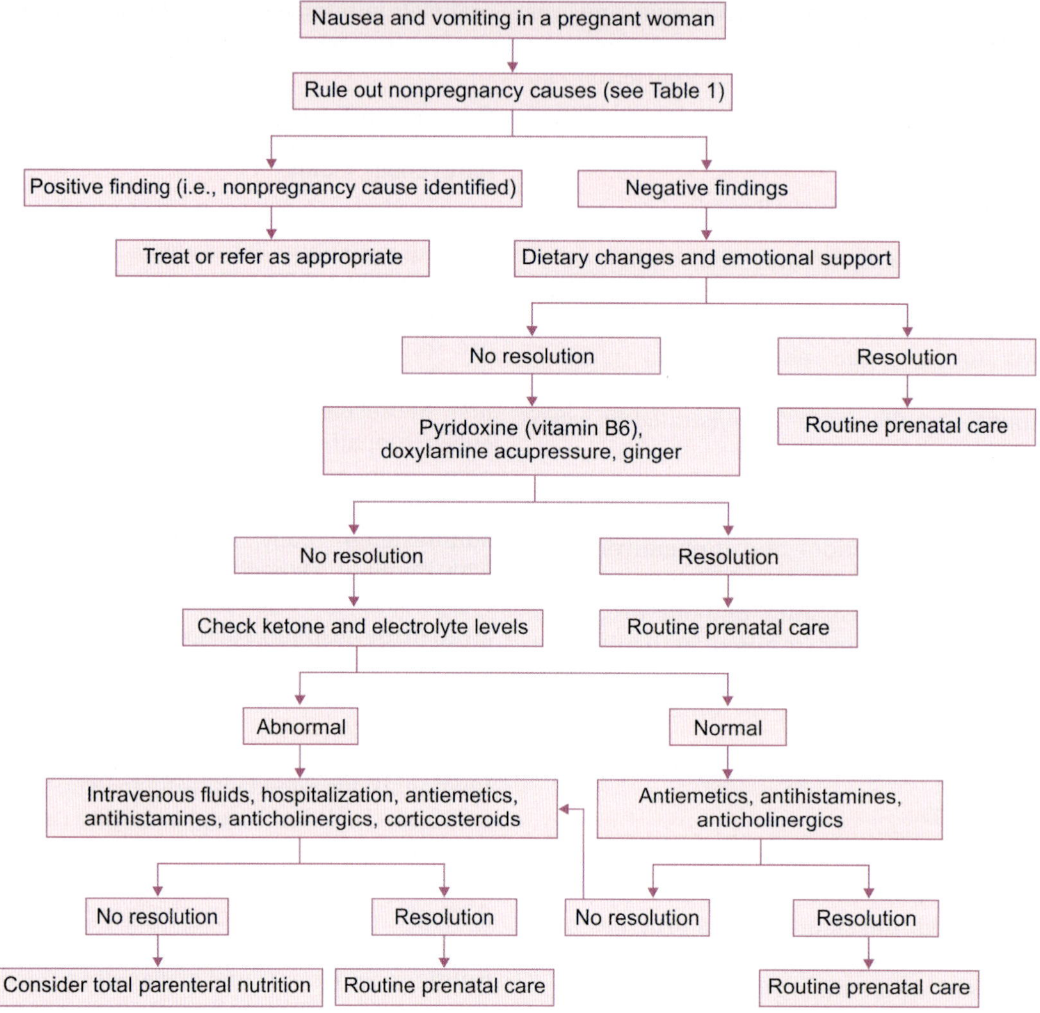

FIGURE 1 Evaluation and management of women with nausea and vomiting during pregnancy.

the exact cause remains unclear. Treatment is individualized. Initial treatment is conservative in the form of dietary changes, emotional support, and alternative therapies. Those who do not respond need medical treatment. Many medicines like pyridoxine and doxylamine, are safe and effective. Patients with severe symptoms may need orally or intravenously administered antiemetic therapy, and hospitalization.

REFERENCES

1. Verberg MF, Gillott DJ, Al-Fardan N, et al. Hyperemesis gravidarum, a literature review. Hum Reprod Update. 2005;11(5):527-39.
2. Tan PC, Tan NC, Omar SZ. Effect of high levels of human chorionic gonadotropin and estradiol on the severity of hyperemesis gravidarum. Clin Chem Lab Med. 2009;47(2):165-71.
3. Panesar NS, Li CY, Rogers MS. Are thyroid hormones or hCG responsible for hyperemesis gravidarum? A matched paired study in pregnant Chinese women. Acta Obstet Gynecol Scand. 2001;80(6):519-24.

4. Tan PC, Omar SZ. Contemporary approaches to hyperemesis during pregnancy. Curr Opin Obstet Gynecol. 2011;23(2): 87-93.
5. Evans AT, Samuels SN, Marshell C, et al. Suppression of pregnancy-induced nausea and vomiting with sensory afferent stimulation. J Reprod Med. 1993;38(8):603-6.
6. Ebrahimi N, Maltepe C, Einarson A. Optimal management of nausea and vomiting of pregnancy. Int J Womens Health. 2010;2:241-8.
7. Boskovic R, Einarson A, Maltepe C, et al. Diclectin therapy for nausea and vomiting of pregnancy: effects of optimal dosing. J Obstet Gynaecol Can. 2003;25(10):830-3.
8. Sheehan P. Hyperemesis gravidarum—assessment and management. Aust Fam Physician. 2007;36(9):698-701.
9. Lacasse A, Lagoutte A, Ferreira E, et al. Metoclopramide and diphenhydramine in the treatment of hyperemesis gravidarum: effectiveness and predictors of rehospitalisation. Eur J Obstet Gynecol Reprod Biol. 2009;143(1):43-9.
10. Matthews A, Dowswell T, Haas DM, et al. Interventions for nausea and vomiting in early pregnancy. Cochrane Database Syst Rev. 2010;(9):CD007575.
11. Chi CC, Lee CW, Wojnarowska F, et al. Safety of topical corticosteroids in pregnancy. Cochrane Database Syst Rev. 2009;(3):CD007346.

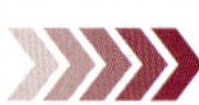

Hyperemesis Gravidarum

6

CHAPTER

S Shantha Kumari, D Vidyadhari

INTRODUCTION

Hyperemesis gravidarum (HG) is defined according to Fairweather's criteria as vomiting occurring in the first 20 weeks of pregnancy with severity that requires patient's admission to hospital, which is unassociated with coincidental medical conditions, such as appendicitis, pyelitis, etc. It is associated with dehydration, weight loss, ketonuria, and electrolyte imbalance (acidosis due to starvation, alkalosis due to loss of hydrochloric acid in vomitus, hypokalemia). It occurs in approximately 0.5–2% of pregnancies and is the most common indication for hospitalization during early pregnancy.[1] The etiology is unknown, but there is a close temporal relationship between onset and peak circulating levels of human chorionic gonadotropin (hCG) and development of HG. The reason for not being seen in all pregnant women is possibly due to the varying biologic activity of different hCG isoforms and differences in their susceptibility.

RISK FACTORS FOR HYPEREMESIS GRAVIDARUM

- Daughters and sisters of women who had the condition
- Multiple pregnancy
- Female fetus
- Obesity
- History of HG in previous pregnancy
- History of motion sickness
- History of migraine.

COMPLICATIONS

Both relatively benign and pernicious complications may be caused by HG[2] (Table 1).

TABLE 1: Complications of hyperemesis gravidarum

Benign complications	*Life threatening complications*
Weight loss	Esophageal rupture
Dehydration	Wernicke's encephalopathy
Acidosis from malnutrition	Central pontine myelinolysis
Alkalosis from vomiting	Retinal hemorrhage
Vitamin deficiencies	Renal damage
Hyponatremia	Spontaneous pneumomediastinum
Hypokalemia	Thrombosis
Muscle weakness	IUGR
ECG abnormalities	Fetal loss
Tetany	
Psychological disturbances	

ECG, electrocardiography; IUGR, intrauterine growth restriction.

Maternal

- *Vitamin deficiencies*: Cyanocobalamin (vitamin B12) and pyridoxine (vitamin B6) deficiencies may lead to anemia and peripheral neuropathy
- Wernicke's encephalopathy is a rare but recognized and distressing complication caused by thiamine deficiency, and can be precipitated by carbohydrate rich food and dextrose infusions. It normally manifests after approximately 7 weeks of vomiting. The classic triad of presentation consists of confusion, ocular abnormalities, and ataxia. Majority of patients exhibit only one of these symptoms. Diagnosis may be confirmed by the finding of low red cell transketolase (thiamine-dependent enzyme). Magnetic resonance imaging (MRI) is the gold standard investigation and typically demonstrates symmetrical lesions around the aqueduct and fourth ventricle
- *Korsakoff's psychosis*: It consists of retrograde amnesia, impaired ability to learn, and confusion
- *Hyponatremia and central pontine myelinolysis*: Hyponatremia (plasma sodium levels <120 mmol/L) presents with anorexia, headache, nausea, vomiting, and lethargy. More pronounced hyponatremia may result in personality changes, muscle cramps, weakness, confusion, ataxia, drowsiness, diminished reflexes, and convulsions. Rapid correction of hyponatremia is dangerous. There is an association between rapid correction of plasma sodium and osmotic demyelination syndrome also known as central pontine myelinolysis, characterized by the loss of myelin in the pontine neurons and in extra pontine sites, such as the internal capsule, basal ganglion, cerebellum, and cerebrum. The classic symptoms of myelinolysis are spastic quadriparesis and pseudobulbar paralysis, which reflects damage to corticospinal and corticobulbar paths
- *Hypokalemia*
- *Depressive illness and psychological morbidity*
- *Mallory-Weiss tears*: Prolonged vomiting may lead to Mallory-Weiss tear of esophagus and episodes of hematemesis[3]
- *Malnutrition*: Protein and caloric malnutrition results in weight loss which may be profound (10–20%), and muscle wasting with consequent weakness
- *Phlebitis*: If total parenteral nutrition (TPN) is required; this is usually given via a central venous catheter and has its own problems like phlebitis and thrombosis
- *Thrombosis*: Since hyperemesis results in dehydration and is usually associated with bed rest, it constitutes a risk factor for thromboembolism.

Fetal

- *Low birth weight*: Infants of mothers with severe hyperemesis associated with abnormal biochemistry and weight loss greater than 5%, have significantly lower birth weight compared to infants of mothers with mild hyperemesis[4]
- *Fetal loss*: Incidence of fetal loss is much higher.

EVALUATION AND DIAGNOSIS

Evaluation includes identification of other causes, as HG is a diagnosis of exclusion. Assessment of severity will determine the management.

Identification of Other Causes

History of onset of vomiting is very important as hyperemesis usually never begins after 9 weeks. In majority, vomiting develop at about 5 weeks gestation, peaks at about 9 weeks, and disappears at about 16–18 weeks. If vomiting begins after 9 weeks of gestation, other causes should be investigated. History should also aim to exclude symptoms of alternative cause of vomiting, such as UTI [urinary tract infection (dysuria or loin pain)], gastrointestinal infection (diarrhea), pancreatitis (abdominal pain), or preceding morbidity (diabetes, Addison's disease). Epigastric pain and hematemesis should be specifically enquired about, which may be either an effect of prolonged vomiting (Mallory-Weiss tear) or suggest other pathology which is causing the symptoms (gastroesophageal reflux and gastric ulceration). Hyperemesis tends to recur in 50% of subsequent pregnancies, so a previous history makes the diagnosis more likely.[5]

Assessment of Severity

Severity can be assessed by physical examination and investigations. Findings at physical examination include weight loss and signs of dehydration like loss of skin turgor, tachycardia, and postural hypotension.

Investigations

- Urinalysis for ketones
- Midstream urine for culture and sensitivity
- Complete blood count
- Serum creatinine, blood urea nitrogen, and electrolytes
- Liver function tests
- Thyroid function tests
- Ultrasound to exclude molar pregnancy and multiple pregnancy.

DIFFERENTIAL DIAGNOSIS

Other, more unusual causes of vomiting should be excluded with the help of history and relevant investigations (Table 2).

TABLE 2: Differential diagnosis

Gastrointestinal diseases • Gastritis • Gastroesophageal reflux • Peptic ulcer disease • Gastroenteritis • Pancreatitis • Appendicitis • Achalasia • Biliary tract obstruction **Genitourinary diseases** • Pyelonephritis • Renal calculi • Renal failure • Red degeneration of fibroid • Ovarian torsion **Obstetric** • Acute fatty liver • Preeclampsia	**Endocrinological diseases** • Diabetic ketoacidosis • Porphyria • Addison's disease • Hyperthyroidism • Hyperparathyroidism **Neurological diseases** • Migraine • Vestibular lesions • Tumors **Miscellaneous** • Drugs • Psychological

MANAGEMENT

The potential maternal and fetal complications of hyperemesis warrant early and aggressive treatment. Treatment is supportive as the condition is self-limiting.

Principles of Management

- Hospitalization: When a patient is stamped as a case of HG, it is desirable to hospitalize the patient even in the early stage[6]
- Cessation of oral feeds: Stop oral feeds for at least 24 hours until after vomiting subside
- Parenteral nutrition: Appropriate parenteral fluid and electrolyte replacement is the initial treatment regimen
- Sedation: Adequate sedation should be given
- Antiemetics: Antihistaminic and antiemetic drugs to control vomiting
- Supplementation: Vitamins to prevent neuropathy
- Steroids in refractile cases: Hydrocortisone only in cases of refractile vomiting not responding to other measures
- Supportive care: Sympathetic caring of the patient is essential. Care of teeth, gums, and oral hygiene is important. With these measures, the condition usually improves and patient is able to take oral feed.

Parenteral Fluids

Adequate and appropriate fluid and electrolyte replacement is the most important component of management. Initial fluid for resuscitation is isotonic saline, 2 liters infused over 3 hours to maintain a urine output more than 100 mL/h (Box 1). For maintenance, dextrose should be given to meet the need of calories. Subsequent fluid requirement varies with patient response, but as much as 125 mL/h may be required. Electrolyte deficiencies are treated and adequate replacement of potassium (K), magnesium (Mg), and phosphorus (P) is done as needed. Potassium chloride supplementation (20 mmol/3 mg per liter of sodium chloride 0.9%) should be given initially with the fluid replacement and then tailored to the serum potassium concentration. Fluid replacement can be tailored according to ketonuria or electrolytes and stopped once these have normalized and oral diet is resumed.[7]

Caution:
- Care must be taken not to correct low plasma sodium levels too quickly as too rapid a correction can cause osmotic demyelination syndrome
- When dextrose is given, thiamine 100 mg should be given first, to prevent Wernicke's encephalopathy.

Box 1: Fluid regimen

Day 1 (replacement)
- 1 liter 0.9% saline over 1 hour with 20 mmol of potassium chloride
- 1 liter 0.9% saline over 2 hours with 20 mmol of potassium chloride
- 1 liter 0.9% saline over 6 hours
- 1 liter 0.9% saline over 8 hours

Day 2 (maintenance)
- 5% dextrose in 0.9% saline as per requirement
- Thiamine 100 mg intravenously, multivitamins added to first liter of fluid
- Correction of electrolyte imbalance

Antiemetics

Various antiemetics are available; the list with dosage and route of administration is given in the table 3. Commonly given antiemetics while patient is on parenteral fluids are ondansetron and promethazine. Later, they can be changed to pyridoxine which is safe and effective.

Principle of antiemetic administration: Stronger antiemetics are given initially to control the acute situation, and milder ones are administered for maintenance.

Corticosteroids

They should be used with caution and are indicated in refractory cases. Methylprednisolone 16 mg, 8 hourly orally or intravenous (IV) can be given for 3 days. Then taper over 2 weeks to lowest effective dose. If symptoms do not improve, discontinue the treatment.

Caution:
- They should be avoided before 10 weeks gestation
- Length of treatment should be limited to not more than 6 weeks, if beneficial.

Vitamin Supplementation

Thiamine supplementation should be given to anyone suffering from prolonged vomiting. If the woman is able to tolerate tablets, thiamine can be given as thiamine hydrochloride tablets 25–50 mg TID. If parenteral treatment is required this is given as thiamine 100 mg diluted in 100 mL of normal saline and infused over 30–60 minutes. The IV preparation is only required weekly. The treatment of Wernicke's encephalopathy requires much higher doses of thiamine. Folic acid 5 mg daily should be prescribed, once oral intake has resumed to make-up for the deficiency induced by vomiting.

TABLE 3: Medical therapy

Drug	Dose	Category
Antiemetics		
Promethazine	12.5–25 mg orally or IM q 4–6 hours	C
Prochlorperazine	5–10 mg orally or IM q 6–8 hours	C
Ondansetron	4–8 mg orally q 12 hours; 0.15 mg/kg IV q 4 hours	B
Motility agents		
Metoclopramide	5–10 mg orally, IM or IV q 6–8 hours	B
Vitamins		
Pyridoxine	10–25 mg orally q 8 hours	A
Thiamine	100 mg/day	A
Antihistaminics		
Droperidol	0.625 1.25 mg IM/IV q 3–4 hours	C
Doxylamine	12.5 mg tid orally	B
Meclizine	25–50 mg orally q 12 hr	B
Dimenhydrinate	50–100 mg orally 4–6 hr	B
Diphenhydramine	25–50 mg orally/IM/IV 4–6 hours	B
Corticosteroids		
Methylprednisolone	16 mg q 8 hours orally or IV then taper	C

IM, intramuscular; IV, intravenous.

DIETARY AND LIFESTYLE ADVICE

After dehydration and acute vomiting resolves, small amounts of oral liquids are given. Once patients tolerate fluids, they can eat small, bland meals, and diet is expanded as tolerated. A summary of the dietary and lifestyle advice to be given to patient is listed below:

- Drink small amount of fluid frequently
- If intolerant to water, alternate fluids like flat lemonade, dilute fruit juice, weak tea and clear soup can be tried
- Eat small frequent meals
- Choose easily digestible bland food
- Avoid an empty stomach and nibble on light snacks between meals
- Early morning nausea may be helped by eating a dry biscuit before getting out of bed
- Salty foods may help. Try potato crisps or salty biscuits
- Avoid fatty, rich, spicy, or very sweet food
- Avoid foul smells and food with strong odors
- Avoid stress.

TOTAL PARENTERAL NUTRITION

Total parenteral nutrition becomes necessary in very severe cases of HG where treatment is ineffective. Metabolic and infectious complications are a risk and strict protocols, and careful monitoring are obligatory. The catheter site must be inspected regularly for signs of infection. Phlebitis and thrombosis are other recognized complications of TPN. Catheter related endothelial disruption may provoke thrombosis but in addition the direct endothelial injury secondary to a hyperosmolar infusate is likely to contribute. Because TPN involves use of high concentration of glucose, thiamine supplementation is mandatory. Enteral feeding with nasogastric tube is an alternative approach after acute symptoms subside with initial therapy.

THROMBOPROPHYLAXIS

Royal College of Obstetricians and Gynaecologists suggests the use of low-molecular-weight heparin in any woman with three recognized risk factors: (1) hyperemesis, (2) immobility, and (3) dehydration. Immobility and dehydration are both associated with hyperemesis.[8]

PSYCHOLOGICAL SUPPORT

All patients with HG require emotional support with frequent reassurance and encouragement from nursing and medical staff. Psychiatric referral may be appropriate in certain cases.

ALTERNATIVE THERAPY

Acupuncture, acupressure, and ginger can be tried to alleviate the symptoms of nausea and vomiting.

Ginger

Though there are no randomized trials there is some evidence that ginger may be beneficial and without adverse effects.

Acupuncture

Acupuncture requires a trained practitioner.

Acupressure

Acupressure may be a cheaper and more readily available option. Acupressure involves stimulation of the P6 Neiguan point, which is on the inside of the wrist, about 2–3 finger breadths proximal to the wrist crease between the tendons about 1 cm deep. Manual pressure is applied to this point for 5 minutes every 4 hours.

CONCLUSION

Medications are underutilized for concerns about treatment safety but American College of Obstetricians and Gynecologists recommends early treatment of symptoms to prevent progression to hyperemesis. Pyridoxine with or without doxylamine is safe and effective and should be considered as first-line treatment. Ginger has shown beneficial effects and can be considered a nonpharmacologic option. Women unable to tolerate oral fluids require admission to hospital. Maintaining hydration is more important than nutrition in the short-term. Severe and prolonged cases may require nasogastric or parenteral therapy. Women should be provided with dietary and lifestyle advice and psychological support.

REFERENCES

1. Verberg MF, Gillott DJ, Al-Fardan N, et al. Hyperemesis gravidarum, a literature review. Hum Reprod Update. 2005; 11(5):527-39.
2. Bashiri A, Neumann L, Maymon E, et al. Hyperemesis gravidarum: epidemiologic features, complications and outcome. EurJ Obstet Gynecol Reprod Biol. 1995;63(2):135-8.
3. Ballit JL. Hyderemesis gravidarium: epidemiologic findings from a large cohort. Am J Obstet Gynecol. 2005;193(3 Pt 1):811-4.
4. Tsang IS, Katz VL, Wells SD. Maternal and fetal outcomes in hyperemesis gravidarum. Int J Gynaecol Obstet. 1996;55(3): 231-5.
5. Verberg MF, Gillott DJ, Al-Fardan N, et al. Hyperemesis gravidarum, a literature review. Hum Reprod Update. 2005; 11:527-39.
6. Fell DB, Dodds L, Joseph KS, et al. Risk factors for hyperemesis gravidarum requiring hospital admission during pregnancy. Obstet Gynecol. 2006;107:277-84.
7. Tan PC, Omar SZ. Contemporary approaches to hyperemesis during pregnancy. Curr Opin Obstet Gynecol. 2011;23(2): 87-93.
8. RCOG Guideline (Green-top 37a). Thrombosis and Embolism during Pregnancy and the Puerperium, Reducing the Risk. 2007.

First Trimester Screening

7

CHAPTER

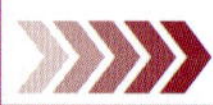

Anita Kaul

INTRODUCTION

Over the last few years due to scientific advances in fields, such as fetal physiology, genetics, imaging, and maternal biochemical testing, there has been a change of thinking regarding screening for maternal and fetal problems. It is now established that most major aneuploidies can be detected at 11–13 weeks of gestation.[1] It is also seen that an integrated hospital visit at 11–13 weeks where maternal characteristics (blood pressure, weight, ethnic origin, and smoking) along with history, ultrasound, and biochemical tests can define the patient at risk for a wide spectrum of pregnancy complications, which include not only chromosomal abnormalities, but also preeclampsia, fetal growth restriction, miscarriage, and stillbirth.[2] Studies are also underway for screening for gestational diabetes and preterm labor in the first trimester.[3,4]

It has, therefore, been proposed that the model of antenatal care needs to be reversed from a mainly third trimester centric care of frequent prenatal visits to concentrating care at the beginning of pregnancy so as to detect, define, and modify maternal and fetal complications. This approach of reversing the pyramid of antenatal care will be better able to triage women to either a high-risk or low-risk group, so that more optimum utilization of the limited health resources will be possible[5] (Fig. 1).

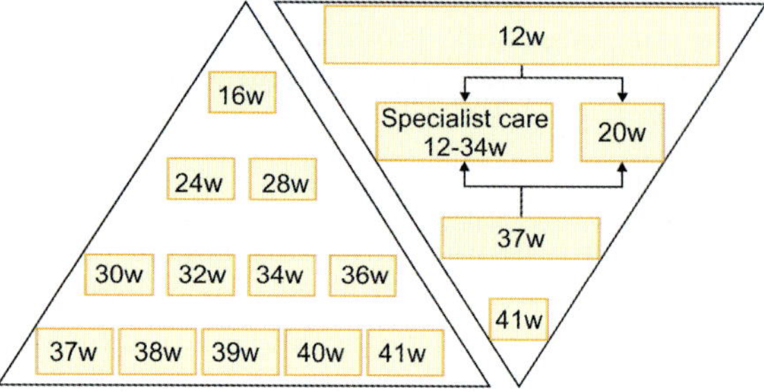

FIGURE 1 Pyramid of prenatal care: past (left) and future (right).

SCREENING FOR FETAL ANEUPLOIDIES

Chromosomal disorders are a cause of perinatal death and childhood handicap. In our country, where infrastructural resources are limited, it may be better to identify aneuploidies early by effective maternal screening and subsequent invasive testing, so that the parents have an option of discontinuing the pregnancy if they choose. Early detection with adequate counseling and adequate time for the parents to consider their choices thoroughly is particularly relevant, in light of the preconception and prenatal diagnostic techniques law in India which prohibits termination of pregnancy after 20 weeks.

The methods of screening for aneuploidies have changed over the decades from maternal age only in the 1970s to nuchal translucency (NT) screening in the first trimester in the 1990s. The addition of more ultrasound markers, e.g., nasal bone, tricuspid regurgitation, ductus venosus pulsatility index (DVPI) to the NT along with first trimester biochemistry, i.e., pregnancy-associated plasma protein A (PAPP-A),[1] and free beta chorionic gonadotropin (β-hCG) has resulted in increasing sensitivity in detecting trisomy 21.

NT is the sonographic appearance of a collection of fluid under the skin behind the fetal neck in the first trimester of pregnancy. The incidence of chromosomal and other abnormalities is related to the size, rather than the appearance of NT. The discovery that NT is a sensitive marker of aneuploidy has been one of the most significant contributions to the advance of prenatal diagnosis.[6]

Essentials for accurate NT measurements:

- Crown-rump length (CRL) between 45 mm and 85 mm
- A good mid-section of the fetus showing the facial profile
- Clear differentiation between the fetal skin and the amnion achieved by spontaneous or induced fetal movement
- Magnification of the image so that the fetal head, neck, and upper thorax occupy three-fourths of the screen
- Placing of the calipers on the border of the white lines (fetal skin and fetal skull) so that the maximal translucent area is measured
- The fetal head should be in a neutral position. Extended head will increase and flexed head will decrease the measurement
- The measurement should be performed in the line of the fetal mandible that usually corresponds to the area of widest NT.

It is imperative, however, that any sonologist who is performing a scan on pregnant women between 11 weeks and 13 weeks, measures the NT correctly as defined by the Fetal Medicine Foundation criteria, otherwise inaccurate risks for aneuploidies will be given to couple (Fig. 2). This is important, as often in our country, the woman may not have repeated ultrasound examinations and may find additional biochemical testing expensive. Hence, it is reliant on the ultrasound examination done at 11–13 weeks to detect anomalies.

In table 1, the detection rates of trisomy 21 are given and it is seen that the detection rates increase from 75% to 80% from just using the NT to 93–96% using the new ultrasound markers such as nasal bone, tricuspid regurgitation, DVPI[7] along with maternal serum biochemistry.

It is also possible to calculate patient risks for trisomy 18 and 13 as well. The biochemical and sonographic features for trisomy 21, 18, and 13 are enumerated in table 2.

Nasal Bone

Absent nasal bone (NB) is another important marker of Down syndrome in the first trimester of pregnancy.[8] The NB is absent in 68.8% of fetuses with Down syndrome and in 32.2 of fetuses with other chromosomal abnormalities. In the normal population, the frequency of absent NB is related to the ethnic origin of the mother, and it is 2.2 in Caucasians, 9.0% in Afro-Caribbeans, and 5% in Asians.[9] These normal variations need to be taken into consideration when evaluating a patient's individual risk of Down syndrome using the NB as a marker.

Requirements for Accurate Nasal Bone Measurements[10]

- The fetus needs to be facing the ultrasound transducer
- The magnification of the image should be such that the head and the thorax occupy the whole image (11–13 weeks scan)
- The angle of insonation should be 90R (face of the transducer should be parallel to the longitudinal axis of the nasal bone and the skin over the nasal bridge)
- In normal fetuses, three echogenic lines should be identified (the skin over the nasal bridge, a line below the skin that corresponds to the nasal bone, and the third line further

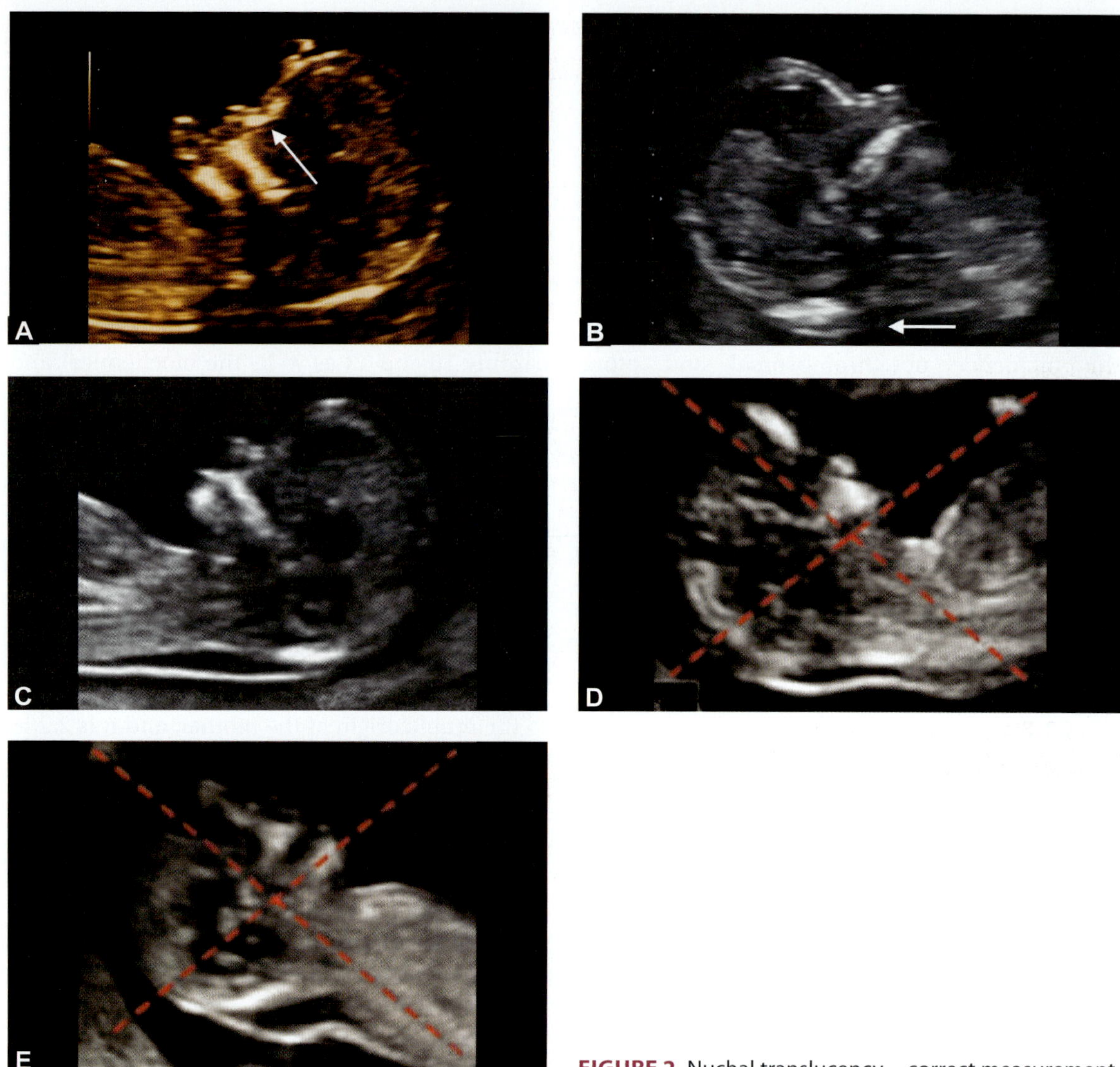

FIGURE 2 Nuchal translucency—correct measurement.

away from the forehead than the nasal bone and at a slightly higher level that corresponds to the skin over the nasal tip)

- The two parallel lines representing the skin over the nasal bridge and the nasal bone compose the so called "equal sign" (=)
- If the bottom part of the equal sign is missing, the nasal bone is considered to be absent.

Free Beta Human Chorionic Gonadotropin

Human chorionic gonadotropin (hCG), is a glycoprotein made up of two alpha and beta subunits that may be bound to each other or free. Both free alpha and beta subunits are increased in Down syndrome but only the free beta subunit has been widely used for screening.

TABLE 1: Performance of different methods of screening for trisomy 21

Method of screening	Detection rate	False-positive rate (%)
Maternal age	30	5
First trimester		
MA + fetal NT	75–80	5
MA + serum free β-hCG and PAPP-A	60–70	5
MA + NT + free β-hCG and PAPP-A (combined test)	85–95	5
Combined test + nasal bone or tricuspid flow or ductus venosus flow	93–96	2.5
Second trimester		
MA + serum AFP, hCG (double test)	55–60	5
MA + serum AFP, free β-hCG (double test)	60–65	5
MA + serum AFP, hCG, uE3 (triple test)	60–65	5
MA + serum AFP, free β-hCG, uE3 (triple test)	65–70	5
MA + serum AFP, hCG, uE3, inhibin A (quadruple test)	65–70	5
MA + serum AFP, free β-hCG, uE3, inhibin A (quadruple test)	70–75	5
MA + NT + PAPP-A (11–13 weeks) + quadruple test	90–94	5

MA, maternal age; NT, nuchal translucency; β-hCG, β-human chorionic gonadotropin; PAPP-A, pregnancy-associated plasma protein-A; AFP, alpha fetoprotein.

TABLE 2: Biochemical and sonographic features of trisomies 21, 18, and 13

	Euploid	Trisomy 21	Trisomy 18	Trisomy 13
NT mixture model				
CRL-independent distribution, %	5	95	70	85
Median CRL-independent NT, mm	2.0	3.4	5.5	4.0
Median serum free β-hCG, MoM	1.0	2.0	0.2	0.5
Median serum PAPP-A, MoM	1.0	0.5	0.2	0.3
Absent nasal bone, %	2.5	60	53	45
Tricuspid regurgitation, %	1.0	55	33	30
Ductus venosus reversed a-wave, %	3.0	66	58	

NT, nuchal translucency; CRL, crown-rump length; β-hCG, beta-human chorionic gonadotropin; MoM, multiple of the median; PAPP-A, pregnancy-associated plasma protein-A.

The increase in free beta-hCG in fetuses with aneuploidy starts at the end of the first trimester and continues during the second trimester, making the test useful for both first and second trimester screening. Total hCG is also increased in aneuploid pregnancies but investigations have demonstrated that is a poor marker in the first trimester of pregnancy.[11] When used alone, free beta-hCG has a detection rate for Down syndrome of 33%, a value that increases to 46% when used in combination with maternal age. When free beta-hCG values are combined with maternal age and PAPP-A the detection rate increases to 67%.[12]

Pregnancy-associated Plasma Protein A

The majority of fetuses with aneuploidy exhibit reduced levels of PAPP-A in the first trimester of pregnancy. PAPP-A concentration is lower in fetuses with aneuploidy but the difference with normal pregnancies becomes smaller with advances in gestational age, making this analyte useful only in the 10–14 week interval. When used alone, it has a detection rate of 38% that increases to 48% when combined with maternal age.[12]

SCREENING FOR FETAL STRUCTURAL ABNORMALITIES

The aim of first trimester scan is not just to screen for trisomy 21 but also to diagnose an increasing number of fetal malformations, which is best assessed around 12 weeks of gestation (Fig. 3). Major fetal abnormalities fall into 3 broad groups when they are detected at 11–13 weeks.[13]

1. Always detectable abnormalities, e.g., body stalk anomaly, anencephaly, alobar holopro-

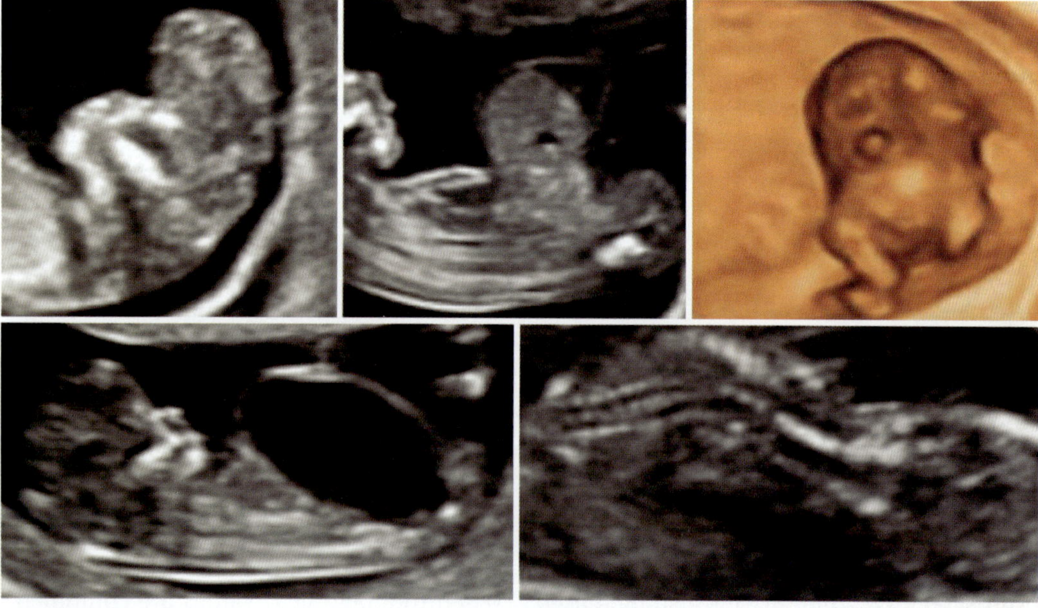

CC, Corpus Callosum; NT, nuchal translucency; DV, ductus venosus; TV, tricuspid value; CHD, congenital heart disease.

FIGURE 3 Abnormalities detected in the first trimester scan.

sencephaly, exomphalos, gastroschisis, and megacystis

2. Undetectable abnormalities because sonographic signs are only manifest during the second or third trimester of pregnancy, e.g., brain abnormalities, such as microcephaly, hypoplasia of the cerebellum or vermis, hydrocephalus and agenesis of the corpus callosum, achondroplasia, echogenic lung lesions, many renal anomalies, and bowel obstruction
3. Abnormalities that are potentially detectable depending on the objectives set for such a scan and consequently the time allocated for the fetal examination, the expertise of the sonographer and the quality of the equipment used. It is also dependent on the presence of an easily detectable marker for an underlying abnormality, e.g., high NT, and abnormal flow in the ductus venosus and across the tricuspid valve in major cardiac defects, and increase in brain stem diameter with decrease in the diameter of the fourth ventricle-cisterna magna complex in open spina bifida.[7,14]

In a study of 12,110 women, 54.5% structural problems were detected, most of these pregnancies were terminated. Those who underwent a second trimester anomaly scan 13.9% defects were detected. Of these, nearly 40% decided to continue the pregnancy as most of them were nonlethal and correctable defects. It was concluded that most of the major structural defects that lead to termination of the pregnancy can be and should be detected at the first trimester scan.[15]

SCREENING FOR PREECLAMPSIA

Preeclampsia is a major cause of maternal and perinatal mortality and it is important to try and identify the women who are at potential risk for developing this condition, in their first visit itself. The woman's risk for preeclampsia should be determined by a series of maternal characteristics, such as maternal age, body mass index, previous and family history of preeclampsia.

By adding mean arterial pressure measurements, uterine artery Doppler measurements and measurement of PAPP-A to the maternal characteristics, in an algorithm, improves the assessment of risk even further[11] (Fig. 4). This is particularly true for the development of preeclampsia (<34 weeks) which is associated with more serious adverse pregnancy outcomes. 77.8% of women will be identified for early preeclampsia, 56.6% for intermediate (34–37 weeks), and 34% with late preeclampsia more than 37 weeks, with a false positive rate of 5%.[16]

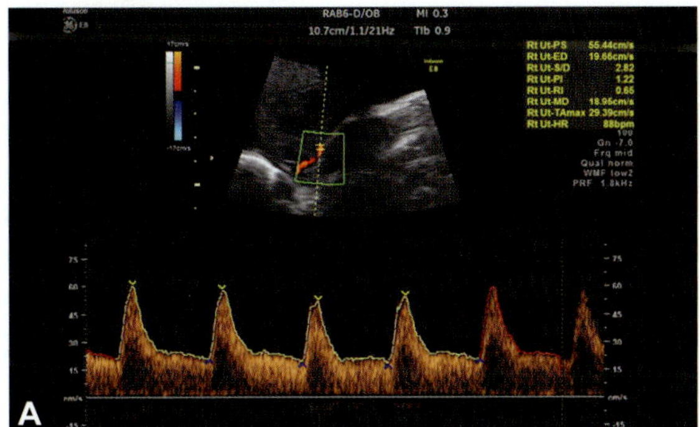

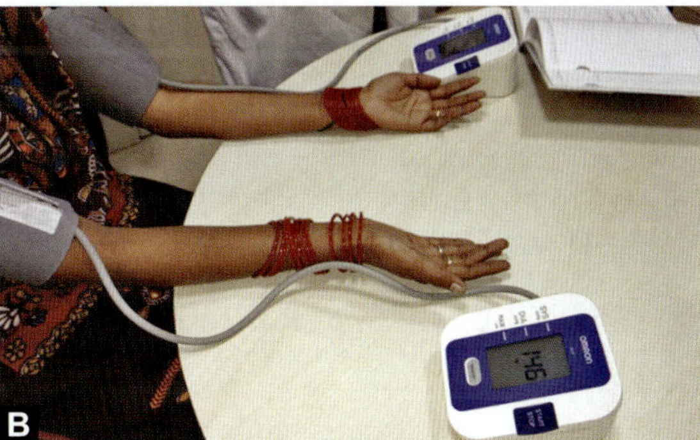

FIGURE 4 Measuring uterine artery and mean arterial pressure.

SCREENING FOR SMALL FOR GESTATIONAL AGE FETUSES

Small for gestational age fetuses can be constitutionally small, or small due to genetic abnormalities, or due to impaired placentation leading to growth restriction. In this latter group the risk of perinatal death and handicap are substantially increased and can be reduced by appropriate monitoring and delivery if identified early. It is seen that an algorithm that combines maternal characteristics, mean arterial pressure, uterine artery Doppler measurements, and PAPP-A at 11–13 weeks could detect 75% of pregnancies without preeclampsia, who delivered small for gestational age neonates before 37 weeks and 45% at term.[17]

SCREENING FOR PRETERM DELIVERY

The vast majority of mortality and morbidity related to preterm births are when they occur before 34 weeks. In two-third of cases, it is due to spontaneous onset of labor or preterm premature rupture of membranes and in one-third, it is iatrogenic and mainly due to preeclampsia. At present there are no useful tools for predicting preterm birth by either history or biophysical or biochemical markers. However, recent studies have shown that the cervical length is shorter in women who go into spontaneous preterm labor.[4] Transvaginal measurement of cervical length with an empty bladder are most accurate, as a full bladder gives an erroneous impression of a long cervix. Screening for preterm birth should be performed along with the early anomaly scan at 11 weeks and repeated at the 20 week anomaly scan. Cervix may be required to be screened periodically thereafter in women at high-risk of preterm birth.

SCREENING FOR MISCARRIAGE AND STILLBIRTH

The rates of miscarriage and stillbirth after demonstration of a live fetus at 11–13 weeks are about 1 and 0.4%, respectively. Increased risk for miscarriage and stillbirth are associated with certain maternal characteristics like older age, increasing maternal weight, and previous miscarriage or stillbirth. Miscarriage and stillbirth are also associated with abnormal results of first trimester screening for aneuploidies, including increased fetal NT thickness, reversed a-wave in the fetal ductus venosus and low maternal serum PAPP-A.[18] At present as there is no useful intervention for avoidance of miscarriage, it may not be justified in using this algorithm in clinical practice. On the other hand, early identification of the group at high-risk for stillbirth could lead to a reduction of this complication through closer monitoring of fetal growth and well-being, and appropriate timing of delivery.

First trimester screening for aneuploidy has multiple advantages. The most important is a detection rate better or similar to that of second trimester screening. Also, majority of women can be reassured early in gestation of the normalcy of the pregnancy and those found to have an affected fetus and who choose to terminate the pregnancy could have it done by a procedure much safer than that used later in gestation. Also, first trimester screening and termination of affected pregnancies protects the privacy of the pregnant women because it is done at a time when the physical manifestations of pregnancy are not apparent. Finally, the decision to terminate or not the pregnancy when the fetus is affected is not influenced by the maternal perception of fetal movements.

First trimester screening is not only an adequate method for early selection of the patients at risk for aneuploidy but also abnormal results in the absence of aneuploidy are associated with obstetrical complications. The National Institute of Child Health and Human Development study on first trimester maternal serum biochemistry and ultrasound and NT screening for trisomy 21 and trisomy 18 demonstrated that PAPP-A and free beta-hCG values below the first percentile were associated with increased risk for fetal growth restriction. PAPP-A less than fifth percentile and NT more than ninety-ninth percentile were associated with increased risk of preterm delivery before 34 weeks.[19] Similar conclusions were found in the FASTER (Fast Assessment of Stroke and Transient Ischemic Attack to Prevent Early Recurrence) trial.[20]

First trimester screening should be performed when the CRL is between 45 mm and 85 mm (10 weeks 4 days and 13 weeks 6 days of gestation). The NT measurement should be performed by a person trained and certified for the performance of the examination. Blood for measurement of the biochemical analytes can be collected by finger stick in specialized filter paper.[21] Follow-up of the first trimester screening results varies depending on the overall strategy adopted for the screening and diagnosis of chromosomal abnormalities.

CONCLUSION

it is clear that we need to change our thinking and provide an early estimation of patient specific risk for a variety of pregnancy complications, which we have seen is possible at 11–13 weeks. This will lead to an improvement in pregnancy outcome by shifting antenatal care from a series of routine visits as was in the past to a more individualized patient and disease specific approach which is more contemporary and meets the need of the mother and fetus effectively.

REFERENCES

1. Nicolaides KH. Screening for fetal aneuploidies at 11 to 13 weeks. Prenat Diagn. 2011;31(1):7-15.
2. Nicolaides KH. Turning the pyramid of prenatal care. Fetal Diagn Ther. 2011;29(3):183-96.
3. Nanda S, Savvidou M, Syngelaki A, et al. Prediction of gestational diabetes mellitus by maternal factors and biomarkers at 11 to 13 weeks. Prenat Diagn. 2011; 31(2):135-41.
4. Greco E, Lange A, Ushakov F, et al. Prediction of spontaneous preterm delivery from endocervical length at 11 to 13 weeks. Prenat Diagn. 2011;31(1):84-9.
5. Nicolaides KH. A model for a new pyramid of prenatal care based on the 11 to 13 weeks' assessment. Prenat Diagn. 2011;31(1):3-6.
6. Nicolaides KH, Azar G, Byrne D, et al. Fetal nuchal translucency: ultrasound screening for chromosomal defects in first trimester of pregnancy. Br Med J. 1992; 304(6831):867-9.
7. Chelemen T, Syngelaki A, Maiz M, et al. Contribution of ductus venosus Doppler in first-trimester screening for major cardiac defects. Fetal Diagn Ther. 2011;29(2):127-34.
8. Cicero S, Curcio P, Papageorghiou A, et al. Absence of nasal bone in fetuses with trisomy 21 at 11-14 weeks of gestation: an observational study. Lancet. 2001;358(9294):1665-7.
9. Cicero S, Rembouskos G, Vandecruys H, et al. Likelihood ratio for trisomy 21 in fetuses with absent nasal bone at the 11-14 week scan. Ultrasound Obstet Gynecol. 2004;23(3):218-23.
10. Sonek JD, Cicero S, Neiger R, et al. Nasal bone assessment in prenatal screening for trisomy 21. Am J Obstet Gynecol. 2006;195(5):1219-30.
11. Aitken DA, McCaw G, Crossley JA, et al. First-trimester biochemical screening for fetal chromosome abnormalities and neural tube defects. Prenat Diagn. 1993;13(8): 681-9.
12. Spencer K, Souter V, Tul N, et al. A screening program for trisomy 21 at 10-14 weeks using fetal nuchal translucency maternal serum free β-human chorionic gonadotropin and pregnancy-associated plasma protein A. Ultrasound Obstet Gynecol. 1999;13:231-7.
13. Syngelaki A, Chelemen T, Dagklis T, et al. Challenges in the diagnosis of fetal non-chromosomal abnormalities at 11-13 weeks. Prenat Diagn. 2011;31(1):90-102.
14. Lachmann R, Chaoui R, Moratalla J, et al. Posterior brain in fetuses with open spina bifida at 11 to 13 weeks. Prenat Diagn. 2011;31(1):103-6.
15. Radhakrishnan P, Venkatesh P, Acharya V, et al. Screening for major fetal defects at 11-13 weeks. Presented at the World Congress in Fetal Medicine. Rhodos. 2010.
16. Akolekar R, Syngelaki A, Sarquis R, et al. Prediction of early, intermediate and late pre-eclampsia from maternal factors, biophysical and biochemical markers at 11-13 weeks. Prenat Diagn. 2011;31(1):66-74.
17. Karagiannis G, Akolekar R, Sarquis R, et al. Prediction of small-for-gestation neonates from biophysical and biochemical markers at 11-13 weeks. Fetal Diagn Ther. 2011;29(2):148-54.
18. Akolekar R, Bower S, Flack N, et al. Prediction of miscarriage and stillbirth at 11-13 weeks and the contribution of chorionic villus sampling. Prenat Diagn. 2011;31(1):38-45.
19. Krantz D, Goetzl L, Simpson JL, et al. Association of extreme first-trimester free human chorionic gonadotropin-beta, pregnancy-associated plasma protein A, and nuchal translucency with intrauterine growth restriction and other adverse pregnancy outcomes. Am J Obstet Gynecol. 2004;191(4):1452-8.
20. Dugoff L, Hobbins JC, Malone FD, et al. First trimester maternal serum PAPP-A and free-beta subunit human chorionic gonadotropin concentrations and nuchal translucency are associated with obstetric complications: a population-based screening study (The FASTER trial). Am J Obstet Gynecol. 2004;191(4):1446-51.
21. Krantz DA, Hallahan TW, Orlandi F, et al. First trimester Down syndrome screening using dried blood biochemistry and nuchal translucency. Obstet Gynecol. 2000;96(2):207-13.

Invasive Procedures

8

CHAPTER

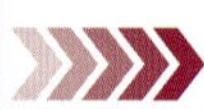

Prashant Acharya, Ashini Acharya

INTRODUCTION

Most women wish to be reassured that their unborn baby is healthy. Ultrasound is the method of choice for detection of anatomical problems (e.g., absent kidneys and spina bifida), but provides no information on the genetic constitution of a fetus. Maternal serum screening, alone or in combination with ultrasound, is often used. The problem of "false positive" screening tests (maternal serum screening and ultrasound) and lack of therapeutic options for chromosomal abnormalities makes couple and the clinician think about karyotyping to get the final result. The aim is, therefore, to select screening and diagnostic tests that are both accurate and safe, and at the same time can be done early in pregnancy to allow to choose termination of pregnancy.

There are limited procedures one can perform in the first trimester for diagnostic and therapeutic purposes. Fetal diagnosis can be from:

- Chorionic villous sampling (CVS)
- Coelocentesis.

Fetal reduction can be helpful in multifetal pregnancy to reduce the number of fetuses or selective fetal reduction in case of one of the fetus being abnormal in multiple pregnancy.

INDICATIONS FOR PRENATAL DIAGNOSIS IN FIRST TRIMESTER

With the introduction of prenatal screening for fetal aneuploidy by ultrasonography (USG) and chemical markers in first trimester, we are able to identify and screen positive patients who are at a higher risk of chromosomal abnormality in the fetus. A positive first trimester screening test for fetal aneuploidy is the most common indication for CVS.

Indications for Chorionic Villous Samples

Chorionic villous sampling is indicated when karyotyping is needed in the following circumstances:

- Positive first trimester USG markers and/or biochemical markers
- Increased maternal age
- Parental abnormal karyotype
- Family history of genetic disorders[1] like:
    - Hematological disorders: thalassemia carrier state of both partners, sickle cell disease carrier state of both partners, hemophilia, and Factor IX and X deficiency
    - Duchene muscular dystrophy
    - Congenital adrenal hyperplasia

- ○ Cystic fibrosis
- ○ Biochemical, metabolic, and amino acid disorders
- ○ Skin disorders: epidermolysis bullosa dystrophica, albinism, and icthyosis.

RECOMMENDATIONS BEFORE PRENATAL PROCEDURES IN FIRST TRIMESTER

Couple counseling is mandatory and has to be individualized. It should address the following:

- Indications for procedure of prenatal testing
- Discussion on the prospective parents' degree of risk for transmitting genetic abnormalities based on factors, such as maternal age, race, and family history
- Prospective parents should be made aware of both the limitations and usefulness of prenatal diagnostic procedure in detecting abnormalities
- Potential serious complications from procedures and the risk for miscarriage attributable to procedures, e.g., the risk from amniocentesis at 15–18 weeks' gestation is approximately 0.25–0.50% (1/400–1/200), and the miscarriage risk from CVS at 11–14 is approximately 0.5–1.0% (1/200–1/100).

METHODS OF INVASIVE PRENATAL DIAGNOSIS IN FIRST TRIMESTER

There are two methods of invasive prenatal testing in the first trimester:

1. Chorionic villous sampling—aspiration of chorionic villi
2. Coelocentesis—aspiration of coelomic fluid.

Chorionic Villous Sampling

Chorionic villous sampling involves aspiration of placental villi and sending the same for either cytogenetic or molecular diagnosis. It is done keeping the following points in mind.

- *Continuous ultrasound guidance*: Continuous ultrasound guidance is mandatory for CVS, as it not only allows one to choose the appropriate site to insert the needle but also permits continuous visualization of the needle tip, during its insertion and during the time that the needle is *in situ*, to avoid damage to the fetus and membranes
- *Sterile techniques*: Sterile techniques including hand-washing, use of sterile gloves, use of antiseptic solution to clean the abdomen, and sterile drapes should be used. A no touch technique (the needle should not be touched anywhere except at the hub) is recommended. It may be noted that infection is the most common cause of procedure associated fetal loss
- *Local anesthesia*: An adequate local anesthesia with 2% lignocaine is provided in the entire path of the needle to make the patient more comfortable as a 18 G needle is required for the CVS
- *Anti-D*: Injection anti-D is indicated in all Rh negative mother after all prenatal diagnostic procedures.

Procedure and Approach

After informed consent and counseling, ultrasound is done for fetal viability, gestational age, number of fetuses, placental site and accessibility, and proposed needle path. CVS can be performed by the transabdominal or the transcervical approach. If the placenta is posterior and low lying, a transcervical route is most appropriate, whereas an anterior placenta is most easily approached abdominally. The approach may also depend on operator's choice and experience. Special needle and approach is required for multiple pregnancies.

Transabdominal CVS is a safer procedure than transvaginal approach. In the latter case, there is a risk of per vaginal spotting or bleeding and also a greater risk of procedure related loss when compared to the transabdominal approach. Since infection is suggested to be a major cause of miscarriage, the greater rate of miscarriage with the vaginal approach could be attributed to the higher rates of infection with this approach. As experience with transabdominal CVS increases, a vaginal approach is rarely indicated. Even a low posterior placenta can be approached by the transabdominal approach.

Timing of the procedure: CVS should be performed after 10 completed weeks. CVS prior to 9 weeks is known to result in hypoglossia and limb reduction abnormalities.[2,3] Therefore, early CVS is not recommended.

An early result is advantageous for the patient as in cases of an unaffected pregnancy, the anxiety is relieved and in cases of affected pregnancy early termination of pregnancy can be undertaken with lower complication rate.

Confined placental mosaicism can occur in about 1% of CVS samples and an amniocentesis or a cordocentesis is then indicated.

Transabdominal Chorionic Villous Sampling

An 18–20 g disposable spinal needle of adequate length (7.5–15 cm) is used. Under aseptic precautions, the needle is passed through anterior abdominal wall into the middle of the substance of chorion frondosum under continuous ultrasound guidance by freehand guide technique (Fig. 1). The stillete is withdrawn and 10 mL syringe with 1 mL saline/media solution is attached to the needle. With gentle up and down movements (not more than twice if possible) while applying continuous negative pressure, villi are aspirated, taking care to avoid puncturing the fetal aspect of amniotic membrane. Needle is withdrawn after applying the negative pressure. Sample is checked with naked eye, but preferably under low power in a microscope. If required it is washed with normal saline and put in to the media solution before transporting it to the laboratory. Fetal heart activity is checked at the end of the procedure.

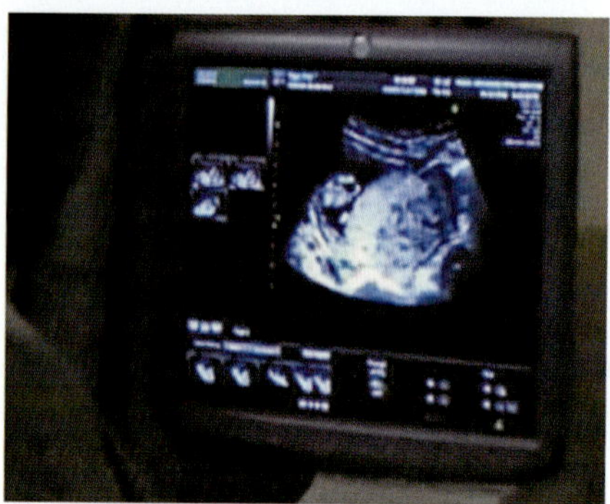

FIGURE 1 Transabdominal chorionic villous sampling under ultrasound guidance.

Advantages and disadvantages of transabdominal CVS: [4]

- Advantages:
  - There is minimal risk of infection
  - It does not cause vaginal bleeding
  - It can be performed in the second and third trimesters
- Disadvantages:
  - The amount of tissue obtained is less than that with transcervical CVS
  - Patient discomfort is greater than that with transcervical CVS or amniocentesis
  - It is difficult to perform if the placenta is posterior
  - It is technically more difficult than transcervical CVS.

Transcervical Chorionic Villous Sampling

Basic principle remains the same, that is, to reach the middle of the substance of the chorionic frondosum and apply negative pressure to obtain the villi from placenta. With all aseptic care, a vaginal speculum is inserted and the cervix is held with a tenaculum. Metal/plastic cannula with metal obturator or Cooks biopsy forceps is passed through the cervix under ultrasound guidance till it reaches into the substance of chorion frondosum, parallel to axis of developing placenta. The obturator is removed and a 10 mL syringe containing 1 mL of saline or media is attached. Negative pressure is applied to the syringe and the cannula is moved up and down several times (preferably not more than twice) through the placenta, and villi are aspirated. Cannula and attached syringe are removed and villi examined.

Advantages and disadvantages of transcervical CVS: [5,6]

- Advantages:
  - Genetic diagnosis is achieved at an early gestational age, minimizing the anxiety of the parents and facilitating termination of pregnancy for patients who choose this option
  - It is comfortable for the patient since no pain or discomfort is involved
  - It is technically simple
- Disadvantages:
  - It has a slightly higher risk of fetal loss (0.8%) than traditional amniocentesis
  - The chromosome composition of the chorionic villous is occasionally (1.3% of the cases) different from the chromosome composition of the fetal cells
  - The enzyme composition of the chorionic villous cells may be different from the fetal cells
  - It is difficult if the placenta is above the lower one-third of the uterus.

Contraindications to transcervical CVS:

- Positive *Neisseria gonorrhoeae* culture of the cervix
- Active genital herpes
- Active bleeding
- Maternal coagulopathy
- Cervical stenosis
- Severe cervicitis
- Uterine myomata
- Intrauterine device inside the pregnant uterus.

Complications of Chorionic Villous Sampling

- *Vaginal bleeding*: Less common after transabdominal procedure
- *Infection*: This can lead to a miscarriage
- *Rupture of membranes*: Rupture of membranes because of mechanical or infective injury to the chorion allowing exposure of amnion to damage or infection. Delayed rupture of membranes may occur in up to 0.3% [5,7]
- *Miscarriage*: Transcervical CVS also increases the total risk to pregnancy compared with a second trimester amniocentesis, mostly because of spontaneous miscarriages.

Transvaginal Chorionic Villous Sampling

There are some patients in whom transabdominal and transcervical CVS are difficult to perform due to extreme uterine retroversion, presence of myomas, or placental localization. In some of these patients, chorionic villi may be obtained using transvaginal aspiration under guidance with an endovaginal probe.[8]

Comparison of Various Approaches of Invasive Prenatal Diagnostic Techniques

Transabdominal Chorionic Villous Sampling versus Second Trimester Amniocentesis

A study in Denmark compared transabdominal CVS with second trimester amniocentesis and found no significant difference in the total pregnancy loss between the two procedures (6.3% versus 7%; relative risk (RR) 0.90; 95% CI 0.66–1.23).

Transabdominal versus Transcervical Chorionic Villous Sampling

Compared with transabdominal CVS, total pregnancy loss and spontaneous miscarriages were higher after transcervical CVS. It is more likely to cause vaginal bleeding immediately after the procedure, in approximately 10% of women.

There was no difference in the incidence of vaginal bleeding later in pregnancy or in amniotic fluid leakage following the procedure and prelabor spontaneous rupture of membranes before 28 weeks. Abdominal CVS may be safer than the transcervical route. Transcervical CVS is also technically more demanding, with more failures to obtain the sample and higher incidence of multiple needle insertions for sample.[9]

Early Amniocentesis versus Transabdominal Chorionic Villous Sampling

There were more spontaneous miscarriages after early amniocentesis than second trimester amniocentesis (7.6% versus 5.9%; RR 1.29; 95% CI 1.03 to 1.61). There was a higher risk of talipes with early amniocentesis compared to CVS (RR 4.61 95% CI 1.82 to 11.66) [10]

Recommendation on choice of method: Second trimester amniocentesis is safer than transcervical CVS and early amniocentesis. If earlier diagnosis is required, transabdominal CVS is preferable to early amniocentesis or transcervical CVS. In circumstances where transabdominal CVS may be technically difficult the preferred options are transcervical CVS in the first trimester or second trimester amniocentesis.[7]

Coelocentesis

Coelocentesis is aspiration of coelomic fluid from the cavity. From 6th week onwards the gestational sac contains amniotic and exocoelomic (chorionic) cavity. Volume of coelomic fluid doubles from 6 weeks to 8 weeks and reaches a maximum of 5–6 mL at 9 weeks and then gradually reduces, and almost disappear by the 13th week. Theoretically, coelocentesis is less traumatic to the fetus and early placenta and may, therefore, be a safer method in early pregnancy. It is especially important in prenatal diagnostic test for sex-linked disorders.[11] However, maternal cell contamination can take place.[12]

Technique of Coelocentesis

Coelomic aspiration is performed under transvaginal guidance. After aseptic precaution 22 G needle is inserted with the needle guide in the coelomic cavity. The needle should be introduced in to the uterus centrally avoiding injury to uterine vessels (Fig. 2). Avoid puncturing the yolk sac and amniotic membrane. Coelomic fluid should be aspirated up to 2 mL with low pressure technique using only 2 mL syringe. The fluid is yellow colored and more viscous in nature than amniotic fluid. Coelomic fluid contains cells that are mostly of hematopoietic origin. The number of viable cell aspirated are maximum around 7 weeks and gradually reduces to 30–40% at around 9 weeks. For prenatal diagnosis, successful culture will be available for genetic testing including fluorescent *in situ* hybridization, karyotyping, and polymerase chain reaction for single gene disorder.

During a relatively short period of time, first trimester screening and diagnosis is surfacing to increase the options available to patients. The new challenges are to develop techniques that can be used during the first trimester of pregnancy to avoid or reduce the phenotypic expression of inherited inborn errors of metabolism. For this reason, experimental *in vivo* ultrasound guided stem cell transplantations have been performed during very early intrauterine development.

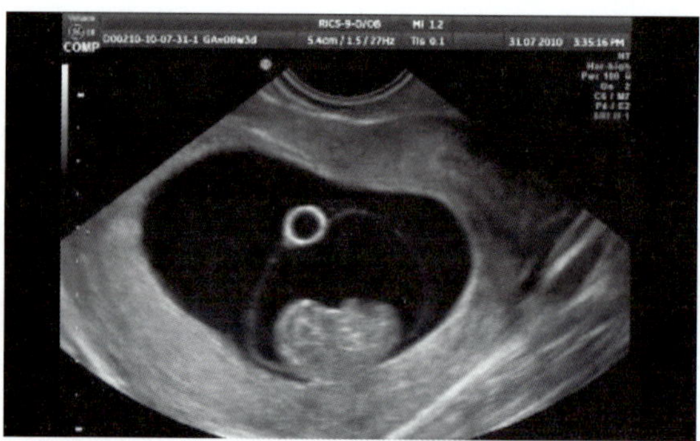

FIGURE 2 Coelocentesis.

One of the approaches for *in utero* stem cell treatment is the coelocentesis procedure. Indeed, coelocentesis has already brought new insights into the composition of coelomic fluid in humans and primates, and some of the biological roles of coelomic fluid in primates are beginning to be elucidated.[13] Parental diagnosis of genetic disorders is feasible and maternal tolerance to xenotransplantations via coelocentesis at 40 days from fertilization has been proven in the baboon animal model.[14] Finally, very recently, it has been reported that the coelomic fluid can be partially replaced *in vivo* by stem cell culture medium opening the doors to transforming the coelomic fluid into a "bio-reactor" that would prolong the survival and permit the expansion of the limited number of stem cells that can be injected into the coelomic cavity.[15]

Coelocentesis is a useful technique for the investigation of early fetal physiology and pathophysiology. Moreover, it offers the possibility for very early prenatal diagnosis, from at least 7 weeks gestation. However, there are three main limitations to the introduction of coelocentesis as an alternative to amniocentesis or CVS, for fetal karyotyping. Firstly, the number of studies examining the safety of the technique is small. Secondly, conventional cytogenetic analysis is not a realistic approach because of the difficulty in culturing coelomic cells. Thirdly, screening for chromosomal defects has shifted from the traditional approach of maternal age to fetal nuchal translucency (NT) and first or second trimester biochemistry. Therefore, further, larger studies are needed to prove the safety of the technique, comparative genomic hybridization or microarrays could be used to examine the fetal karyotype and new ultrasound or biochemical markers for chromosomal abnormalities should be identified in the early first trimester. Nevertheless, for the diagnosis of conditions, such as beta thalassemia where the risk for an affected fetus is 25%, coelocentesis may be a realistic alternative.

MULTIPLE PREGNANCY AND SELECTIVE FETAL REDUCTION

Since the advent of assisted reproductive technology (ART), multiple pregnancies, which constitute a significant risk to both fetuses and the mother, have become increasingly common. The fraction of multiple pregnancies accounted for by ART continues to increase from 28% in 1986 to almost 50% in 1993. The trend is even more significant with higher order multiple pregnancies (triplets and up), which now constitute from 0.1% to 0.3% of all pregnancies. Multiple pregnancies are known to be associated with an increased rate of maternal and perinatal complications. Medical concerns aside, the socioeconomic impact of providing care for such high-risk pregnancies cannot be underestimated. Selective multifetal reduction can be offered as an option, where one or more babies are aborted in order to improve perinatal outcome for the remaining fetuses.

Timing, Technique, and Outcome

Multifetal reduction is usually carried out in the first trimester. It can be done by transvaginal or transabdominal route under USG guidance. This procedure is best performed as a transabdominal procedure between 10–12 weeks of gestational age, under local anesthesia. Fetus with an increased NT should be selected; otherwise the fetus nearest to the ultrasound probe is selected. Spinal needle no. 21 with stylet is advanced through the abdominal and uterine wall into the fetal sac. Stylet is removed. Syringe is loaded with 2 mL of 2 mEq potassium chloride solution. The needle is visualized on ultrasound and advanced into the fetal thorax and potassium chloride is injected. Needle is removed after confirming fetal cardiac asystole. Cardiac activity of other fetus is confirmed. Postprocedural second look ultrasound is done after few hours and another scan a few days later.

Complications

- Leaking per vaginum
- Bleeding per vaginum
- Abortion or loss of remaining fetuses
- Infection.

Weighing Risks Versus Benefits

Multifetal reduction in higher-order multiple gestations has many benefits for the remaining fetuses, including substantially increasing the duration of pregnancy, reducing the incidence of prematurity, reducing neonatal mortality, and shortening the neonatal intensive care stay. As the number of fetuses increase, so does the risks of preterm labor and delivery. For singletons, the average length of gestation is 40 weeks, compared with 36 weeks for twins, 33 weeks for triplets, and about 29 weeks for quadruplets. Each additional viable fetus present in the first trimester shortens the duration of gestation by about 3.6 weeks. Thus, each fetus reduced, either spontaneously or medically, can potentially prolong gestation by about 3 weeks. With quadruplet and higher-order pregnancies, which have high rates of neonatal mortality and morbidity, the advantages of selective fetal reduction outweigh the risks of the procedure. Whether triplet pregnancies benefit from selective reduction to twins also is the subject of ongoing debate. Most studies done to date suggest an improved perinatal outcome for triplet pregnancies reduced to twins compared with non-reduced triplet pregnancies.[16-18] Reduction of twin pregnancy to singleton is not often considered. However, a comparative analysis showed that the loss rate is lower in twins that are reduced to singleton.[19]

Prenatal diagnostic tests help in filling up the gaps in biochemical screening and ultrasound scan. They are useful for establishing a definitive diagnosis. They help in the final decision making as to whether the pregnancy should be terminated. Reduction of multifetal pregnancy is best performed at 11 weeks when early anomalies can be visualized by checking the NT and nasal bone. Reduction of triplets to singleton and even twins to singleton improves the pregnancy outcome by prolonging gestation.

REFERENCES

1. Verp MS. Prenatal diagnosis of genetic disorders. In: Gleicher N, editor. Principles and practice of medical therapy in pregnancy, 2nd ed. Norwalk,CT: Appleton and Lange; 1992. pp. 159-70.
2. Schloo R, Miny P, Holzgreve W, et al. Limb reduction defects following chorion villous sampling. Amer J Med Genet. 1991;42:4040-413.
3. Report of National Institute of Child Health and Human Development Workshop on Chorionic Villus Sampling and Limb and Other Defects. Am J Obstet Gynecol. 1993;169(1):1-6.
4. Saura R, Longy M, Horovitz J, et al. Risks of transabdominal chorionic villus sampling before the 12th week of amenorrhea. Prenat Diagn. 1990;10(7):461-7.
5. Rhoads GG, Jackson LG, Schlesselman SE, et al. The safety and efficacy of chorionic villus sampling for early prenatal diagnosis of cytogenetic abnormalities. N Engl J Med. 1989;320(10): 609-17.
6. Multicentre randomised clinical trial of chorion villus sampling and amniocentesis. First report. Canadian Collaborative CVS-Amniocentesis Clinical Trial Group. Lancet 1989;1(8628):1-6.
7. Kuliev AM, Modell B, Jackson L, et al. Risk evaluation of CVS. Prenat Diagn. 1993;13(3):197-209.
8. Sidransky E, Black SH, Soenksen DM, et al. Transvaginal chorionic villus sampling. Prenat Diagn. 1990;10(9):583-6.
9. Jackson LG, Zachary JM, Fowler SE, et al. A randomized comparison of transcervical and transabdominal chorionic-villus sampling. The U.S. National Institute of Child Health and Human Development Chorionic-Villus Sampling and Amniocentesis Study Group. N Engl J Med. 1992;327(9): 594-8.
10. Alfirevic Z, Sundberg K, Brigham S. Amniocentesis and chorionic villus sampling for prenatal diagnosis. Cochrane Database Syst Rev. 2003;(3):CD003252.
11. Jouannic JM, Costa JM, Ernault P, et al. Very early prenatal diagnosis of genetic diseases based on coelomic fluid analysis:a feasibility study. Hum Reprod. 2006;21(8):2185-8.
12. Jouannic JM, Tachdjian G, Costa JM, et al. Coelomic fluid analysis: the absolute necessity to prove its fetal origin. Reprod Biomed Online. 2008;16(1):148-51.
13. Santolaya-Forgas J, Roman W, Edwin S et al. (2006) Concentration of soluble VEGF-RI and VEGF-R-2 in extra-embryonic celomic fluid in primates. Available from: www.med.miami.edu.
14. Santolaya-Forgas J, Galan I, Deleon- Luis J, et al. A study to determine if human umbilical cord hematopoietic stem

cell can survive in baboon extra-embryonic celomic fluid: a Prerequisite for determining the feasibility of in-utero stem cell Xeno transplantation via celocentesis. Fetal Diagn Ther. 2007;22(2):131-5.

15. Santolaya-Forgas J, Deleon-luis J, Galan I. Can extra-embryonic celomic fluid be partially replaced with stem cell culture medium? Ultrasound Obstet Gynecol. 2006;28(2):232-3.
16. Mansour RT, Aboulghar MA, Serour GI, et al. Multifetal pregnancy reduction: modification of the technique and analysis of the outcome. Fertil Steril. 1999;71(2):380-4.
17. Yaron Y, Bryant-Greenwood PK, Dave N, et al. Multifetal pregancy reduction of triplets to twins: comparison with nonreduced triplets and twins. Am J Obstet Gynecol. 1999; 180(5):1268-71.
18. Boulot P, Vignal J, Vergnes C, et al. Multifetal reduction of triplets to twins: a prospective comparison of pregnancy outcome. Human Reprod. 2000;15(7);1619-23.
19. Evans MI, Kaufman MI, Urban AJ, et al. Fetal reduction from twins to singleton: a reasonable consideration? Obstet Gynecol. 2004;104(1):102-9.

Vaccination

9

CHAPTER

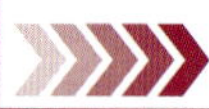

Sangeeta Tejpuria

INTRODUCTION

Vaccination is one of the most effective strategies employed to prevent morbidity and mortality from infectious diseases. The single most effective mean of disease prevention is active vaccination. Preferably, vaccination status should be reviewed prior to conception. However, this goal is difficult to accomplish taking into consideration that many pregnancies are unplanned. Pregnancy is considered to be a time when women have consistent contact with their healthcare providers and it presents an opportunity for providers to review their immunization status and to advocate for appropriate vaccination antepartum and in the immediate postpartum period. All forms of immunization, with the exception of live viral or live bacterial vaccines are generally considered to be safe for administration during pregnancy. It is important that healthcare providers counsel pregnant women about the benefits of receiving vaccines that are recommended during pregnancy as well as the potential risks to the developing fetus. It is imperative that obstetricians and primary care providers are aware of, and implement the vaccination guidelines for women, both during pregnancy and in the postpartum period.

IMMUNIZATION DURING PREGNANCY

Ideally, all women should have their immunization status up to date prior to conception. However, owing to suboptimal vaccine administration in adult women and the fact that many pregnancies are unplanned, this goal is difficult to accomplish. Pregnancy provides an opportunity for healthcare professionals to provide primary prevention measures as well as to increase awareness of health-related issues as a component of routine prenatal care with the added benefit of the availability of support services and often insurance coverage. Vaccination during pregnancy and the puerperal period includes vaccines routinely recommended to all pregnant women. Vaccines administered for certain medical or exposure indications and postpartum immunizations. The use of mother as a vehicle to protect her fetus and newborn infant against recognized pathogens through transplacental passive antibody transfer is another advantage of immunization during pregnancy.[1,2] Obstetricians and primary care providers should be aware of the vaccination guidelines published by US Center for Disease Control and Prevention and Advisory Committee on Immunization Practices (ACIP).[3]

Immunologic and anatomic changes during pregnancy alter the pregnant patient's response to infection. These changes can result in increased susceptibility to infection or increased severity of certain infections. The effects of maternal infection on fetus are dependent on multiple factors, including the type of organism, the inoculum, pre-existing host immunity, and host defenses. These factors among others help to determine whether the infectious agent can infect and traverse the placenta. Also, fetuses vary from their mothers and one from another in their ability to avoid or overcome infection. Overwhelming infection usually result in abortion or fetal death. Less frequently, infection can result in structural or developmental abnormalities.

A decision to vaccinate during pregnancy should be based on the woman's relative risk of exposure to the disease, susceptibility to the disease, gestational age, and the relative risk of the vaccine being considered.

All forms of immunization, except live-viral and live-bacterial vaccines are considered to be safe during pregnancy.

ATTENUATED VIRUS VACCINE

Administration of live virus vaccines are contraindicated during pregnancy, this includes vaccines against measles, mumps, rubella, poliomyelitis, yellow fever, varicella, and influenza.

Measles-Mumps-Rubella Vaccine

Measles-mumps-rubella (MMR) vaccine and its component vaccine should not be administered to women considering pregnancy. MMR vaccine or rubella vaccine is a live vaccine, if given, women should be advised to delay pregnancy for 1–3 months. Pregnancy is a contraindication to live vaccination; however, if administered inadvertently during pregnancy, it is not an indication for termination of pregnancy as no deleterious reports on the fetus have been documented.[4] Every women should be checked for rubella immunity during her antenatal check up and if found unimmunized, she should be immunized in the postpartum period. Live vaccines are not contraindicated during breast feeding.

In the "Vaccine in Pregnancy Registry" data from 1971–1989 of 286 women who were vaccinated with rubella vaccine between 3 months before to 3 months after conception are documented. There was no evidence of congenital rubella syndrome in any of the offspring.[5]

Polio Vaccine

Polio vaccines are available in two forms:

1. Live attenuated oral vaccine
2. Inactivated vaccine.

Neonatal mortality is documented to be 40% if a woman is infected with polio virus in pregnancy. Both live and inactivated polio vaccine administrations were studied during pregnancy and were found to be safe.[6] It is better to avoid vaccination during pregnancy.[7] If, however, a pregnant woman still requires immunization, she should be advised vaccination with inactivated vaccine. It is given in three dose series, second dose 4–8 weeks after the first dose, and the last dose 6–12 months after the second one.

Yellow Fever

Yellow fever vaccination during pregnancy is contraindicated. The vaccine should be administered only if travel to an endemic area is unavoidable and if an increased risk of exposure exists.[8] Despite the apparent safety of this vaccine, infants born to these women should be monitored closely for evidence of congenital infection and other possible adverse effects from vaccinations.

Varicella

Varicella infection although uncommon in adults and may result in significant maternal and fetal morbidity. Infection during pregnancy may result in congenital varicella syndrome, neonatal varicella, or herpes zoster during infancy.[9] Varicella vaccine is contraindicated during pregnancy. It is recommended atleast 28 days prior to conception. In nonimmune women it should be given in postpartum period. However, varicella vaccination during pregnancy should not be regarded as a reason to terminate the pregnancy.

Influenza

The inactivated influenza vaccine has been administered during pregnancy in the developed countries since the 1960s.[10] As the influenza vaccine has minimal immunogenicity prior to 6 months of age, maternal vaccination during pregnancy has the potential to decrease neonatal influenza. In fact, in one study, immunization during pregnancy was shown to reduce the incidence of laboratory-confirmed influenza in infants up to 6 months of age by 63% as well as lessen febrile influenza-like illness by approximately a third in both young infants and mothers.[11] Only five women, therefore, would need to be vaccinated during pregnancy to prevent a single case of febrile influenza-like illness in a mother or an infant.

Advisory Committee on Immunization Practices and American College of Obstetricians and Gynecologists (ACOG) recommend administration of the trivalent-inactivated influenza vaccine to women who will be pregnant during the influenza season (October to May) regardless of gestational age.[12,13] Immunization is especially important for women who will be in their third trimester or who will have infants under the age of 6 months during the influenza season.[10] Immunization with the live-attenuated influenza vaccine is not advised during pregnancy.[7]

The influenza A (H1N1) virus is a specific subtype of influenza A that was determined to be responsible for a worldwide influenza pandemic that began in 2009. The viral strain responsible for the pandemic originated from a reassortment of several swine strains, a human strain, and an avian strain.[14] The genetic shift involved in the emergence of the novel H1N1 strain limits the ability of the immune system to recognize and destroy the virus. As with seasonal influenza, cough, fever, headache, sore throat, rhinorrhea, chills, and muscle aches are the most common symptoms.[15] Pregnant women might be at an increased risk of complications from pandemic H1N1 virus infection which could prove fatal particularly if infection occurs in the third trimester. Hence, they should be promptly treated with anti-influenza drugs if infection is confirmed.[16]

Vaccines for H1N1 became available in 2009 in both live-attenuated and inactivated formulations, and pregnant women were one of the initial target groups for immunization with the inactivated vaccine.[15] The USA 2010-2011 influenza vaccine will protect against an influenza A virus subtype H3N2 virus, an influenza B virus and the 2009 H1N1 influenza.[17]

INACTIVATED OR ASSEMBLED VIRUS VACCINE

Hepatitis A

Hepatitis A vaccine is an inactivated vaccine, so it is considered safe during pregnancy.[18] Vertical transmission of hepatitis A has been documented; and pregnancy complications like preterm birth is also associated with hepatitis A virus infection.

Hepatitis B

There is 90% risk of infants getting chronically infected with hepatitis B virus infection. Apart from perinatal transmission, infection from household contacts are the sources of infection to the newborns. Women at risk are counseled for vaccination during pregnancy as recommended by ACIP[19] (having more than one sex partner during the previous 6 months, been evaluated or treated for an sexually transmitted diseases, recent or current injection drug use, or having an hepatitis B surface antigen positive sex partner) should be vaccinated. Pregnancy is not a contraindication to vaccination.

Human Papilloma Virus Vaccine

Quadrivalent human papilloma virus vaccine is not recommended for use in pregnancy.[20] It is pregnancy category B agent and no adverse effects upon the fetus have been reported with inadvertent use. If a women is found to be pregnant after initiating the vaccination series, the remainder of the 3-dose regimen should be delayed until after completion of the pregnancy. If a vaccine dose has been administered during pregnancy, no intervention is needed.

Rabies

Rabies vaccination in pregnant women is considered as safe since a long time. Any pregnant patients who are bitten by wandering animal are at risk. They need proper post-exposure management.

Arya and Agarwal studied the safety of post-exposure rabies immunization in pregnancy and reported on the high safety of this vaccine during pregnancy.[21] Moreover, modern rabies vaccine containing inactivated virus by beta propiolactone are considered safe. Additionally, rabies exposure during pregnancy should not be considered as an indication for termination of pregnancy.

LIVE ATTENUATED BACTERIAL VACCINE

Bacillus Calmette–Guérin Vaccine

Although no harmful effects to the fetus have been associated with BCG vaccine, its use is not recommended during pregnancy.[22]

INACTIVATED BACTERIAL VACCINE

Pneumococcal Polysaccharide Vaccine

Morbidity from pneumonia is increased during pregnancy and is likely due to the physiological respiratory and cardiovascular changes associated with parturition.[7]

Women who are at high risk for contracting *Pneumococcus* (e.g., who are immune suppressed, had a splenectomy, or sickle cell disease) are candidates for vaccination during pregnancy.[7]

Safety of pneumococcal polysaccharide vaccine (PPV23) during the first trimester has not been evaluated hence should be avoided, although no adverse effect have been reported. It is safe to administer the PPV23 to women in the 3rd trimester of pregnancy.[23]

Meningococcal Conjugate Vaccine

Studies of vaccination with meningococcal polysaccharide vaccine (MPSV4) during pregnancy have not documented adverse effects among either pregnant women or newborns. On the basis of these data, pregnancy should not preclude vaccination with MPSV4, if indicated.[24]

Typhoid

Pregnancy complications like transplacental infection, miscarriage, and intrauterine fetal demise are associated with typhoid infection during pregnancy. Pregnant women anticipating travel to endemic areas like Africa, Asia, and Latin America are advised vaccination during pregnancy. Typhoid vaccination is considered safe during pregnancy, and the use of parenteral capsular polysaccharide vaccine[7] is recommended.

Anthrax

As no trial has been conducted documenting the safety of anthrax vaccine during pregnancy, it is contraindicated during pregnancy. Composition of anthrax vaccine is a sterile, cell free bacterial vaccine hence no complications are expected. If a woman is exposed to anthrax infection during pregnancy as a life saving measure, she would be advised vaccination.

TOXOIDS

Tetanus

This vaccine is routinely recommended for pregnant women; it is safe and given universally in many countries of the world to prevent neonatal tetanus. Although no evidence exists that tetanus toxoids are teratogenic, waiting until second trimester of pregnancy to administer is a reasonable precaution for minimizing any concern about the theoretical possibility of such reactions.

IMMUNOGLOBULINS

No known risk exists for the fetus from passive immunization of pregnant women with immunoglobulin preparation.

Hepatitis B

Maternal screening, and active and passive immunoprophylaxis have reduced the perinatal, or vertical, transmission of hepatitis B virus (HBV) dramatically. Multiple injections of hepatitis B immune globulin (HBIG) in HBV carrier mothers with a high degree of infectiousness in late pregnancy, effectively and safely prevent HBV intrauterine transmission.

Rabies

The currently available equine rabies immunoglobulins (ERIG) are highly purified (enzyme refined and heat treated) and are known to be safe in pregnancy.

Tetanus

Controlled clinical trial documenting safety of human tetanus immunoglobulin in pregnant women has not been documented; hence it is used with caution. Safety of immunoglobulins during pregnancy can be advocated by clinical experience, as no harm to mother and fetus are expected.

Varicella

Varicella zoster immune globulin (VZIV) should be strongly considered for susceptible, pregnant women who have been exposed.[25] Greatest effectiveness of treatment is to be expected when it is begun within 96 hours after exposure.

Hepatitis A

Immunoglobulin (Ig) is safe for women who are pregnant. Ig is a safe, inexpensive, and effective means of preventing the spread of hepatitis A virus (HAV) infection.

The sooner you get a shot of Ig after being exposed to HAV, the greater the likelihood that infection will be prevented.

NEW DEVELOPMENTS

Exciting advancements in the creation of vaccines to prevent other infections that may affect pregnant women and their newborn infants are underway. For example, congenital cytomegalovirus (CMV) infection may result in permanent hearing, cognitive, and motor impairments in affected infants. A CMV vaccine composed of recombinant CMV envelope glycoprotein B has recently undergone a phase II placebo-controlled randomize double-blinded trial in nonpregnant subjects with favorable results suggesting that it may have the potential to prevent CMV in young women and congenital CMV in infants.[26]

On another front, vaccines against *malaria* are currently being developed. Pregnant women are more susceptible to malaria, particularly in the first and second trimesters.[27] Furthermore, malaria infection during pregnancy confers greater maternal as well as neonatal risk, including anemia and a reduction in birth weight.[28] Vaccines targeting the dominant variant surface antigen, VAR2CSA, as well as other *Plasmodium falciparum* erythrocyte membrane protein variants are under investigation.[28]

Group B streptococcus (GBS) infection is another target for potential immunization. Despite a substantial increase in antibiotic prophylaxis during delivery, the incidence of late-onset disease in infants has not decreased.[29] Approximately 25% of infants with late-onset GBS present with meningitis, and those affected by meningitis are at risk for permanent neurological impairment, including cerebral palsy, hydrocephalus, and mental retardation. GBS conjugate vaccines have undergone phase I and II testing, including a phase 1 randomized double-blinded controlled trial conducted in pregnant women at 30–32 weeks gestation.[29] Immunization against GBS has the potential to improve both maternal and neonatal outcomes.

Finally, respiratory syncytial virus (RSV) has been studied as an infection that could be reduced through maternal immunization. RSV is the most frequent cause of lower respiratory tract disease in infants worldwide. Infection typically occurs early in life and is more severe in the younger pediatric population. Low umbilical cord RSV titers are associated with the increased risk for neonatal disease, while breast feeding is noted to be protective against infection. These latter observations led Munoz and colleagues[30] to undertake a study examining the safety and immunogenicity of an RSV purified protein subunit vaccine in women in their third trimester of pregnancy. They demonstrated that the experimental vaccine was safe, well tolerated, and immunogenic in these pregnant women. Infants born to vaccine recipients did not display any adverse events related to maternal vaccination and had significant concentrations of neutralizing antibody in their bloodstream. Vaccine-specific antibodies were also detected in maternal breast milk. Given the preliminary nature of this study, clinical efficacy was not detected in infants of vaccinated mothers but the findings did support the need for further investigations in this regard.

MEDICOLEGAL AND ETHICAL CONSIDERATIONS

Studies have not conclusively established an association between the vaccines discussed above and maternal or fetal harm, it is worth noting that, there is not a single vaccine specifically Food and Drug Administration (FDA) approved for use in pregnancy primarily due to the absence of industry-sponsored trials in pregnant subjects. Therefore, critical efficacy and safety data are lacking and most clinically based vaccine recommendations extrapolate these presumptive outcomes.[31] However, immunization during pregnancy is fraught with numerous hypothetical risks. These risks include:

- Transmission of an attenuated virus to the placenta or fetus
- Reproductive effects including miscarriage, congenital malformations, and growth retardation
- Unpredictable or idiosyncratic reactions
- Ineffectiveness of the vaccine during pregnancy
- Embryotoxicity of immunoglobulins produced after vaccination.

There are complicated liability issues in the setting of vaccination during pregnancy. Not only is there a potential for adverse events concerning the mother, but there is a possibility of harm to her unborn fetus. In the USA, three types of claims may be retained when an adverse reaction is associated with a vaccination:

1. Failing in advising
2. Failing in the conception of the product
3. Failing in the manufacturing of the product.[32]

Healthcare providers must remember that even though explicit recommendations exist concerning vaccination during pregnancy and the immediate postpartum period, maternal autonomy must be respected. After appropriate counseling, a woman has the right to accept or decline a vaccination, despite what may be in the best interest of her or her child. Furthermore, pregnant women are considered a vulnerable population. Particular attention, therefore, must be paid to informed consent in the setting of maternal vaccination.

CONCLUSION

The ACIP of the Center for Disease Control and Prevention has issued guidelines in Oct 1998 (Updated May 2007) which recommends that killed vaccines are safe in pregnancy but the live ones are best avoided. Box 1 outlines the vaccines contraindicated in pregnancy, box 2 gives the vaccines that can be safely administered during pregnancy, and box 3 gives a list of vaccines that may be used in pregnancy if the risk of infection is high, i.e., on special recommendation.

Box 1: Vaccines to be avoided during pregnancy

- Influenza live virus vaccine (nasal spray)
- Oral polio vaccine
- Measles vaccine
- Measles-mumps-rubella vaccine
- Small pox vaccine
- Typhoid vaccine oral
- Varicella live virus vaccine
- Yellow fever vaccine
- Bacillus Calmette–Guérin (BCG) vaccine
- Pneumococcal vaccine

Box 2: Vaccines safe during pregnancy

- Tetanus toxoid
- Hepatitis B
- Influenza killed vaccine
- Meningococcal vaccine against *Neisseria meningitidis*
- Rabies

Box 3: Vaccines administered on special recommendation only

- Anthrax
- Hepatitis A
- Inactivated polio vaccine
- Parenteral typhoid vaccine
- Yellow fever

REFERENCES

1. Englund JA. The influence of maternal immunization on infant immune responses. J. Comp. Pathol. 2007;137 (Suppl. 1): S16-9.
2. Munoz FM, Englund JA. A step ahead, Infant protection through maternal immunization. Pediatr. Clin North Am. 2000; 47(2):449-63.
3. Centres for Disease Control and Prevention. Guidelines for vaccinating pregnant women. [online] Available from: www.cdc.gov/vaccines/pubs/prfeg-guide.htm [Accessed October, 2013].
4. Gruslin A, Steben M, Halperin S, et al. Immunization in pregnancy. J. Obstet. Gynaecol Can. 2009;31(11):1085-101.
5. Watson JC, Hadler SC, Dykewicz CA, et al. Measles, mumps, and rubella—vaccine use and strategies for elimination of measles, rubella, and congenital rubella syndrome and control of mumps: recommendations of the Advisory Committee on Immunization Practices (ACIP). MMWR Recomm Rep. 1998;47(RR-8):1-57.
6. Harjulehto-Mervaala T, Hovi T, Aro T, et al. Oral poliovirus vaccination and pregnancy complications. Acta Obstet Gynecol Scand. 1995;74(4):262-5.
7. Carroll ID, Williams DC. Pre-travel vaccination and medical prophylaxis in the pregnant traveler. Travel Med Infect Dis. 2008;6(5):259-75.
8. Cetron MS, Marfin AA, Julian KG, et al. Yellow fever vaccine. Recommendations of the Advisory Committee on Immunization Practices (ACIP), 2002. MMWR Recomm Rep. 2002;51(RR-17):1-11.
9. Marin M, Güris D, Chaves SS, et al. Prevention of varicella recommendations of the Advisory Committee on Immunization Practices (ACIP). MMWR Recomm Rep. 2007;56(RR4):1-40.
10. MacDonald NE, Riley LE, Steinhoff MC. Influenza immunization in pregnancy. Obstet Gynecol. 2009;114(2 Pt 1):365-8.
11. Zaman K, Roy E, Arifeen SE, et al. Effectiveness of maternal influenza immunization in mothers and infants. N Engl J Med. 2008;359(15):1555-64.
12. Tamma PD, Ault KA, del Rio C, et al. Safety of influenza vaccination during pregnancy. Am J Obstet Gynecol. 2009;201(6): 547-52.
13. ACOG Committee on Obstetric Practice. ACOG committee opinion number 305, November 2004. Influenza vaccination

and treatment during pregnancy. Obstet Gynecol. 2004; 104(5Pt 1):1125-6.
14. Carison A, Thung SF, Norwitz ER. H1N1 influenza in pregnancy: What all obstetric care providers ought to know. Rev Obstet Gynecol. 2009;2(3):139-45.
15. Sullivan SJ, Jacobson RM, Dowdle WR, et al. 2009 H1N1 influenza. Mayo Clin Proc. 2010;85(1):64-76.
16. Jamieson DJ, Honein MA, Rasmussen SA, et al. H1N1 2009 influenza virus infection during pregnancy in the USA. Lancet. 2009;374(9688):451-8.
17. Centers for Disease Control and Prevention (2013). Vaccine information statements, influenza vaccine – seasonal inactivated [online] Available from: www.cdc.gov/vaccines/pubs/vis/downloads/vis-flu.pdf [Accessed, October, 2013].
18. Advisory Committee on Immunization Practices (ACIP), Fiore AE, Wasley A, et al. Prevention of hepatitis A through active of passive immunization: recommendations of the Advisory Committee on Immunization Practices (ACIP). MMWR Recomm Rep. 2006;55(RR-7):1-23.
19. Mast EE, Margolis HS, Fiore AE, et al. A comprehensive immunization strategy to eliminate transmission of hepatitis B virus infection in the United States: recommendations of the Advisory Committee on Immunization Practices (ACIP) part 1: immunization of infants, children, and adolescents. MMWR Recomm Rep. 2055;54(RR-16):1-31.
20. Markowitz LE, Dunne EF, Saraiya M, et al. Quadrivalent human papillomavirus vaccine: recommendations of the Advisory Committee on Immunization Practices (ACIP). MMWR Recomm Rep. 2007;56(RR-2):1-24.
21. Arya SC, Agarwal N. Assessing the safety of post-exposure rabies immunization in pregnancy. Hum Vaccin. 2007;3(5):155.
22. The role of BCG vaccine in the prevention and control of tuberculosis in the United States. A joint statement by the Advisory Council for the Elimination of Tuberculosis and the Advisory Committee on Immunization Practices. MMWR Recomm Rep. 1996;45(RR-4):1-18.
23. Munoz FM, Englund JA, Cheesman CC, et al. Maternal immunization with pneumococcal polysaccharide vaccine in the third trimester of gestation. Vaccine. 2001;20(5-6):826-37.
24. Bilukha OO, Rosenstein N, National Center for Infectious Diseases, et al. Prevention and control of meningococcal disease. Recommendations of the Advisory Committee on Immunization Practices (ACIP). MMWR Recomm Rep. 2005;54 (RR-7):1-21.
25. Prevention of varicella: Recommendations of the Advisory Committee on Immunization Practices (ACIP). Centers for Disease Control and Preventions. MMWR Recomm Rep. 1996; 45(RR-11):1-36.
26. Pass RF, Zhang C, Evans A, et al. Vaccine prevention of maternal cytomegalovirus infection. N Engl J Med. 2009;360(12):1191-9.
27. Sharma S. Pathak S. Malaria vaccine: a current perspective. J Vector Borne Dis. 2008;45(1):1-20.
28. Tuikue Ndam N, Deloron P. Towards a vaccine against pregnancy-associated malaria. Parasite. 2008;15(3):515-21.
29. Edwards MS. Group B streptococcal conjugate vaccine: a timely concept for which the time has come. Hum Vaccin. 2008;4(6):444-8.
30. Munoz FM, Piedra PA, Glezen WP. Safety and immunogenicity of respiratory syncytial virus purified fusion protein-2 vaccine in pregnant women. Vaccine. 2003;21(24):346-7.
31. Brent RL. Risks and benefits of immunizing pregnant women: the risk of doing nothing. Reprod Toxicol. 2006;21(4):383-9.
32. Trannoy E. Will ethical and liability issues and public acceptance allow maternal immunization? Vaccine. 1998;16(14-15): 1482-5.

Supportive Drug Use

10

CHAPTER

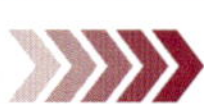

Sunita Tandulwadkar, Bhavana Mittal, Pooja Lodha

INTRODUCTION

First trimester of pregnancy has immense importance and peculiarities. So much interest has been generated in this phase of pregnancy that specialized units called early pregnancy units which have been established that deal with problems specific to this period. The era of assisted reproductive technology (ART) has laid further importance to the first trimester of pregnancy in the form of luteal support. In patients with threatened abortion and recurrent pregnancy loss, the treatment options are limited and mostly empirical. This chapter reviews the role of some of these commonly used drugs.

HUMAN CHORIONIC GONADOTROPIN

Human chorionic gonadotropin (hCG) is produced by cytotrophoblast during early pregnancy. It mediates its action through the luteinizing hormone (LH)/hCG receptor, and its major function is to maintain the progesterone production of corpus luteum during early pregnancy. Known and putative functions of hCG have recently been extensively reviewed.[1] It is administered in a dose of 5,000 IU every third week. It is used in women with unexplained recurrent miscarriage, and a Cochrane review suggests that the use of hCG in recurrent miscarriage is equivocal and further studies are required to show benefit of its use.[2] However, Food and Drug Administration (FDA) classifies hCG as a pregnancy category X drug, which means it has the potential to cause birth defects in the baby. The use of hCG can lead to ovarian hyperstimulation syndrome in women with polycystic ovary syndrome. Also in patients with ovarian cysts, it can stimulate the growth of these cysts and cause problems, such as bleeding in these patients.

With the increasing awareness regarding importance of universal first trimester aneuploidy screening (double marker plus a nuchal scan between 11–13 completed weeks gestational age), increasing number of ART conceived women are being seen for the same. Such women are frequently on supportive hCG injections, and care should be taken that they don't give blood for dual marker within 72 hours of taking the hCG injection. One of the components of dual marker is beta-hCG, which may be falsely high due to the exogenously administered hCG, and this in turn can give false positive screen for aneuploidies.

PROGESTERONE

Progesterone and estradiol are required for successful pregnancy, both to prepare the uterus for embryo implantation and to stabilize the endometrium during pregnancy. Progesterone is the sine qua non of the luteal phase. It probably acts as an immunological suppressant blocking T-helper 1 (Th1) activity and induces release of Th2 cytokines. It can be given prophylactically to all patients or only those with inadequate luteal phase. Luteal phase support is given to all patients with threatened abortion and recurrent miscarriages to provide additional hormonal support with various degrees of success. A recent meta-analysis has shown trends for improved live birth rates in these women.[3]

In vitro fertilization (IVF) ovarian stimulation protocols routinely include the use of gonadotropin-releasing hormone (GnRH) agonists or antagonists to suppress the pituitary and prevent a premature endogenous LH surge. However, because LH is suppressed by GnRH agonists/antagonists, it is important to supplement progesterone in the luteal phase of IVF cycles to maximize clinical pregnancy rates.[4] Numerous studies have confirmed that ovarian stimulation used in assisted reproduction is associated with luteal phase insufficiency and progesterone supplementation resulting in a trend toward improved ongoing and clinical pregnancy rates.

The US FDA label for a progesterone product reads: "If pregnancy occurs, treatment may be continued until placental autonomy is achieved, up to 10–12 weeks."[5,6]

Route of Administration

Various routes are used and common ones are shown in box 1.

Box 1: Progesterone options

- Progesterone gel 8% vaginally, once or twice daily
- Micronized progesterone 200–400 mg twice daily preferably vaginally
- Progesterone injection in oil 50/100 mg/day.

Oral Route

The development of the micronization process allowed for much improved absorption of progesterone. However, the systemic level of progesterone is too low after oral administration. The first passage of progesterone through the liver after oral ingestion leads to massive metabolism, such that only 10% of the administered dose circulates as active progesterone. Any effort to increase the oral dose sufficiently to achieve the requisite serum progesterone levels produces a degree of somnolence unacceptable to most patients. Therefore, oral progesterone supplementation should not be relied upon for support of pregnancy.

Intramuscular Route

The intramuscular (IM) route delivers progesterone with high efficacy and bypasses the first pass metabolism. However, the drawbacks of IM method are discomfort to the patient, need for trained personnel to administer injection, and side effects, such as abscess and allergic response. Also, menses are delayed as long as progesterone therapy continues. The usual dose is 25–100 mg daily. Another option may be 17 alpha hydroxyl progesterone with the advantage of twice a week administration. The efficacy is similar to daily IM injections but theoretical concerns about teratogenesis remains.

Vaginal Route

The advantages of vaginal route are acceptability of the patient, no need for special equipment or training, and lack of allergic reactions. Vaginal progesterone therapy does not delay menses past the normal expected date beyond 3 days. Various studies have demonstrated that vaginal route is as good as (if not better) IM therapy and clearly better than oral.[7] This is despite the fact that serum progesterone levels are abnormally low as targeted delivery from the vagina to the uterus occurs. The various formulations that are used are micronized progesterone tablets, 8% bioadhesive gel, suppositories, sialistic rings, and gelatin capsules. Advantages of gel over other vaginal therapies are a longer half-life and lower patient to patient variability.

Duration of Administration

The duration of supplementation is not entirely clarified. However, most clinicians empirically continue the supplementation till about 8–10 weeks, when placenta takes over.

A shift from ovarian to placental production of gonadal steroids occurs over a period of weeks. In one study, placental progesterone was detected as early as 50 days of gestational age. Lutectomy led to miscarriage in almost every case if performed before 7 weeks of gestational age, and almost never if performed after that time.[8]

DOCOSOHEXANOIC ACID

Most dramatic neurodevelopmental changes occur prenatally and early postnatally. Clinically established as a nutrient essential for the development of an infant's brain and central nervous system, docosohexanoic acid (DHA) occurs naturally in breast milk, and is added to infant formula.[9] In the last trimester of pregnancy, the fetal brain increases in size while rapidly accumulating DHA.[9] Maternal and neonatal concentrations of DHA and arachidonic acid are associated with improved outcomes in early infancy, and concentrations of DHA are associated with favorable neurodevelopmental outcome beyond early infancy. However, in some studies DHA supplementation in women with singleton pregnancies did not enhance infant visual acuity, did not lower levels of postpartum depression in mothers, and did not improve cognitive and language development in their offspring during early childhood.[10,11] The March of Dimes[12] recommends that the pregnant woman consumes at least 200 mg DHA per day. Natural sources of DHA are dietary polyunsaturated fatty acids, sea weed, anchovies, sardines trout and other oily fish.

FOLIC ACID

Neural tube defects (NTDs) which comprise open spina bifida, anencephaly, and encephalocele, complicate 1.5/1000 pregnancies and represent the first congenital malformations to be preventable through public health measures. The effect of periconceptional folic acid on reducing the incidence of both, occurrence and recurrence of NTDs has been confirmed in quality randomized controlled trials.[13] Prophylaxis commenced after pregnancy has been diagnosed, is unlikely to prevent these serious handicapping malformations, as adequate folic acid is needed at the time of embryogenesis. As many women do not plan a pregnancy, in particular, those at nutritional risk because of poor dietary habits and/or poor socioeconomic status, the only reasonable approach to maintaining adequate periconceptional levels of folic acid would appear to be through food fortification. In the United States, all cereal-based products have been fortified since 1998.

A Department of Health Expert Advisory Group has recommended that women with a history of NTD take 4 mg (usually prescribed as 5 mg tablets) of folic acid preconceptionally and for the first 8 weeks of pregnancy. To prevent the first occurrence of NTD, they recommended a folic acid supplement of 400 µg per day for all women planning a pregnancy.

Biological plausibility of folate action:

- Hyperhomocysteinemia, either of dietary or metabolic origin [i.e. Methylenetetrahydrofolate reductase (MTHFR) homozygosity], could exert a teratogenic effect through its ability to act as N-methyl-D-aspartate (NMDA) blocker in early embryonic neural ectoderm
- Folate deficiency could have a direct effect on neural epithelium, which unlike most embryonic cells express very high levels of folate receptors

- By exerting a pharmacological effect, perhaps on cell proliferation or cell death.

ASPIRIN

Use of low dose aspirin in early pregnancy is shown in table 1.

HEPARIN

Use of heparin in early pregnancy is shown in Table 2.

ANTIOXIDANTS

Pregnancy is an inflammatory state exhibiting increased susceptibility to oxidative stress such that the balance between reactive oxygen species and antioxidants can be easily disrupted. Increased DNA damage has been shown to be involved in many pathological states including pregnancy complications. Modern lifestyles like exposure to pollutants, poor diet, and lack of exercise cause excess inflammation, oxidative stress, and ultimately DNA damage increasing the risk of infertility, miscarriage, and late-pregnancy complications. Moreover, baseline DNA damage rises with age and couples in developed societies are delaying childbirth, placing them at further risk.[14] However, there is insufficient evidence to examine the effects of different combinations of vitamins on miscarriage, stillbirth, or other maternal and infant outcomes.

AYURVEDIC OR HERBAL PREPARATIONS

The ancient system of ayurveda has its own therapy for early pregnancy in the form of sattvic food (balanced diet), healthy environment, transcendental meditation, and ayurvedic oil massage (abhyanga). There are herbal therapies for problems of pregnancy, e.g., nausea, vomiting, bleeding, anemia, etc. The clever and scientific use of this system of therapy can be an adjunct to the modern day treatments.

TABLE 1: Use of low dose aspirin in early pregnancy

Condition	*Intervention*	*Result*	*Reference*
Early pregnancy loss + antiphospholipid syndrome	LDA (75 mg/day) and heparin	Significantly improves live birth rate	RCOG Consensus views arising from the 48th Study Group: implantation and early development
Recurrent miscarriage and APL	LDA and heparin	Significantly improves the live birth rate	RCOG Guideline No 17, May 2011. The investigation and treatment of couples with recurrent miscarriages
Preeclampsia IUGR Perinatal death	LDA initiated in early pregnancy (<16 weeks)	Reducing incidence, particularly for women at high risk	RCOG preeclampsia—study group consensus statement 2003
Kidney disease	LDA	Prophylaxis against preeclampsia	Study group consensus statement 2008
Severely obese	LDA	Research is required	Study group consensus statement 2007
Mechanical heart valves	LDA	Decreased risk of intracardiac thrombosis	Study group consensus statement 2006

LDA, low dose aspirin; RCOG, Royal College of Obstetrics And Gynaecologists; APL, antiphospholipid; IUGR, intrauterine growth restriction.

TABLE 2: Use of heparin in early pregnancy

Condition	*Intervention*	*Result*	*Reference*
Early pregnancy loss + antiphospholipid syndrome	Low dose aspirin (75 mg/day) and heparin	Significantly improves live birth rate	RCOG Consensus views arising from the 48th Study Group: Implantation and Early Development
Recurrent miscarriage and APL	LDA and heparin	Significantly improves the live birth rate	RCOG Guideline No 17, May 2011. The investigation and treatment of couples with recurrent miscarriages
Preeclampsia IUGR Perinatal death	Heparin	Randomized trials should assess the role	Preeclampsia study group consensus statement 2003
Nephrotic syndrome	Heparin	Thromboprophylaxis	Study group consensus statement 2008
Severely obese	Heparin	Research is required	Study group consensus statement 2007
Heart disease	Heparin	Decreased risk of intracardiac thrombosis	Study group consensus statement 2006
More than 4 hours air flight + risk factor for DVT	Heparin	Thromboprophylaxis	Study group consensus statement 2011
Thrombophilia /idiopathic venous thromboembolism	Heparin in early pregnancy	Thromboprophylaxis	Study group consensus statement 2011

LDA, low dose aspirin; APL, antiphospholipid; IUGR, intrauterine growth restriction, DVT, deep venous thrombosis.

The problems and complications faced in the first 12 weeks of pregnancy are unique to this period. Hence, supportive drugs like hCG, progesterone, folic acid, aspirin, and heparin where indicated, are essential for a successful outcome in pregnancies conceived with ART or in patients with recurrent miscarriages.

REFERENCES

1. Filicori M, Fazleabas AT, Huhtaniemi I, et al. Novel concepts of human chorionic gonadotropin: reproductive system interactions and potential in the management of infertility. Fertil Steril. 2005;84(2):275-84.
2. Morley LC, Simpson N, Tang T. Human chorionic gonadotropin (hCG) for preventing miscarriage. Cochrane Database Syst Rev. 2013;1:CD008611.
3. Nardo LG, Sallam HN. Progesterone supplementation to prevent recurrent miscarriage and to reduce implantation failure in assisted reproduction cycles. Reprod Biomed Online. 2006;13(1):47-57.
4. Pritts EA, Atwood AK. Luteal phase support in infertility treatment: a meta-analysis of the randomized trials. Hum Reprod. 2002;17(9):2287-99.
5. Committee for Medicinal Products for Human Use (CHMP) guideline on the choice of the non-inferiority margin. Stat Med. 2006; 25(10):1628-38.
6. International Committee for Monitoring Assisted Reproductive Technology (ICMART), de Mouzon J, Lancaster P, et al. World collaborative report on Assisted Reproductive Technology, 2002. Hum Reprod. 2009;24(9):2310-20.
7. Smitz J, Devroey P, Faguer B, et al. A prospective and randomized comparison of intramuscular or intravaginal natural progesterone as a luteal phase and early pregnancy supplement. Hum Reprod. 1992;7(2):168-75.
8. Csapo AI, Pulkkinen MO, Ruttner B, et al. The significance of the human corpus luteum in pregnancy maintainance. I. Preliminary studies. Am J Obstet Gynecol. 1972;112(8):1061-7.

9. Nancy L.Morse. Benefits of Docosahexaenoic Acid, Folic Acid, Vitamin D and Iodine on Foetal and Infant Brain Development and Function Following Maternal Supplementation during Pregnancy and Lactation. Nutrients. 2012;4(7):799-840.
10. Smithers LG, Gibson RA, Makrides M. Maternal supplementation with docosahexaenoic acid during pregnancy does not affect early visual development in the infant: a randomized controlled trial. Am J Clin Nutr. 2011;93(6):1293-9.
11. Makrides M, Gibson RA, Mc Phee AJ, et al. Effect of DHA supplementation during pregnancy on maternal depression and neurodevelopment of young children: a randomized controlled trial. JAMA. 2010;304(15):1675-83.
12. Nutrition and Pregnancy (Part II) – March of Dimes. Available from URL: www/marchofdimes.com/pdf/...CA_Nutrition_and_Pregnancy_Part_II.p
13. RCOG. Periconceptional Folic Acid and Food Fortification in the Prevention of Neural Tube Defects (Scientific Impact Paper 4), 2013.
14. Furness DL, Dekker GA, Roberts CT. DNA damage and health in pregnancy. J Reprod Immunol. 2011;89(2):153-62.

Prescription Writing

11

CHAPTER

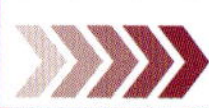

Ashis K Mukhopadhyay, Sagnika Dash

INTRODUCTION

Prescription of medications during the first trimester of pregnancy is a subject of debate. Except for a few, almost all commonly used drugs have some side effects. Their role in maintaining the well-being of the mother and the child, however, cannot be ignored. About 8% of pregnant women need permanent drug treatment due to chronic diseases like epilepsy, diabetes, bronchial asthma, thyroid disorders, severe depression, etc.[1]

Most women would receive transient drug treatment for common ailments like nausea and vomiting, acute respiratory infection, urogenital infection, headache, nervousness, constipation, etc.[2]

Proper prescription of drugs in pregnancy is a challenge and should provide maximal safety to the fetus as well as therapeutic benefit to the mother. Double-blind, randomized and prospective drug trials are generally impossible to perform during pregnancy. For obvious ethical considerations, no studies of teratogenicity are conducted during embryogenesis in humans. The studies are, therefore, either retrospective in nature (case reports, case series, and case control studies) or prospective cohort studies. For the rarer malformations, usually case reports are commonly used for study of teratogenicity, but they can neither prove nor disprove teratogenicity.

STAGES OF DEVELOPMENT IN RELEVANCE TO TERATOGENECITY

Gestational age is calculated from the first day of the last menstrual period. Thus, "pregnant women" are not pregnant in the first 2 weeks of their pregnancies. The third week covers the preimplantation period when the zygote travels from the ampulla of the fallopian tube to the uterus. The fourth week comprises the implantation period when the blastocyst finds its place in the uterus. However, the zygotes and blastocysts have continuous mitoses producing totipotent stem cells during this period. Serious damage can cause their death; on the other hand, they have a complete recovery following minor damage. These facts explain the rule of "all-or-none effect" or in other words the consequences of these damages have only two outcomes: complete loss of zygotes/blastocysts, which causes only some delay in the onset off menstrual bleeding, or a healthy birth.

Therefore, human teratogenic drugs cannot induce congenital anomalies in the first month of gestation because the specific activation of DNA in the stem cells and the so-called differentiation of specific cells and organs of the body starts on the 29th day. The main organ-forming period lasts from the 29th day to the 84th day of gestation. On the other hand, we know that the critical period for some congenital anomalies exceeds the end of the third month, e.g., the critical period for posterior cleft palate and hypospadias covers the 12th weeks to 14th weeks and 14th weeks to 16th weeks of gestation, while the critical period of undescended testis and patent ductus arteriosus is 7–9 months and 9–10 months, respectively. Thus, the optimal approach is to consider the specific critical period of each congenital anomalies separately.

Note: First month of gestation is resistant to teratogenic influences, and only the second and third months represent the critical period of most major congenital anomalies.

The stages in development of a fetus are recognized as discussed below (Fig. 1).

Implantation Phase

The time from conception until implantation known as the "all or none" period, when insults to the embryo are likely to result in death of the conceptus and miscarriage (or resorption), or in intact survival. At this stage, the embryo is undifferentiated, and repair and recovery are possible through multiplication of the still totipotent cells to replace those which have been lost. Exposure of embryos to teratogens during the preimplantation stage usually does not cause congenital malformations, unless the agent persists in the body beyond this period.

Embryonic Phase

The embryonic period, 18 days to 56 days after conception, is the period when the basic steps

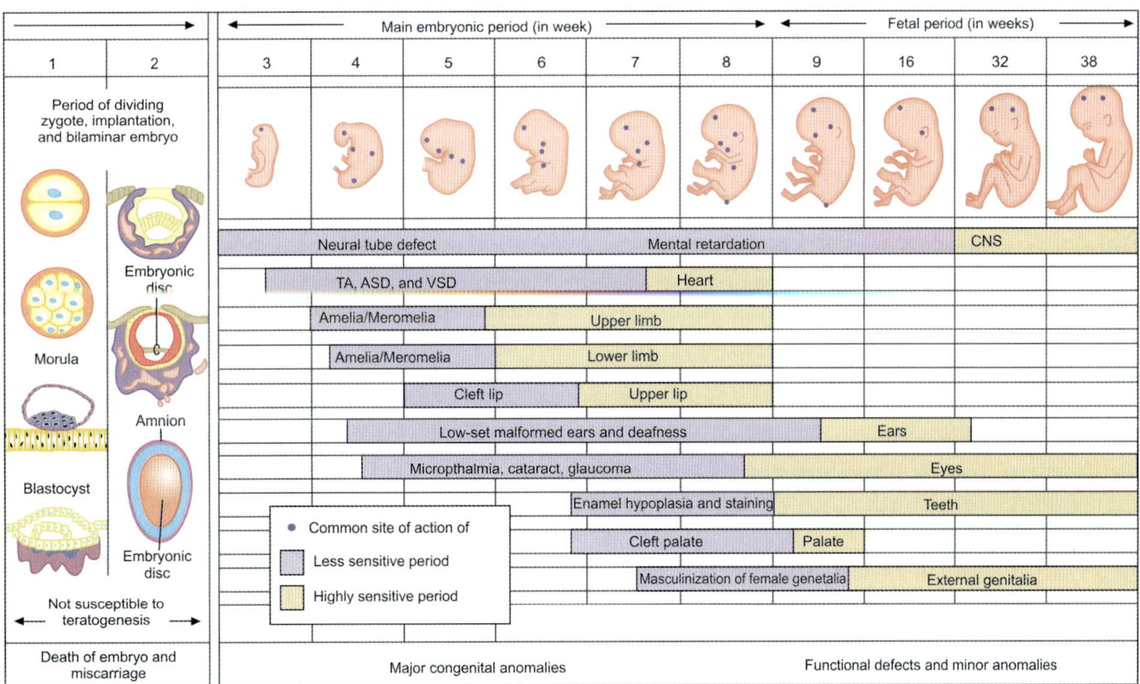

CNS, central nervous system; TA, truncus arteriosus; ASD, atrial septal defect; VSD, ventricular septal defect.

FIGURE 1 Period of gestation and teratogenicity.

in organogenesis occur. This is the period of maximum sensitivity to teratogenicity since not only are tissues differentiating rapidly but damage to them becomes irreparable. Exposure to teratogenic agents during this period has the greatest likelihood of causing a structural anomaly. Since teratogens are capable of affecting many organ systems, the pattern of anomalies produced depends upon which systems are differentiating at the time of teratogenic exposure.

Fetal Phase

The fetal phase, from the end of the embryonic stage to term, is the period when growth and functional maturation of organs and systems already formed occurs. Teratogenic exposure in this period will affect fetal growth (e.g., intrauterine growth restriction), the size of a specific organ, or the function of the organ, rather than cause gross structural anomalies. The term fetal toxicity is commonly used to describe such an effect. Of particular interest is the potential effect of psychoactive agents (e.g., antidepressants, antiepileptics, alcohol, and other drugs of abuse) on the developing central nervous system, which has led to a new field of *behavioral teratology*.

In contrast to the above stages, it is a well-recognized fact that certain anomalies occur long after the exposure of the offending agent, such as adenocarcinoma of cervix and vagina, as seen in the offspring if the mother is exposed to estrogenes during pregnancy. Such association is attributed to structural and functional maturation that continues after birth.

PRINCIPLES OF PRESCRIBING IN PREGNANCY

Try nonpharmacological treatments first where possible

- When selecting drugs:
  - Consider the one with the best safety record over time
  - Avoid newer drugs, unless safety has been clearly established
  - Do not assume that over-the-counter and herbal drugs are safe
  - Check the latest advice from the manufacturer about cautions and contra-indications in pregnancy
- When considering dosage and duration of treatment:
  - Avoid first trimester
  - Use the lowest effective dose
  - Limit the duration to the minimal period required
  - If possible, use intermittently rather than continuously
  - Consider reducing or withdrawing the drug before expected date of delivery.

DEFINING PREGNANCY RISK

Teratogenic medications can be characterized as *high-risk teratogens* (e.g., isotretinoin, which is thought to affect approximately 20–30% of exposed fetuses)[3] or *moderate-risk teratogens*, which increase the risk of a birth defect to a smaller degree.[4] Potential fetal effects after exposure to teratogenic medications include spontaneous miscarriage, malformations, visible developmental impairment, small size for gestational age, impaired intellectual development, carcinogenesis, and increased risk of genetic mutations.[5] These fetal effects are modified by a variety of factors including medication dose and duration of exposure,[6] gestational age at exposure,[6,7] and genetic susceptibility. Adequate nutrition (e.g., folate intake) may be able to decrease the risk of teratogenicity of some medications, e.g., in animal studies, folic acid attenuates the risk of valproic acid-related birth defects.[8]

Unfortunately, the most significant adverse effects of medications occur early in pregnancy, before many women realize that they are pregnant. From conception to 2 weeks after fertilization, teratogens increase the risk of early fetal death and spontaneous abortion.[7] Organogenesis occurs during weeks 3–8, and during this time the fetus is at risk of developing major morphologic abnormalities.[7] During later weeks of gestation, teratogenic exposures increase the risk for more subtle morphologic abnormalities and can produce biochemical, behavioral, or reproductive abnormalities. However, the consequences of later exposures can still be of great clinical significance (e.g., renal impairment from angiotensin-converting enzyme inhibitor use, which can be fatal for the fetus).[6]

REPRODUCTIVE HEALTH NEEDS OF WOMEN ON TERATOGENIC MEDICATIONS

The fundamental initial steps in caring for women of reproductive age who are candidates for teratogenic medications include recognition of a medication as a potential teratogen, and assessing a woman's pregnancy status and fertility intentions.

Identifying Teratogens

Providers must consider teratogenicity each time they prescribe medications to women of reproductive age, just as they should counsel women about fertility goals and preconception or contraceptive counseling. Information resources available to providers including drug labels, draw on information from pregnancy registries, retrospective cohort studies, case-control studies, and pregnancy surveillance programs.

Assessing Fertility Intentions

Any woman of reproductive age who is taking or considering taking a teratogenic medication should be encouraged to articulate her fertility goals. Particularly for women with chronic medical conditions, regardless of her stated fertility intentions, the implications of a patient's medical condition for her pregnancy, including the risk of teratogenic medications, must be regularly discussed. Pregnancy intentions should be assessed regularly as they may charge with time. When possible, pregnancy intentions should be assessed in an open-ended way, which may be more consistent with women's actual experience. For example, questions can be phrased as "How would you feel about becoming pregnant?" Or "Would you mind becoming pregnant?"[5]

Preconception Counseling and Pregnancy Testing

For women desiring pregnancy, the teratogenicity of a given medication must be discussed in detail and documented, with acknowledgement of the uncertainty surrounding these issues. In addition, the risks and benefits of stopping a given medication must be discussed. Of note, women who have depression or anxiety may be more likely to have inflated concerns about the teratogenic risks associated with medications. Providers should be particularly aware of this, given the risk of depression during pregnancy; physician reassurance can often mitigate patients' concerns.[9,10]

For patients of reproductive age who are sexually active and have no history of surgical sterilization, a pregnancy test should be conducted prior to initiation of a teratogenic medication. Some experts recommend monthly pregnancy testing for sexually active women who are not using prescription contraception.[5]

Prescribing for Women who are Pregnant or Desiring Pregnancy

For acute, relatively mild medical conditions that do not pose a significant risk to a woman or her pregnancy (e.g., a viral upper respiratory infection), medications should be avoided during the first trimester if possible. When the benefit of a medication is felt to outweigh potential risks, clinicians should consider prescribing the lowest effective dose or the medication with the most data on safety in pregnancy. Older medications with good safety records are generally preferred to newer medications with less supporting data.[5] For chronic medical conditions or conditions that pose a risk to the woman or fetus if untreated, safer alternatives to a medication should be sought if they exist. For example, pregnant women or women desiring pregnancy with severe hypertension, oral agents of choice include methyldopa, labetalol, and metoprolol. Some women with severe depression will need to continue receiving pharmacologic therapy while pregnant. Selective serotonin reuptake inhibitors are considered to be safer than tricyclic antidepressants, but paroxetine should be avoided since it has the strongest association with fetal cardiac malformations.[11] Many women with rheumatoid arthritis are transitioned from disease-modifying antirheumatic drugs, such as methotrexate to higher doses of steroids during, or in anticipation of pregnancy. While steroids carry risks for pregnant women and fetuses, they are probably safer than many disease-modifying antirheumatic drugs.[12]

Improving Providers' Ability to Address Women's Reproductive Health Needs

A number of types of evidence suggest that providers are not adequately meeting the reproductive health needs of women who are considering use of potentially teratogenic medications. Diverse interventions are needed to address this problem.

First, the need for better data on drug safety in pregnancy is clear. A solid evidence base could help prevent women with chronic medical conditions from stopping or under dosing necessary medications, and help other women avoid medications that could be harmful to the fetus.

Second, healthcare providers need better education in identifying potentially teratogenic medications, evaluating the risks and benefits of such medications, counseling patients appropriately, and prescribing effective contraception. This is particularly important for primary care physicians, who not only prescribe majority of teratogenic medications but may also find themselves at the center of coordinating care while weighing the views of multiple specialists who may be involved in managing a patient's chronic medical condition, and the clinicians who are focused on the well-being of the pregnancy.

Third, changes in healthcare finance and delivery systems can support providers in meeting patients' needs. Since primary care providers have identified limited clinical time and lack of reimbursement for time spent counseling patients as barriers to preconception and contraceptive counseling,[13] health reform legislation should consider increasing reimbursement for these important preventive activities. Clinics may wish to designate mid-level providers or counselors to assist with these services, for example, through documentation of a "contraceptive vital sign" that assesses and records patients' contraceptive use prior to meeting with a physician.[14]

EFFECTS OF PREGNANCY ON DOSE REQUIREMENT OF DRUGS

Changes in the maternal physiology during pregnancy have a profound impact on the pharmacokinetics of the drugs administered. This is relevant for drugs that have a narrow therapeutic index. For most of the drugs, the absorption is reduced and elimination increased, thus leading to decreased plasma concentration. Nevertheless, the impact of other parameters like total body water changes, alteration in serum proteins, hepatic metabolism, and alteration in renal clearance has to be considered before any alteration in the dosing is planned.

Total Body Water Changes

Maternal body water level rises rapidly during the second trimester to increase by 15% at 12 weeks. It then reaches a plateau level during the last several weeks of pregnancy with an approximate total gain of 8 liters. This has the effects discussed below.

Total Drug Concentration

It creates a larger space for hydrophilic drugs to get distributed, thus reducing the maximum plasma concentration of the drug.

Free Drug Concentration

Because of hemodilution, there is a fall in plasma protein concentration decreasing the total plasma concentration of albumin-bound drugs. In addition, steroid and placental hormones displace drugs from their protein-binding sites. There is thus the possibility of a rise in free (active) drug concentration of agents that are normally albumin-bound. This would be expected to produce an exaggerated drug effect. However, unbound drug is distributed or metabolized, and excreted, and so free concentration of drug is minimally influenced.

Precaution: Changes in protein binding due to hemodilution are of clinical importance, when monitoring plasma concentrations of drugs, for example, phenytoin, as most laboratories report total (rather than free) drug concentration.

Serum Protein

There is a progressive fall in the concentration of serum proteins to the order of 7–8% of the normal prepregnancy level. There is evidence of fall followed by plateauing and ultimately an abrupt rise prior to delivery. The plasma protein reaches the prepregnant value by 12 weeks postpartum. Though there is a reduction in total protein concentration, the synthesis of globulin is increased (except gamma globulins) altering the albumin globulin ratio. Pregnancy has the greatest effect on protein binding of sulfonamides, diazepam, and salicylic acid. The magnitude of this effect is such that quantitatively significant changes in the pharmacokinetic and pharmacodynamic characteristics of certain drugs may be expected to occur during pregnancy (in addition to possible changes caused by other pregnancy related effects such as altered activity of drug-metabolizing enzyme systems). Most drugs (except a few like dexamethasone) exhibit significant negative correlations between free fraction values and serum albumin concentrations during pregnancy.

Note: Albumin:globulin ratio decreases and has effects on the pharmacokinetics of drugs. The fraction of free drug (unbound portion) is increased and so is the activity of the drug.

Liver Metabolism

Alteration of liver metabolism can affect drugs in different ways:

- *Induction of enzymes*: Some enzymes of the hepatic cytochrome P-450 system are induced by estrogen/progesterone, resulting in a higher rate of metabolism, and hence elimination of drugs (for example, phenytoin)
- *Inhibition of enzymes*: Some isoenzymes are competitively inhibited by progesterone and estrogen, leading to impaired elimination (for example, theophylline)
- *Cholestasis*: Clearance of drugs, such as rifampicin, that are secreted via the biliary system, may be diminished due to the cholestatic property of estrogen
- *Altered activity of extrahepatic enzymes*: Some extrahepatic enzymes, such as cholinesterase, have diminished activity during pregnancy.

Note: The inhibition or induction of hepatic enzymes by estrogen or progesterone and their effect on cholestasis will cause the concentration of drugs to increase or decrease.

Renal Clearance

Renal blood flow is increased by 60–80% during pregnancy, and glomerular filtration rate rises by 50%, leading to enhanced elimination of drugs that are normally excreted unchanged, for example penicillin and digoxin. This leads to slightly lower steady-state drug concentrations, although this rarely necessitates escalation in the dosage.

Note: Increased renal blood flow and glomerular filtration rate accompanied by hemodilution leads to lower concentration of some drugs eliminated by the kidney.

MONITORING THERAPEUTIC LEVELS IN PREGNANCY

The indications for therapeutic drug level monitoring are shown in box 1. During pregnancy a number of continuously changing circumstances exist which might be expected to modify the relation between plasma drug levels and dosage. Dose titration for protein bound drugs should be based on free drug monitoring. Most of the drugs are monitored on the basis of plasma concentration. A few important ones are anticonvulsants, magnesium sulfate, digoxin, mood stabilizers, and antipsychotics. The safe therapeutic level of magnesium sulfate used in the treatment of eclampsia is between 4 meq/L and 7 meq/L. Side effects tend to increase when the magnesium level goes beyond 7 meq/L. Therefore, estimation of magnesium level in the blood is desirable whenever toxic features are encountered.

Box 1: Indications for therapeutic drug level monitoring

- There is established relationship between plasma drug concentration and pharmacologic effect
- Knowledge of drug levels influence the further management
- The drug has narrow therapeutic index
- Prevention of life threatening side effects which increase beyond a certain therapeutic drug level
- Poor patient compliance
- The drug dose cannot be optimized by clinical observation alone

PASSAGE OF DRUGS TO FETUS AND CATEGORY OF DRUGS

Drug transfer across placenta occurs mainly by diffusion. Thus small lipophilic unionized agents can readily pass across this barrier. The rate limiting steps being the placental blood flow. Drugs having large molecular weight like heparin and those which are highly protein bound agents cannot cross the barrier. The placenta and fetal liver have the capacity of metabolizing drugs. Both phase I and phase II reactions can be performed by fetus as early as 8 weeks post conception. Fetal drug accumulation may occur because:

- Metabolic enzyme activity in fetus is low
- Fifty percent of the fetal circulation from the umbilical vein bypasses the fetal liver to the cardiac and cerebral circulations
- Elimination from the fetus is by diffusion back to the maternal compartment. Since, most drug metabolites are polar, this favors accumulation of metabolites within the fetus, although as the fetal kidney develops, more drug metabolites are excreted into the amniotic fluid
- Another process leading to accumulation of drugs within the fetus is the phenomenon of "ion trapping". The basis for this is the (slightly) more acidic nature of fetal plasma pH compared to maternal plasma. Weak bases, which are mainly nonionized (lipophilic), diffuse across the placental barrier and become ionized in the more acidic fetal blood; all these lead to a net increase movement of drugs from the maternal to fetal systems.

Note: While drugs with large molecular weight cannot cross the placental barrier, there is accumulation of certain drugs which cross the placenta because of low metabolic enzyme activity of fetus, bypassing of the fetal liver, polarity of metabolites, and ion trapping.

The definitions for drugs used in pregnancy by the US Food and Drug Administration is given in table 1.

TABLE 1: United States Food and Drug Administration pharmaceutical pregnancy categories

Pregnancy category A	Adequate and well-controlled human studies have failed to demonstrate a risk to the fetus in the first trimester of pregnancy (and there is no evidence of risk in later trimesters)
Pregnancy category B	Animal reproduction studies have failed to demonstrate a risk to the fetus and there are no adequate and well-controlled studies in pregnant women or animal studies have shown an adverse effect, but adequate and well-controlled studies in pregnant women have failed to demonstrate a risk to the fetus in any trimester
Pregnancy category C	Animal reproduction studies have shown an adverse effect on the fetus and there are no adequate and well-controlled studies in humans, but potential benefits may warrant use of the drug in pregnant women despite potential risks
Pregnancy category D	There is positive evidence of human fetal risk based on adverse reaction data from investigational or marketing experience or studies in humans, but potential benefits may warrant use of the drug in pregnant women despite potential risks
Pregnancy category X	Studies in animals or humans have demonstrated fetal abnormalities and/or there is positive evidence of human fetal risk based on adverse reaction data from investigational or marketing experience, and the risks involved in use of the drug in pregnant women clearly outweigh potential benefits

SAFE AND UNSAFE DRUGS

The most commonly used classes of drugs in pregnancy are analgesics, spasmolytic, anti-anemics, antacids, systemic, local antibiotics, etc. Though every drug prescribed should be individualized and a risk-benefit analysis done by the treating physician, it is imperative that category X should not be administered at any point during pregnancy (Table 2).

Prescribing in pregnancy should be done only after full knowledge of the effects the drug may have on pregnancy. The obstetrician should have in depth understanding about the pharmacokinetics of drug, its placental transfer, and ability of fetus to eliminate it.

TABLE 2: Safe and unsafe drugs in pregnancy

Drug groups	*Safe*	*Unsafe*
Antiemetic	• Promethazine • Cyclizine • Dicyclomine • Prochlorperazine • Metoclopramide • Doxylamine • Ondansetron	• Domperidone (X)
Gastroesophageal reflux disease and peptic ulcer	• Ranitidine • Famotidine • Cimetidine • Pantoprazole • Lansoprazole	• Mosapride • Omeprazole • Cisapride (X)

Contd...

Contd...

Drug groups	*Safe*	*Unsafe*
Laxative	• Dietary fiber • Ispaghula • Lactulose	• Senna • Bisacodyl • Docusate • Saline purgative
Antidiarrheal	• Oral rehydration salt	• Diphenoxylate-atropine • Loperamide
Cold and cough	• Nasal drops • Xylometazoline • Cromoglycate	• Codeine • Dextromethorphan • Bromhexine • Expectorant • Budesonide • Oxymetazoline
Antiallergic	• Chlorpheniramine • Cetrizine	• Promethazine • Loratadine • Fexofenadine • Astemizole (X)
Antibacterial	• Penicillin-G • Ampicillin • Amoxicillin-clavulanate • Cloxacillin • Piperacillin • Cephalosporin • Erythromycin • Azithromycin • Clindamycin • Vancomycin • Nitrofurantoin	• Clotrimazole • Fluoroquinolones • Tetracycline • Doxycycline • Chloramphenicol • Gentamicin • Streptomycin • Kanamycin • Tobramycin • Clarithromycin
Antitubercular	• Isoniazid • Rifampicin	• Pyrazinamide • Ethambutol • Streptomycin
Antiamoebic	• Diloxanide furoate • Metronidazole	
Antimalarial	• Chloroquine • Proguanil • Mefloquine	• Quinine • Primaquine • Pyrimethamine + sulfadoxine • Artemether • Artesunate

Contd...

Contd...

Drug groups	*Safe*	*Unsafe*
Antihelminthic	• Piperazine • Niclosamide • Praziquantel	• Albendazole • Mebendazole • Ivermectin • Pyrantel pamoate • Diethycarbamazine
Antifungal	• Clotrimazole • Tolnaftate • Terbinafine	• Amphotericin B • Fluconazole • Itraconazole • Ketoconazole • Griseofulvin • Nystatin
Antiretroviral	• Nevirapine • Nelfinavir • Saquinavir • Didanosine • Ritonavir	• Lamivudine • Abacavir • Indinavir • Zidovudine • Efavirenz
Antihypertensive	• Methyldopa • Hydralazine • Nifedipine • Pindolol • Labetalol	• ACE-inhibitor • Angiotensin antagonist (X) • Thiazide diuretics • Furosemide • Propranolol • Nitroprusside • Atenolol • Metoprolol • Clonidine • Prazosin
Antianemic	• Iron salt (oral) • Iron dextran (intramuscular) • Folic acid • Vitamin B12	
Antidiabetic	• Insulin • Metformin • Sulfonylurea • Acarbose	• Nateglinide • Repaglinide • Pioglitazone • Rosiglitazone
Corticosteroid	• Prednisolone (inhaled and topical low dose)	• Betamethasone • Dexamethasone (high dose and prolonged use)
Thyroid hormone	• Thyroxine	

Contd...

Contd...

Drug groups	*Safe*	*Unsafe*
Antithyroid drugs	• Propylthiouracil	• Carbimazole • Radioactive iodine (X) • Iodide
Antipsychotic	• Clozapine • Haloperidol	• Chlorpromazine • Fluphenazine • Trifluoperazine • Olanzapine • Risperidone
Antimanic		• Lithium carbonate • Valproate • Carbamazepine
Antidepressants	• Imipramine • Fluoxetine	• Trimipramine • Dothiepin • Sertraline • Paroxetine • Citalopram • Trazodone • Venlafaxine • Amitriptyline • Clomipramine • Moclobemide
Anticoagulants	• Heparin (low molecular weight and unfractionated)	• Warfarin • Acenocoumarol
Antiasthmatic	• Salbutamol/salmeterol (inhaled) • Ipratropium bromide (inhaled) • Beclomethasone/budesonide (inhaled) • Sodium cromoglycate (inhaled) • Montelukast • Zafirlukast	• Phenindione • Theophylline • Ketotifen • Systemic corticosteroids

REFERENCES

1. Yang T, Walker MC, Krewski D, et al. Maternal characteristics associated with pregnancy exposure to FDA category C, D, and X drugs in a Canadian population. Pharmacoepidemiol Drug Saf. 2008;17(3):270-7.
2. Malm H, Martikainen J, Klaukka T, et al. Prescription of hazardous drugs during pregnancy. Drug Saf. 2004;27(12):899-908.
3. Sladden MJ, Harman KE. What is the chance of a normal pregnancy in a woman whose fetus has been exposed to isotretinoin? Arch Dermatol. 2007;143(9):1187-8.
4. Mitchell AA. Systematic identification of drugs that cause birth defects—a new opportunity. N Engl J Med. 2003;349(26): 2556-9.
5. Schwarz EB, Borrero S, Chireau MV. Safe prescribing for women of reproductive age: treatment recommendations for the VA Fed. Pract. 2009;26(2):38-45.
6. US Department of Health and Human Services, Food and Drug Administration, Center for Drug Evaluation and Research (CDER), et al. (2005). Reviewer Guidance: Evaluating the Risks of Drug Exposure in Human Pregnancies. [online] Available from www.fda.gov/downloads/scienceresearch/specialtopics/

womenshealthresearch/ucm133359.pdf. [Accessed October, 2013].

7. Moore KL, Persaud TVN. The Developing Human: Clinically Oriented Embryology, 8th Edition. PA, USA: Saunders/Elsevier; 2008.
8. Hsieh CL, Wang HE, Tsai WJ, et al. Multiple point action mechanism of valproic acid-teratogenicity alleviated by folic acid, vitamin C and N-acetylcysteine in chicken embryo model. Toxicology. 2012;291(1-3):32-42.
9. Behringer T, Rollman BL, Herbeck-Belnap B, et al. Impact of physician counseling and perception of teratogenic risks: a survey of 96 nonpregnant women with anxiety. Prim Care Companion CNS Disord. 2011;13(2).
10. Walfisch A, Sermer C, Matok I, et al. Perception of teratogenic risk and the rated likelihood of pregnancy termination: association with maternal depression. Can J Psychiatry. 2011;56(12):761-7.
11. Stewart DE. Clinical practice. Depression during pregnancy. N Engl J Med. 2011;365(17):1605-11.
12. Kuria B, Hemanxez-Diaz S, Liu J, et al. Patterns of medication use during pregnancy in rheumatoid arthritis. Arthritis Care Res (Hoboken). 2011;63(5):721-28.
13. Howard TB, Tassinari MS, Feibus KB, et al. Monitoring for teratogenic signals: pregnancy registries and surveillance methods. Am J Med Genet C Semin Med Genet. 2011;157(3): 209-214.
14. Schwarz EB, Santucci A, Borrero S, et al. Perspectives of primary care clinicians on teratogenic risk counseling. Birth Defects Res. A Clin Mol Teratol. 2009;85(10):858-63.
15. Schwarz EB, Parisi SM, Williams SL, et al. Promoting safe prescribing in primary care with a contraceptive vital sign: a cluster-randomized controlled trial. J Gene Int Med. 2012;10(6):516-22.

Effect of Tobacco, Substance Misuse and Alcohol Abuse

12
CHAPTER

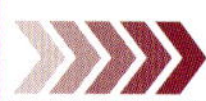

Shashi Prateek, Ananya Banerjee, Deepali Dhingra

INTRODUCTION

The 26th of June is celebrated globally every year as International Day against drug abuse and illicit trafficking in an effort to apprise the people in general and the youth in particular, of this evil. With a turnover of around $500 billion, it is the third largest business in the world, next to petroleum and arms trade. About 190 million people all over the world consume one drug or the other. Drug addiction causes immense human distress, and the illegal production and distribution of drugs have spawned crime and violence worldwide. India too, is caught in this vicious circle of drug abuse, and the numbers of drug addicts are increasing day by day. According to one United Nation (UN) report, one million heroin addicts are registered in India, and unofficially there are as many as five million.[1]

Globalization has taken a toll in every aspect. Multidrug abuse has become rampant in reproductive population and is becoming extremely common in the pregnant population. The effects of smoking, alcohol, and habit forming drugs are acting as a double edged sword affecting not only mothers but also having detrimental effects on the baby. The various effects in the first trimester are listed in box 1.

Box 1: Effects of alcohol, smoking, and habit forming drug

- Disinhibited behavior of mother
- Lack of balanced diet
- Increased incidence of pregnancy complications
- Many substances cross the placenta and cause permanent malformations or agenesis
- Avoidance of prenatal care
- Increased risk of associated infections and psychiatric disorders[2,3]

There are drugs that modify the user's traits and character, which pose a particular problem in the management of these patients and also pose significant challenges for care providers. It has been seen that multidrug abuse is common in pregnancy and that these pregnant woman are less likely to receive prenatal care. Though, drug abuse is seen across all strata of women, but an increased incidence is seen in women who are younger, unmarried, and have lower education levels.

IMPACT ON CHILDREN

The effect of this lifestyle on previous pregnancies and children (if involved) is important. Children who are exposed to drugs prenatally are also at higher risk of involvement with child protection agencies.[4] Children of drug-using parents are at increased risk of neglect, physical and emotional abuse, and up to 50% of drug users do not live with their children.[5] There is often a fear that detection of substance misuse in pregnancy will lead to the child being taken into custody by social services after child birth. The confidential enquiry into maternal mortality in the UK noticed an increase in maternal mortality around the time case conferences were held and children taken into custody.[6] Women may sometimes not declare substance misuse if they believe that this will lead to the baby being removed by child protection services. It is also important to ascertain the status of the partner's children (if relevant) and history of contact with them. The safe storage of take-home substitute medication (methadone/buprenorphine) needs to be clarified to minimize the risk of access and potential overdose by children.

SPECIFIC SUBSTANCE ABUSE IN PREGNANCY

Alcohol

Ethyl alcohol is one of most potent teratogens known and historically most studied because of its long and unfortunate association with human civilizations. Excessive consumption was finally accepted to be harmful by scientific community during early 1970s There is no dose-response relationship, but binge drinking appears to be worse than smaller, more frequent amounts of alcohol.[2] High parity and absence of maternal alcohol dehydrogenase 1B, for which the gene is located on chromosome 4. Single nucleotide polymorphism in this gene is related to alcohol consumption and having reduced risk of alcoholism allele are among other risk factors.[2]

There is conclusive scientific evidence that certain patterns of drinking during pregnancy can be harmful to the unborn child, particularly heavy chronic and episodic consumption.[7, 8] The effects of other maternal drinking patterns are less well understood, but in recent years there have been an increase in research examining the effects of low-moderate consumption. While much of the recent evidence has failed to show an association between maternal drinking and fetal effects [including intelligence quotient (IQ), fetal growth, miscarriage, and stillbirth].[9-11] A 2012 study found that among children with particular genetic variants, low-moderate levels of maternal alcohol consumption was associated with lower IQ.[12] As a result there is no consensus on whether there is a "safe" limit for alcohol consumption during pregnancy and if so where this limit should be defined.[8]

Public Health Concerns

Among the children of women whose alcohol consumption during pregnancy was heavy and chronic, several conditions have been described and linked to the maternal drinking pattern. The best known of these is "fetal alcohol syndrome" (FAS), recognized since the 1970s[13] followed by "fetal alcohol effects" (FAE), a term originally used for a milder spectrum of harm found at lower levels of maternal alcohol consumption. However, as "FAE" is considered confusing and inaccurate by experts, [14] it has since been replaced with the concept of "partial fetal alcohol syndrome (PFAS) with confirmed maternal alcohol exposure."[7]

Infants with FAS are characterized by at least one feature in each of the four following categories:[15,16]

1. *Pre- and postnatal growth deficiencies*: Intrauterine growth retardation, including smaller than normal head circumference, small size at each term of gestation; continuing growth below the tenth percentile after birth, and failure to thrive.
2. *Physical anomalies*: A cluster of facial features, including short upturned nose, receding

forehead and chin, smaller than normal eye apertures, absent groove in upper lip (philtrum), and asymmetrical ears. Other problems include cardiac, gastrointestinal, and limb and joint anomalies.

3. *Central nervous system dysfunction*: Moderate to severe learning difficulties, cognitive hearing, and visual disabilities.
4. *Identifiable drinking problem of the mother*: In many cases, a drinking problem can be identified in the mother of children born with FAS symptoms. Where this cannot be established, the impairment is generally inconsistent with familial factors or environment.

Another term has been used more recently to cover a broad range of categories from individual, less serious factors to full-blown FAS. This is the so-called "fetal alcohol spectrum disorder" (FASD).[17] While the symptoms in infants with FASD are not as severe as those found in babies with FAS, they include poor sucking reflex, sleep disorders, behavioral problems, and fine and gross motor dysfunction,[8,18] More specific categories, such as alcohol-related birth defects (ARBD) and alcohol-related neurodevelopmental disorder (ARND) have also been identified.[11,19] Mothers of infants with these conditions have drinking patterns that include heavier alcohol intake in pregnancy. These conditions are a serious public health issue with significant implications for the growth and development of the affected children before and after birth, persisting into adulthood.

Fetal alcohol syndrome: Heavy alcohol consumption affects the embryogenesis which is manifested later as FAS (Box 2).

Fetal alcohol spectrum disorder: It is an umbrella term that includes the full range of prenatal alcohol damage that may or may not meet the criteria for FAS and is estimated to occur in up to 1 in 100 children.[21]

Box 2: Fetal alcohol syndrome* diagnostic criteria: Centre for Disease Control and Prevention (CDC) classification 2005[20]

- Dysmorphic facial features
  - Small palpebral fissures
  - Thin vermilion border
  - Smooth philtrum
- Prenatal and/or postnatal growth impairment
- Central nervous system abnormalities
  - *Structural:* Head size <10th percentile, significant brain abnormality on imaging
  - *Neurological*
  - *Functional:* Global cognitive or intellectual deficits, in atleast three domains

*All criteria must be fulfilled.

Smoking/Tobacco Consumption

Maternal smoking during pregnancy has long been considered an important risk factor for low birth weight (LBW). The reduction in infant weight is not attributable to earlier gestation, because infants of smokers exhibit growth retardation at all gestational ages.[22] In a recent study of pregnant teenagers,[23] more than one-half of whom were smokers, prenatal tobacco exposure was significantly related to reduced birth weight, birth length, head circumference, and chest circumference. These reductions were even more pronounced than those found in a similar cohort of children of adult women.[24] Two key ingredients of cigarette smoke that are known to affect fetal growth are carbon monoxide and nicotine. Carbon monoxide causes fetal hypoxia, a reduction in the amount of oxygen available to the fetus,[25,26] whereas nicotine can lead to a decrease in the flow of oxygen and other nutrients across the placenta by constricting uterine arteries. In addition, nicotine itself can cross the placenta to affect the fetal cardiovascular system (CVS) and central nervous systems (CNS).[27] Other constituents of tobacco smoke (e.g., cadmium and toluene) have also been shown to cause fetal growth retardation (Office of Environmental Health Hazard Assessment).[28]

In the literature on humans, prenatal tobacco exposure has also been linked to CNS effects, including cognitive and neurobehavioral outcomes, although the reports are inconsistent. At birth, prenatal tobacco exposure has been associated with poorer auditory orientation and autonomic regulation,[29] and increased tremors and startles.[30] In a recent race-matched study of cocaine exposed and non-cocaine-exposed infants, neurological exams showed that prenatal tobacco exposure was significantly related to muscle tone abnormalities when controlling for other variables, including head circumference and prenatal care.[31] The authors concluded that maternal cigarette smoking, rather than cocaine exposure, might be the major predictor of tone abnormalities. Associations between prenatal tobacco exposure and increased activity, inattention, and impulsivity has also been reported. Behavioral and psychological problems have also been linked to prenatal tobacco exposure.

Overall approximate prevalence of tobacco addiction during pregnancy is around 20%. Tobacco is complex, containing almost 2,000 individual constituents of which nicotine is the main compound responsible for pleasurable response and the addictive action. Tobacco must be consumed as such or in the form of smoking. Exposure to cigarette smoke poses serious health risks to anyone who indulges in or is surrounded by it (passive smokers). Smoking during pregnancy can lead to a plethora of health risks to both the mother and the fetus. Exposure leads to an increased risk of lung cancer, pulmonary, and cardiovascular diseases. Exposure to cigarette smoke decreases the fertility of both men and women. It can lead to many effects in the first trimester (Box 3).

Box 3: Effects of tobacco consumption in first trimester

- Spontaneous abortion
- Ectopic pregnancy
- Subchorionic hemorrhage
- Birth defects, such as cleft lip or cleft palate

Cannabis

Cannabis is the most commonly used illicit drug in surveys reported in Australia (36.1%), USA (40%), and UK (20.9%). Consumption is said to reach a peak among teenagers and young adults (15–30 years).[32] Cannabis use is often comorbid with tobacco and alcohol use, and women who report regular cigarette smoking are 4.5–9.5 times more likely to report cannabis misuse and dependence.[33] The active ingredient in cannabis is d9-tetrahydrocannabinol (THC), and it acts on the cannabinoid 1 and 2 receptors, part of a cannabinoid system in the human brain. Cross-placental transfer of THC is approximately a third of maternal plasma levels.[32] Increasing evidence suggests that developmental exposure to cannabinoids induces subtle neuro-functional alterations in the offspring.[33] The endocannabinoid system is thought to influence neural systems governing mood, cognition, and reward.[34] Most studies on the effects of cannabis in pregnancy are confounded by sociodemographic variables and the comorbidity of other drugs, especially nicotine.

Cocaine/Crack Cocaine

The reported prevalence of cocaine use during pregnancy varies from 0.3% to 9.5%.[35] *In utero* cocaine exposure has been reported to produce a continuum of obstetric complications and reproductive casualty. Cocaine use in pregnancy can lead to spontaneous abortion, preterm births, placental abruption, and congenital anomalies.[36]

Cocaine in all its forms specifically acts by constricting blood vessels. Consequently, one mechanism by which cocaine exerts a teratogenic influence on fetal development is through the vasoconstrictive effects of cocaine on maternal blood flow, which impair placental blood flow and may lead to maternal hypertension, fetal vasoconstriction, and episodes of fetal hypoxia.[37]

Cocaine also alters the developing monoaminergic neurotransmitter systems, which include dopamine, norepinephrine, and serotonin.[38] This disruption may affect brain development globally, as well as impact the structural and functional aspects of specific systems.

Cocaine is a local anesthetic and a potent, short-acting stimulant of the CNS. It can be consumed by inhalation of powder or intravenous injection. It is a potent vasopressor and fetotoxic. During early pregnancy, cocaine may increase the risk of miscarriage. Whether cocaine causes fetal malformations is still controversial. Several studies of the offspring of women who abused cocaine during pregnancy have described an increased incidence of cranial defects, including exencephaly, encephalocele, partial bone defects, limb reduction defects, urogenital abnormalities, and intestinal perforation, obstruction, or atresia.[39,40]

Box 4: Obstetric complications due to cocaine

- Spontaneous abortion
- Low birth weight
- Intrauterine growth restriction
- Preeclampsia
- Placental abruption
- Premature rupture of membranes
- Preterm birth
- Fetal distress
- Fetal demise

Opioids

Most studies show association of opiate use with LBW, preterm births, and reduced fetal growth parameters.[41,42] However, for opioid intake in early months of pregnancy, data is relatively limited compared to alcohol and tobacco. Opiate use is not associated with fetal malformations. The observed adverse pregnancy outcomes are secondary to withdrawal and parallel high-risk behaviors. Opiate use in pregnant women ranges anywhere from 1% to 21%.[41,42] Obstetric complications increase up to six-fold[43] (Box 4).

A significant percentage of pregnant drug users presenting to drug services are dependent on opioids, which include heroin, illicit methadone, and buprenorphine.[44] All drugs cross the placenta and are secreted in breast milk. Pregnant opioid-dependent women experience a six-fold increase in maternal obstetric complications, such as LBW, toxemia, malpresentation, puerperal morbidity, fetal distress, and meconium aspiration.[44] Women who are opioid dependent have higher rates of miscarriage compared with non-drug users.[45] Among pregnant women who continue illicit intravenous heroin consumption, the risks of medical complications, such as infectious diseases, endocarditis, abscesses, and sexually transmitted diseases are increased.[46] Opioid users, particularly those abusing heroin frequently have menstrual irregularities that include oligomenorrhea and amenorrhea. The disruption is postulated to be due to the effect on the hypothalamic-pituitary-ovarian axis via changes in gonadotropin levels. This can lead to unplanned or unexpected pregnancies as women may not be aware when they are ovulating.[47] Opioids, unlike alcohol, cocaine, or benzodiazepines, have not been specifically linked to any teratogenic effects.[46] Neonatal complications documented include opioid withdrawal, postnatal growth deficiency, microcephaly, neurobehavioral problems, and a 74-fold increase in sudden infant death syndrome.[44] High rates of intrauterine growth retardation and LBW have been reported in heroin-addicted mothers.[42]

Maternal opioid and methadone use during gestation predisposes the infant to signs and symptoms of central and autonomic nervous system regulatory dysfunction, traditionally defined as neonatal abstinence syndrome, which frequently results in significant morbidity and prolonged hospital stays.[48] It is characterized by irritability, gastrointestinal disturbances, sleep, and feeding disturbances, and can disrupt mother-child bonding. The onset, duration, and severity varies, and are mainly influenced by the type of drug used, the severity of maternal drug dependence, the timing of the last drug intake, and fetal metabolic factors. It is important to recognize that many opioid-exposed infants are in actuality polydrug exposed, and the contributory effect of other licit and illicit substances, including alcohol and nicotine, to the signs and symptoms of physiologic and behavioral dysregulation after birth, must be considered.[49]

Note: Many opiates particularly heroin passes through placenta to fetus within 1 hour of administration, accumuates in amniotic fluid and causes placental insufficiency.

While caring for women with drug abuse during pregnancy, the role of counseling, for individual drugs, environmental stressors, as well as individual personality traits should be reviewed. The treatment is initiated in an empathetic yet directive fashion with the involvement of obstetricians, neonatologists, psychiatrists, and psychologists. Sometimes, physician intervention may be needed in acute crises as a result of either overdose or withdrawal. Legal enforcement and social institutions have their unique yet defining role in curbing this menace of substance abuse in pregnancy.

REFERENCES

1. Murthy P. Women and Drug use in India. Substance, Women and High risk Assessment Study: United Nations Office on Drugs and Crime, Ministry of Social Justice and Empowerment, Government of India and United Nations Development Fund for Women; 2008.
2. Bauer CR, Shankaran S, Bada HS, et al. The Maternal Lifestyle Study: drug exposure during pregnancy and short-term maternal outcomes. Am J Obstet Gynecol. 2002;186(3):487-95.
3. Helmbrecht GD, Thiagarajah S. Management of addiction disorders in pregnancy. J Addict Med. 2008;2(1):1-16.
4. Gilchrist G, Taylor A. Drug-using mothers factors associated with retaining care of their children. Drug Alcohol Rev. 2009;28(2):175-85.
5. Advisory Council on the Misuse of Drugs (ACMD). Hidden Harm: Responding to the Needs of Children of Problem Drug Users. London: Home Office; 2003.
6. Lewis G. Saving Mothers Lives: Reviewing maternal deaths to make motherhood safer 2003-2005. London, UK: CEMACH Publications; 2007.
7. Institute of Medicine. Fetal alcohol syndrome: Diagnosis, Epidemiology, Prevention, and .Treatment Washington, DC: The National Academy Press; 1996.
8. Plant ML., Abel EL., Guerri C. Alcohol and pregnancy. In: I Macdonald, editor. Health issues related to alcohol consumption, 2nd edition. Oxford, U.K.: Blackwell Science. pp. 182-213.
9. Kesmodel U, Bertrand J, Støvring H, et al. The effect of different alcohol drinking patterns in early to mid pregnancy on the child's intelligence, attention, and executive function. BJOG. 2012;119(10):1180-90.
10. Kesmodel US, Eriksen HL, Underbjerg M, et al. The effect of alcohol binge drinking in early pregnancy on general intelligence in children. BJOG. 2012;119(10):1222-31.
11. Patra J, Bakker R, Irving H, et al. Dose-response relationship between alcohol consumption before and during pregnancy and the risks of low birth weight, preterm birth and small for gestational age (SGA)- a systematic review and meta-analyses. Brit J Obstet Gynaecol. 2011;118(12):1411-21.
12. Lewis SJ, Zuccolo L, Davey Smith G, et al. Fetal Alcohol Exposure and IQ at Age 8: Evidence from a Population-Based Birth-cohort Study. PloS One. 2011;7(11):e 49407.
13. Jones KL, Smith DW. Recognition of the fetal alcohol syndrome in early infancy. Olancet. 1973;2(7836):999-1001.
14. Kaskutas, LA. Interpretations of risk: The use of scientific information in the development of the alcohol warning label policy. Int J Addict. 1995;30:1519-48.
15. Streissguth AP, O Malley K. Neuropsychiatry, implications and long-term consequences of fetal alcohol spectrum disorders. Sem in Clin Neuro. 2000;5(3):177-190.
16. Warren KR, Calhoun FJ, May PA, et al. Fetal alcohol syndrome an international perspective. Alcoholism. Clin Exp Res. 2001;25(5 Suppl ISBRA):202S-6S.
17. Sokol RJ, Delaney-Black V, Nordstrom B. Fetal alcohol spectrum disorder. J Am Med Asso. 2003;290 (22):2996-9.
18. Nayak RB, Murthy P. Fetal alcohol spectrum disorder. Ind Pediat. 2008;45(12):977-83.
19. Kelly YJ, Sacker A, Gray R, et al. Light drinking during pregnancy. Still no increased risk for socioemotional difficulties or cognitive deficits at 5 years of age. Journ Epid Comm Health. 2012;66(1):41-8.

20. Bertrand J, Floyd RL, Weber MK. Fetal Alcohol Syndrome Prevention Team, Division of Birth Defects and Developmental Disabilities, Centre of Disease Control and Prevention (CDC).
21. Burd L, Cotsonas-Hassler TM, Martsolf JT, et al. Recognition and management of fetal alcohol syndrome. Neur Ter. 2003;25:681.
22. National Cancer Institute (NCI). Health Effects of Exposure to Environmental Tobacco Smoke: The Report of the California Environmental Protection Agency. Smoking and Tobacco Control Monograph No.10. NIH Pub. No.9904645. Bethesda, MD: U.S. Department of Health and Human Services. National Institutes of Health, National Cancer Institute; 1999.
23. Corneliu MD, Goldschmidt L, Taylor PM, et al. Prenatal alcohol use among teenagers: Effects on neonatal outcomes. Alcohol Clin Exp Res. 1999;23(7):1238-44.
24. Day N, Cornelius M, Goldschmidt L, et al. The effects of prenatal tobacco and marijuana use on offspring growth from birth through age 3 years. Neurotoxicol and Teratol. 1992;14(6):407-14.
25. Lambers DS, Clark KE. The maternal and fetal physiologic effects of nicotine. Semin Perinatol. 1996;20(2):115-26.
26. U.S. Department of Health and Human Services (USDHHS). The Health Consequences of Smoking for Women. HHS Pub. No. 396. Rockville MD: USDHHS; 1980.
27. Stillman RJ, Rosenberg MJ, Sachs BP. Smoking and reproduction. Fertil Steril. 1986;46(4): 545-66.
28. Office of Environmental Health Hazard Assessment (OEHHA). Evidence of Developmental and Re-productive Taxicity of Cadmium. Reproductive and Cancer Hazard Assessment Section. OEHHA. California Environmental Protection Agency; 1996.
29. Picone TA, Allen LH, Olsen PN, et al. Pregnancy outcome in North American women. II. Effects of diet, cigarette smoking, stress, and weight gain on placentas, and on neonatal physical and behavioral characteristics. Am J Clin Nutr. 1982;36(6):1214-24.
30. Fried PA, Makin JE. Neonatal behavioural correlates of prenatal exposure to marihuana. Cigarettes and alcohol in a low risk population. Neurotoxicol Teratol. 1987;9(1):1-7.
31. Dempsey DA, Hajnal BL, Partridge JC, et al. Tone abnormalities are associated with maternal cigarette smoking during pregnancy in utero cocaine-exposed infants. Pediatrics. 2000;106(1 Pt 1):79-85.
32. Kennare R, Heard A, Chan A. Substance use during pregnancy: risk factors and obstetric and perinatal outcomes in South Australia. Aust. N Z J Obstet Gynaecol. 2005;45(3):220-5.
33. Campolongo P, Trezza V, Palmery M, et al. Developmental exposure to cannabinoids causes subtle and enduring neurofunctional alternations. Int Rev Neurobiol. 2009;85:117-33.
34. Jutras-Aswad D, DiNieri JA, Harkany T, et al. Neurobiological consequences of maternal cannabis on human fetal development and its neuropsychiatric outcome. Eur Arch Psychiatry Clin Neurosci. 2009;259(7):395-412.
35. Day E, George S. Management of drug misuse in pregnancy. Adv Psychiatr Treat. 2005;6(4):253-61.
36. Keegan J, Parva M, Finnegan M, et al. Addiction in pregnancy. J Addict Dis. 2010;29(2):175-91.
37. Kuczkowski KM. Peripartum care of the cocaine-abusing parturient: are we ready? Acta Obstet Gynecol Scand. 2005;84(2):108-16.
38. Harvey JA. Cocaine effects on the developing brain: current status. Neurosci Biobehav Rev. 2004;27(8):751-64.
39. Bateman DA, Chiriboga CA. Dose-response effect of cocaine on newborn head circumference. Pediatrics. 2000;106(3):E33.
40. Fares I, McCulloch KM, Raju TN. Intrauterine cocaine exposure and the risk for sudden infant death syndrome: a meta-analysis. J Perinatol. 1997;17:179-82.
41. Schempf AH. Illicit drug use and neonatal outcomes: a critical review. Obstet Gynecol Surv. 2007;62(11):749-57.
42. Binder T, Vavøinková B. Prospective randomized comparative study of the effect of buprenorphine, methadone and heroin on the course of pregnancy, birth weight of newborns, early postpartum adaptation and course of the neonatal abstinence syndrome in women followed up in the outpatient department. Neuro endocrinol Lett. 2008;29(1):80-6.
43. Kakko J, Heilig M, Sarman I. Buprenorphine and methadone treatment of opiate dependence during pregnancy: comparison of fetal growth and neonatal outcomes in two consecutive case series. Drug Alcohol Depend. 2008;96(1-2):69-78.
44. Minozzi S, Amato L, Vecchi S, et al. Maintenance agonist treatments for opiate dependent pregnant women. Cochrane Database Syst Rev. 2008;(2):CD006318.
45. Mayet S, Groshkova T, Morgan L, et al. Drugs and pregnancy—outcomes of women engaged with a specialist perinatal outreach addictions service. Drug Alcohol Rev. 2008;27(5): 497-503.
46. Winklbaur B, Kopf N, Ebner N, et al. Treating pregnant women dependent on opioids is not the same as treating pregnancy and opioid dependence: a knowledge synthesis for better treatment for women and neonates. Addition. 2008;103(9):1429-40.
47. Schmittner J, Schroeder JR, Epstein DH, et al. Menstrual cycle length during methadone maintenance Addiction. 2005;100(6):829-36.
48. Jansson LM, Velez M, Harrow C. The opioid-exposed newborn: assessment and pharmacologic management. J Opioid Manag. 2009;5(1),47-55.
49. Farid WO, Dunlop SA, Tait RJ, et al. The effects of maternally administered methadone, buprenorphine and naltrexone on offspring: review of human and animal data. Curr Neuropharmacol. 2008;6(2):125-150.

Travel Guidelines

13

CHAPTER

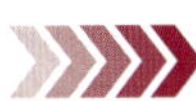

Pratap Kumar, Alok Sharma

INTRODUCTION

Travel is becoming more prevalent in this era of globalization and is considered a part of leading a normal life. Pregnant women need to observe some precautions during travel. Schedules need to be rarely changed unless there are pregnancy complications. However, many airlines do not allow travel after 32 weeks and this should be borne in mind when women plan to travel for their delivery.

TRAVEL DURING PREGNANCY

Travel is not a contraindication during the first 8 months of pregnancy. The main concerns with travel during pregnancy are complications due to pregnancy, access to medical care, getting good and hygienic food and fluids. Caution is given to a pregnant woman with medical and obstetrical problems. Travel during the first trimester, though safe, may aggravate nausea and vomiting, and may even be embarrassing.

According to the American College of Obstetrics and Gynecology, the safest time for a pregnant woman to travel is during the second trimester. Third trimester is the time where one should be advised to defer overseas travel because of concerns about access to medical care in case of problems, such as hypertension, phlebitis, or premature labor. Travel decisions should be discussed with the health care provider.

Preparation for Travel during Pregnancy

Once a pregnant woman has decided to travel, a number of issues need to be considered:

- An ectopic pregnancy should be ruled out before beginning any travel
- Pregnant travelers should enquire about what their general health insurance policies cover and, if needed, obtain a supplemental policy for their trip
- She should check medical facilities at the destination to manage complications of pregnancy, pregnancy-induced hypertension, cesarean sections, and premature or sick neonates
- Determine whether prenatal care will be required while abroad and who will provide it
- The pregnant traveler should make sure that she does not miss antenatal visits requiring specific timing
- She should be routinely screened for human immunodeficiency virus, and hepatitis B and C at the destination. The pregnant traveler should also be advised to know her blood type, and Rh-negative pregnant women should receive anti-D immune globulin prophylactically at about 28 weeks' gestation.

The immunoglobulin dose should be repeated after delivery if the infant is Rh positive

- Determine if the traveler risks influenza on this trip, and recommend influenza vaccine accordingly.

Traveling By Air during Pregnancy

If there is a normal healthy pregnancy, air travel during pregnancy is safer. Pregnant mothers with medical conditions or a high-risk pregnancy may not be allowed to travel by any mode of transport. A written consent to travel is required mentioning the expected due date and a health certificate from an obstetrician.[1] The common risk factors indicating special precautions who should not travel by air are listed in box 1.[2]

The Effects of Barometric Pressure on Pregnancy

Condition most commonly associated with changes in barometric pressure involve pain in joints. Many pregnant women report nausea, flatulence, and headaches. Some evidence exists to suggest a sudden change in barometric pressure can even induce premature labor pains but this has not been scientifically proven.

The first month of pregnancy has feelings of fatigue, nausea, and general exhaustion which will become more prevalent in this time, and travel may or may not be comfortable. According to the University of Pennsylvania Health System, air travel is not necessarily contraindicated for the first trimester, unless existing conditions suggest that the experience may be unhealthy for the mother or the fetus.[3]

The risk for miscarriage and ectopic pregnancy during the first trimester are increased. It is good to verify the integrity of blood banks at the destination(s) in case a transfusion is required in an emergency. One needs to carry medical records, and have them available during the trip. The Royal College of Obstetricians and Gynecologists advises that women after 37 weeks of gestation should not travel as delivery could occur at this stage. For women with uncomplicated multiple pregnancies, it is 34 weeks.[2]

Box 1: Risk factors in pregnant women for air travel[2]

- Severe anemia
- Obstetric hemorrhage
- Nephrotic syndrome
- Wearing a cast from a recent fracture in the leg
- Otitis media and sinusitis
- Asthma and respiratory problems marked by breathlessness
- Previous deep venous thrombosis
- Severe obesity
- Sickle cell crisis

Seat and Exercise

It is advisable to have an aisle seat with sufficient leg room that will help in stretching the legs and also aid in moving around or visiting the washroom with ease. It is good to go up and down on the aisle to boost blood circulation and stretch muscles. Simple measures of sitting exercises, such as rotating ankles, wiggling toes, and gently flexing calf muscles will also help as stretching exercises and this will avoid any risk of thrombosis.[4]

Seat Belts

When fastening seat belt, the same should be put under the belly and across thighs to prevent any undue pressure on the uterus.

Food Choices

Raw foods, such as salads, cut fruits, and foods which contain raw eggs like mayonnaise, mousse or soufflés should be avoided at all times, as there is a risk of food poisoning or infections. It is good to have plenty of water and hot food. Women should consume small frequent meals to avoid air sickness. If nauseous, she can suck on a mint or lozenges. Liquids should be consumed frequently to prevent dehydration as that will increase the risk of deep venous thrombosis (DVT).

Fear of Decreased Oxygen

All planes have oxygen pressurized cabins in which one will not suffer from shortness of breath at high altitudes unless there is a medical condition.[5]

Deep Venous Thrombosis

Deep venous thrombosis is of great concern. The risk of DVT is increased during air travel because of the long periods of immobility and restricted space to stretch. A properly fitted graduated elastic compression stockings during the flight and exercising ankles and legs while sitting to reduce the risk of DVT is recommended in all long haul flights.

Direct estimates of the risk of travel-related venous thromboembolism in pregnancy were seen in the literature. The overall incidence of symptomatic venous thrombosis after a long-haul flight has been estimated to be around 1/400 to 1/10,000. The figure rises to ten times when asymptomatic venous thrombosis is concerned.[6]

Precautions for Prevention of DVT

- Repeated movement of ankles and calves while sitting
- Elastic compression stockings
- Avoid dehydration
- A tablet of baby aspirin has been recommended on the day of travel as it prevents platelet aggregation and clot formation.

Airline Policy

When it comes to airline travel, all the airlines have different policies for pregnant women. Some of the common airline policies include:

- Most airlines allow women till 28th week of their pregnancy
- After the 28th week of pregnancy, the pregnant travelers have to get a medical certificate from their obstetrician[7]
- Airlines don't allow pregnant women to travel in their last 4 weeks of pregnancy
- Most airlines restrict the length of flight for pregnant women to 4 hours, especially in the later stages of pregnancy.

Traveling By Car during Pregnancy

Traveling by land during pregnancy is generally safe whether one is going in a car, bus, or train. Certain precautionary measures can help keep the pregnant woman and the baby safe.

Car Travel (as a Passenger)

Even though car travel is seen as generally safe; with bad roads, there will be constant vibrations and bumps which can cause concern. Long distance travel should not be undertaken at a stretch. Constant movements of all joints and legs should be done to avoid thrombosis. Travel should be avoided on full stomach as it may aggravate motion sickness.

Wearing the Seat Belt

Seat belts are all the more important during pregnancy as two lives need protection, the mother and the baby. In an older study on 208 pregnant women who had road accidents, death was seen in 3.6% among those wearing a lap belt compared with 7.8% among those not wearing a seat belt. Fetal mortality was 16.7% among women wearing a lap belt compared with 14.4% among women not wearing a seat belt.[7] In UK, the confidential enquiry into maternal deaths provides information on the correct use of seat belts in pregnancy.[8] The advice is as follows:

- A seat belt should never pass over the belly as a sudden jerk may cause complications
- Use three-point seat belts which consists of two belts; one is the shoulder belt which runs from one side of the shoulder and buckles up near the waist while the other belt is a lap belt, which runs across the waist or pelvis. The lap

belt should run beneath the abdomen across the pelvis while the shoulder belt should pass over the abdomen and in between the breasts
- Adjust the fit to be as snug as comfortably possible.

Car Travel (as a Driver)

There are generally no major problems to drive when pregnant, so long as some general guidelines are followed.
- Seat belt is to be used as described above
- Driving can cause discomfort in legs during late pregnancy
- Avoid traveling for long hours.

Traveling By Bus

A journey by a bus during pregnancy can be quite uncomfortable as it tends to be crowded, noisy, and the trip itself can be bumpy. Also access to toilets is restricted.

Traveling By Train

Traveling during pregnancy by train is safe. Certain precautionary measures can help protect against unforeseen circumstances and make the trip comfortable.

Appropriate Luggage

Pregnant women should not carry or lift any heavy objects. A suitcase with wheels or a stroller is preferable. It may be better to hire a porter.

Time Management

Trains can get unpredictable. It is always better to be before time to catch a train in order to minimize any confusion and to avoid the crowd.

Choice of Lower Berth

It is always better to book a lower berth as it not only aids in easy movement but also reduces any risk of a fall.

Movement

Trains have enough space for exercising legs.

Washroom Visits

There are only a few washrooms in a train and that too are small in size. One needs to be careful about maintaining balance as the train's rocking movement especially in the bathroom can make a person disoriented. The woman should always hold on to some kind of support and wash hands after visiting a bathroom.

Sea Travel

When traveling by sea, the motion of the ship can make one feel nauseous, dizzy, and prone to stomach problems. Sea sickness is very common. There are also concerns of limited access to healthcare if an acute emergency arises. Hence, it is best avoided.

International Travel

Before planning an international travel, discussion with the health care provider is essential. The woman should be cautious about food and water since infectious diarrhea may be a problem. Diarrhea can cause dehydration, which reduces the blood flow to the conceptus. It is important to make sure all the essential vaccinations needed for the countries which are planned have been given. Some immunizations cannot be given to pregnant woman (*See* Chapter 9: Vaccination).

Vaccination against Communicable Diseases for the Pregnant Traveler

The following is a list of immunizations and when they need to be given:
- Diphtheria and tetanus vaccine can be offered after the first trimester
- Hepatitis A and B vaccinations might be given in the second trimester
- Pulmonary influenza vaccine should be provided to a pregnant traveler susceptible

to persistent respiratory illness. However, the influenza live virus vaccine (nasal spray) should not be administered

- Measles, mumps, and rubella vaccinations should not be given in pregnancy
- Yellow fever should not be offered to a pregnant lady unless she is traveling to an endemic region
- Typhoid (oral vaccine) is not usually offered to pregnant patients as it is a live attenuated vaccine. Parenteral capsular polysaccharide vaccine may be administered. However, it is not advised unless the threat of typhoid is unavoidable (*See* Chapter 9: Vaccination)
- Japanese encephalitis vaccine is not suggested in pregnancy at all. Keeping away from journey to contaminated locations ought to be considered.

Prophylaxis against Malaria

Travel to malaria-endemic places calls for private protective measures since no prophylaxis is hundred percent successful. For malaria prophylaxis, permethrin-impregnated bed nets and electrical citronella coils ought to be utilized. Chloroquine and proguanil have been employed for decades in UK with no documented birth defects. It is recommended that in case of proguanil, 5 mg of folic acid/day should be given. However, administration in the first trimester is a problem for any drug. Mefloquine has been provided in the second trimester with no adverse effects and it may be considered for travel to chloroquine-resistant areas. Pyrimethamine with dapsone can be given in pregnancy.

Travel Insurance

One should make sure that the health insurance done should be valid abroad and during pregnancy. It must be ensured that the policy covers a newborn if one were to give birth during travels.[9] The policy should also cover complications and adverse outcomes like miscarriage.[10] They should provide cover till term. There are a few that cover up to 32 weeks and some covers up to 28 weeks.[11] Travel insurance agencies should be contacted directly for more comprehensive information.

Traveling during pregnancy should be carefully planned in consultation with the obstetrician. It may be restricted if there are pregnancy complications like threatened miscarriage or any other problems that need special care. Travel to another country has risk issues like exposure to endemic communicable diseases and insurance coverage which needs to be dealt with.

REFERENCES

1. Hezelgrave NL, Whitty CJ, Shennan AH, et al. Advising on travel during pregnancy. BMJ. 2011;342:d2506.
2. NICE's guidance on air travel and pregnancy. (2008) Antenatal care: routine care for healthy pregnant women. Section 5.14, pp.101-2.
3. ACOG Committee on Obstetric Practice. ACOG Committee Opinion No. 443: Air travel during pregnancy. Obstet Gynecol. 2009;114(4):954-5.
4. Royal College of Obstetricians and Gynecologists. (2008). Air travel and pregnancy. Scientific advisory committee paper. [online] Available from: www.rcog.org.uk/womens-health/clinical-guidance/air-travel-and-pregnancy [Accessed october, 2013].
5. Magann EF, Chauvan SP, Dahlke JD, et al. Air travel and pregnancy outcomes, a review of pregnancy regulations and outcome for passengers, flight attenders and aviators. Obstet Gynecol Surv. 2010;65(6):396-402.
6. Royal College of Obstetricians and Gynaecologists. Advice on preventing deep vein thrombosis for pregnant women travelling by air; 2009.
7. Crosby WM, Costiloe JP. Safety of lap-belt restraint for pregnant victims of automobile collisions. New Engl J Med. 1971;284(12):632-6.
8. Johnson HC, Pring DW. Car seatbelts in pregnancy: the practice and knowledge of pregnant women remain causes for concern. BJOG. 2000;107(5):644-7
9. World Health Organization. Travellers with special needs. In: Martinez L, editor. International Travel and Health. Geneva: World Health Organization; 2002.
10. Pearce G. Travel insurance and the pregnant woman. MIDIRS Midwifery Digest. 1997;7:164.
11. Rose SR. Pregnancy and travel. Emerg Med Clin North Am. 1997;15(1):93-111.

Role of Exercise and Bed Rest

14

CHAPTER

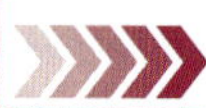

Maninder Ahuja

INTRODUCTION

Historically, bed rest has been prescribed in pregnancy for problems of threatened abortion, premature rupture of membranes, intrauterine growth restriction, pregnancy induced hypertension (PIH), placenta previa, pregnancy with hypertension or heart disease, and bad obstetric history. However, scientific data point in the opposite direction. Rest is no longer recommended for normal pregnancy, rather exercise in pregnancy, is important. Various scientific studies have highlighted that bed rest has no role to play in normal pregnancy, threatened abortion, multiple pregnancy, or recurrent pregnancy loss.

CURRENT EVIDENCE ON BED REST IN PREGNANCY

- *Bed rest in singleton pregnancies for preventing preterm birth*: Cochrane review has shown that at present to prevent preterm birth there is no evidence, either supporting or refuting the use of bed rest at home or in hospital[1]
- *In multiple pregnancies*: Routine hospitalization to give a better outcome, does not help the patients. Rather some evidence is pointed toward increased risk of preterm birth. So we should not recommend routine bed rest in multiple pregnancies[2]
- *Bed rest to prevent miscarriage*: If we have a viable pregnancy and there is bleeding per vaginum in the first half of pregnancy, bed rest does not improve pregnancy outcome. Also outcome does not change if women are allowed their routine activity at home[3]
- *Advantage of exercise*: There is optimum weight gain in fetuses born to mothers who exercised during pregnancy[4]
- Various studies have proved that bed rest leads to significantly increased ultra-distal bone loss.[5,6]

It has been observed that pregnant women who are participating in both aerobic and strength building exercises during pregnancy have advantage of less late pregnancy complications, good growth of fetus, less chances of early miscarriages, and neonatal outcomes are better as compared to women who are not involved in any exercise routine.

Various investigators have concluded that it is better for fetal and pregnancy outcomes to involve women in some sort of physical activity.[7]

RISKS OF SEDENTARY LIFE STYLE IN PREGNANCY

If women do not do regular physical activity or exercise then they are prone to the following complications in pregnancy.

- Loss of muscle tone and strength

- Backache
- Excessive weight gain
- Varicose veins
- Deep venous thrombosis.

It is seen that women who are regularly involved in physical activity have less chances of developing diabetes mellitus and are better prepared mentally to cope with physical changes of pregnancy.[7]

BARRIERS TO EXERCISE DURING PREGNANCY[8]

National Institute for Health and Care Excellence (NICE) guidelines of 2010 suggest 30 minutes of moderate exercise per day during pregnancy. They also suggest that not only friends and relatives but even health professionals tend to discourage women regarding physical activity during pregnancy.

Routine hospitalization and best rest did not reduce the risk of preterm birth in multiple pregnancies. However it may improve the growth of the infants and prevent low birth weight.[2]

There are many barriers to exercise during pregnancy. It has been observed in many studies that even active women are found to reduce their prepregnancy activity because of following barriers:

- Advice from friends, that exercise or physical activity may be harmful, and bed rest and less activity is advisable
- Some women get misinformation from some magazines
- Sometimes women feel so tired and exhausted that they don't have the energy to do any structured exercise besides routine household work
- Ill-informed family members sometimes can give wrong advice or even physical instructors may tell them to go slow
- Many a times because of their physical appearance women feel shy to participate in these activities.

Therefore, proper counseling is required before a pregnant woman can be motivated to the advantages of exercise during pregnancy.

During the childbearing year, from conception through postpartum recovery, a woman's body undergoes extensive changes which frequently necessitate many adaptations. Physical and hormonal changes occur gradually throughout the 9 months of pregnancy, and these are reversed in a matter of weeks during postpartum recovery. Skeletal tissue, muscle and connective tissue, blood volume, cardiac output, body weight, and posture are affected.

As more pregnant women engage in demanding occupations, physical activities, and sports, the obstetricians and midwives who take care of them must become knowledgeable about the physical changes of pregnancy and the effects of exercise on the mother and fetus. Because prevention is the best approach to healthcare, understanding both the bodily stresses that may result from pregnancy changes and the means to prevent unnecessary problems enables healthcare to be instituted early in pregnancy and continued through the postpartum period.

HISTORICAL PERSPECTIVE

The value and possible hazards of physical exercise and sports activities during pregnancy have been debated for years. Early observers correlated an uneventful pregnancy and easy labor with physical activity. In Exodus, Biblical writers observed that Hebrew slave women had an easier time giving birth than their sedentary Egyptian mistresses[9] and in 9 BC, Plutarch urged Spartan women to harden their bodies with exercise to decrease the pain of childbearing.[10]

In Victorian times, pregnant women were encouraged to remain indoors and keep themselves "confined."[11] With more women in the workplace in the 1930s and their apparent ease of birthing, physicians once again advocated "strong body movements" for sedentary pregnant women.

Based on her work in India in the 1930s, Vaughan instituted antenatal exercise classes in England. She wrote that "flexible hips and spine are conducive to ease of labor," and women were encouraged to squat. Exercise classes taught by physiotherapists became popular in Great Britain and Sweden, where they were valued for their effects on back and abdominal muscles.[12]

During the mid-1950s, despite the lack of scientific proof of benefits, "keep fit" exercises introduced by obstetric physiotherapist `Helen Herdman in Britain were included with relaxation and breathing skills in Grantly Dick-Read's book on pain management for labor. In fact, Herdman's own book delineated an excellent program of prenatal exercises which form the basis of the best of many prenatal exercise programs today. The Lamaze method, popularized in the United States in 1959 by Elizabeth Bing[13] focused on both physical and psychological preparation for child birth. From the mid-1970s through the 1990s, the emphasis on health and the public's renewed involvement in exercise caught the interest of the "pregnant population." Numerous books on prenatal exercise, as well as videotapes and audio cassettes, flooded the market,[14] and community centers, hospitals, health maintenance organizations, and industries began to offer exercise classes for expectant women. Physicians and midwives must be aware that some of these book authors and some instructors of prenatal exercise classes lack adequate training, and may neither have sufficient knowledge of the physiologic changes of pregnancy nor of the cautions expectant women should follow while exercising. Many expectant women enroll in regular aerobics classes and try to keep up with the nonpregnant participants or instructor, often to their detriment.

Before enrolling in a pregnancy exercise class, it is recommended that the expectant women be past her first trimester, be under medical supervision, and be warned of any medical reason that either precludes her from taking the classes or warrants limitations. As outlined by the American College of Obstetrics and Gynecology (ACOG),[15] these conditions include heart disease, toxemia, ruptured membranes, risk of premature labor, intrauterine growth retardation, poor weight gain, vaginal or uterine bleeding, anemia, hypertension, and fetal distress. Consultation with healthcare providers or some degree of caution is necessary for expectant women with respiratory conditions, such as asthma[16] or orthopedic conditions, such as back and hip pain or joint problems. The qualifications of the instructor of the prenatal exercise program should include a medical background; knowledge of obstetrics, muscle physiology, and kinesthesiology; and experience working with expectant mothers.[15] Physician should make enquiries regarding the qualifications of instructors before signing approval notes for their patients to attend classes. Two-way communication between the obstetrician and prenatal exercise instructors should be instituted to ensure the safety of the patient.[15] There is as yet no scientific evidence of tangible results of physical preparation in pregnancy in the reduction of the length of labor; however, observers feel that effective abdominal expulsive efforts by the mother can shorten the second stage. No reduction in uterine inertia or episiotomies (which are performed routinely in the United States) has been documented, but there has been a lower incidence of cesarean birth correlated with physical fitness.

No relation has been noted between physical fitness of the mother and the newborn's birth, weight, length, head circumference, or 1-minute apgar score, but recent studies have found that strenuous maternal exercise in pregnancy may negatively affect the mother's weight gain and in some cases causes decreased weight of newborn infant.[17]

PSYCHOLOGICAL AND PHYSICAL BENEFITS

Birth is a normal, natural, and physiologic process. Supporting the premise that pregnancy is a state of health, both physical and mental aspects of body image must be considered. With an increase in body weight and a protuberant abdomen, most women feel heavy, unattractive, and cumbersome; their movements seem clumsy, uncoordinated, and lacking in agility. The pregnant woman's body image may reach an all-time low; her posture sags, and she loses her self-esteem and confidence.[18] There is a strong relation between physical and mental health, and exercise is generally thought to have tremendous psychological value and boosts self-esteem.[19]

With a well-regulated, non-strenuous exercise program instituted in the fourth month of pregnancy through the postpartum period, a pregnant woman is able to maintain good physical condition, to develop a sensible, healthy approach to exercise to increase her comfort in pregnancy, to prepare for postpartum recovery, and to sustain the necessary muscular activity for the work of child-birth. Feelings of well-being and confidence that result from whole-body exercise on a regular basis enable her to approach childbirth with positive expectations.

Physical activity improves circulation, appetite, digestion, and elimination, all of which are affected during pregnancy and in turn are mirrored in the pregnant woman's mental attitude.[18,19]

Self-esteem is reduced immeasurably after childbirth, when the woman is upset by her "ruined figure and additional folds of flesh." Exercise during pregnancy and reinstituted soon after delivery ensures quicker postpartum healing and recuperation with renewal of positive body image and self-esteem. These feelings of well-being and additional energy allow the new mother to feel that she is doing something for herself and enable her to better face the responsibilities of parenting.[14]

MATERNAL EXERCISE AND PERINATAL AND FETAL OUTCOME

Studies on maternal exercise and birth outcome indicate that most fetuses are able to tolerate moderate maternal exercise programs that women continue throughout pregnancy.[20,21] Studies of endurance exercises (i.e., running and aerobics) over the course of pregnancy monitored exercisers every 6–8 weeks. Before the end of the first trimester, one-third of study subjects stopped intensive exercising and forming two new groups (i.e., exercisers and nonexercisers). In each group, 9% experienced preterm labor before 37 weeks. Exercisers started labor 5 days earlier than nonexercisers and had lower incidences of obstetrical interventions, need for labor stimulation, episiotomy, cesarean birth, and epidural anesthesia as well as shorter active stage of labor.[21]

Decreases in birth weight and less maternal weight gain have been noted in women who continued high-performance activities[18] during pregnancy. Other studies contradict these findings of low birth weight, finding instead a higher rate of fetal anomalies, which could be related to hyperthermia experienced during intense exercise in early pregnancy.[20]

THERMOREGULATORY SYSTEM IN PREGNANCY

Basal metabolic rate, increases during pregnancy, and necessitates a 300 kcal increase in the pregnant woman's caloric intake. The physiologic changes and increase in adipose tissue insulation makes pregnant women feel warmer even at rest. Research studies on maternal thermoregulation suggest that hyperthermia, specifically in the first trimester, can produce adverse effects on fetal development. As maternal temperatures increase, so does the fetal temperature. Teratogenic effects of heat on the fetus have been demonstrated in animal research.

When exercising, pregnant women must be reminded to wear loose-fitting clothing and drink fluids before, during, and after exercise.[20] Women who are fit tend to maintain a cooler temperature because of their more efficient cardiovascular system. Avoiding hyperthermia is one of the primary rationales for both the ACOG and American College of Sports Medicine in establishing safety guidelines for prenatal exercise intensity and duration.

A regimen of regulated exercises, done slowly and deliberately and without strain or to the point of fatigue, includes all areas of the body and assists with the postural correction described previously.These exercises improve tone and elasticity of slackened or stretched muscles (abdominals, rhomboids, upper back, and neck muscles); stretch shortened muscles (lower back and pectorals); reduce tension in joints of the pelvis, shoulders, hips, and knees; support breasts by strengthening pectorals; and improve posture and increase vital capacity of lungs. Although in many childbirth preparation classes a variety of exercises are taught,[14] the following basic examples can be easily explained by the physician or midwife at the prenatal visits. Guidelines for exercise during pregnancy/postpartum are as follows:

- Regular exercise (3 times/week) is preferable to intermittent activity[15]
- All exercises should be done slowly and deliberately. Jerking bouncing movements that strain joints should be avoided. Wooden and securely carpeted surfaces will reduce body shock and provide sure footing
- Activities requiring jumping, jarring motions, or rapid change of direction should be avoided because of joint instability
- Vigorous exercise should be avoided in very hot, humid weather, and during periods of febrile illness
- It is vitally important to begin any exercise session with the period of warm up exercises, such as arm circling, shoulder and neck rotations, trunk flection, and gentle knee bends. This should be followed by stretching of the various muscle groups in the arms, legs, and trunk to prevent the damage of muscle fibers and joint strain[15]
- Similarly, each session ends with muscle and joints stretches done slowly, without bouncing or jerky movements. Cooling down should be accompanied by slow and comfortable breathing and followed by relaxation period
- Heart rate should be measured before the exercise session and at time of peak activity, and the target level of 140 beats per minute should not be exceeded except in strong athlete who have consulted and established their own target rates with their positions
- Strenuous exercise should not exceed 15 minutes in duration, and exercises that employ or produce the valsalva maneuver should be avoided
- Caloric intake should be adequate to meet the extra energy needs of pregnancy and lactation as well as the exercise performed. Liquid should be taken liberally before, during, and after exercise to prevent dehydration
- Maternal core temperature should not exceed 38.5°C.[20]

PRECAUTIONS DURING EXERCISE

Medical practitioners who are looking after pregnant women or her exercise schedule have to be careful that while exercising they should have enough fluid intake as it is very important the women is not dehydrated so either energy drinks or plain water can be taken.

Group exercises or contact exercises where women can fall down or can suffer trauma or injury should be avoided.

In the first trimester, because of nausea and vomiting, it is not advisable to start routing exercise program but it can be started after 3 months when she feels better.

In the third trimester any lying down exercises should not be done so that blood supply to fetus is not compromised due aortocaval compression.

Third trimester women are so much incapacitated because of weight of gravid uterus that except for walking and stretching exercises not much activity would be possible.

Conditions where moderate exercise should be done under medical supervision are listed below:

- Cardiac disease
- Restrictive lung disease
- Preeclampsia or pregnancy induced hypertension
- Intrauterine growth restriction
- Preterm prelabor rupture of membranes
- Heavy smoker (more than 20 cigarettes a day)
- Orthopedic limitations
- Poorly controlled hypertension
- Unevaluated maternal cardiac arrhythmia
- Chronic bronchitis
- Multiple gestation (individualized and medically supervised)
- Poorly controlled thyroid disease
- Morbid obesity (body mass index >40)
- Malnutrition or eating disorder
- Poorly controlled diabetes mellitus
- Poorly controlled seizures
- Anemia (hemoglobin <10 g/L).

The healthcare professionals take decisions in the above mentioned conditions, for starting a mild exercise programme.

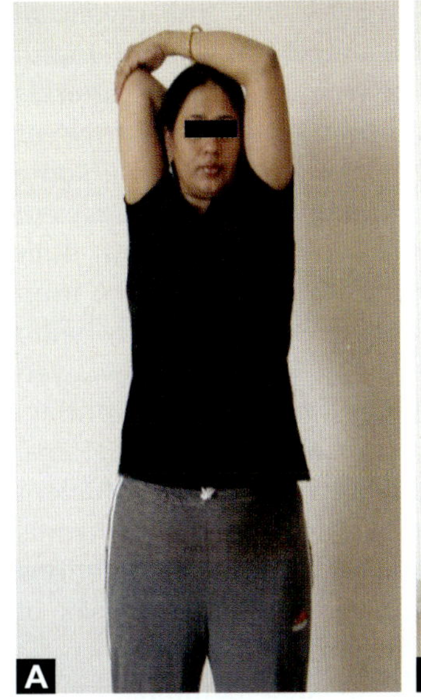
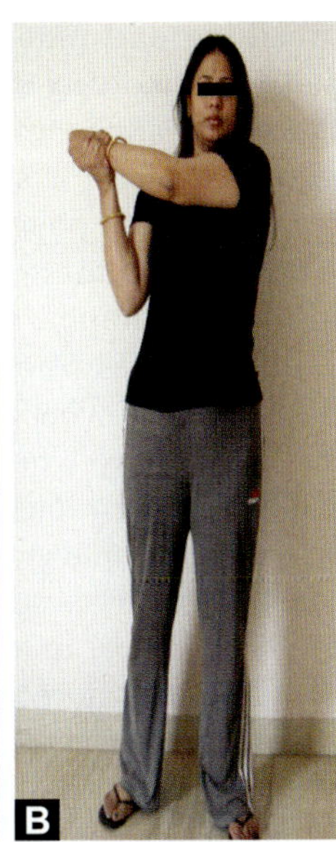

FIGURE 1 **A,** Triceps stretch; **B,** Shoulder stretch.

TYPES OF EXERCISES

Exercise has to be in combination of stretching, aerobic, strength building and resistance exercise. The duration and intensity varies from person to person. After 20 weeks no lying down exercises should be done and walking lunges should not be done after second trimester.

Stretching exercises can be done throughout pregnancy (Fig. 1). If any of the following symptoms appear during exercise then patient should immediately stop exercise and seek medical attention, these are RCOG Guidelines:

- Excessive shortness of breath
- Chest pain or palpitations
- Presyncope or dizziness
- Painful uterine contractions or preterm labor
- Leakage of amniotic fluid
- Vaginal bleeding
- Excessive fatigue
- Abdominal pain, particularly in back or pubic area
- Pelvic girdle pain
- Reduced fetal movement
- Dyspnea before exertion
- Headache
- Muscle weakness
- Calf pain or swelling.

COCHRANE REVIEW OF EXERCISE DURING PREGNANCY

Regular aerobic exercise during pregnancy appears to improve physical fitness, but the evidence is insufficient to infer important risks or benefits for the mother or baby. Aerobic exercise is physical activity that stimulates a person's breathing and blood circulation. The review of 14 trials, involving 1,014 pregnant women, found that pregnant women who engage in vigorous exercise at least 2-3 times per week improve (or maintain) their physical fitness, and there is some evidence that these women have pregnancies of the same duration as those who maintain their usual activities. There is too little evidence from trials to show whether there are other effects on the woman and her baby. The trials reviewed included noncontact exercise, such as swimming, static cycling, and general floor exercise programs. Most of the trials were small and of insufficient methodological quality, larger, and better trials are needed before confident recommendations can be made about the benefits and risks of aerobic exercise in pregnancy.

Preeclampsia is a dreaded complication of pregnancy, and etiologies and hypothesis about eclampsia are oxidative stress and endothelial dysfunction leading onto various pathological changes in various organs.

It is observed that women who are exercising during pregnancy have a less risk of developing preeclampsia.[22]

A very interesting hypothesis supporting exercise during pregnancy to prevent pre-eclampsia is that aerobic exercise reduces oxidative stress by giving more oxygen supply to tissues and this leads to more growth of placenta and increased vascularity and at the same time causes reversal of endothelial dysfunction.[23,24,25] As same mechanism has been seen working in cardiac, diabetes, and aging where we find endothelial dysfunction.[26,27]

CONCLUSION

A review of the evidence and NICE[28] and RCOG[29] guidelines suggests that, in most cases, exercise is safe for both mother and fetus during pregnancy and women should, therefore, be encouraged to initiate or continue exercise to derive the health benefits associated with such activities.

REFERENCES

1. Sosa C, Althabe F, Belizán J, et al. Bed rest in singleton pregnancies for preventing preterm birth. Cochrane Database Syst Rev. 2004;(1):CD003581.
2. Crowther CA, Han S. Hospitalisation and bed rest for multiple pregnancy. Cochrane Database Syst Rev. 2010;(7):CD000110.
3. Aleman A, Althabe F, Belizán JM, et al. Bed rest during pregnancy for preventing miscarriage. Cochrane Database of Syst Rev. 2005;(2):CD003576.
4. Owe KM, Nystad W, Bø K. Association between regular exercise and excessive newborn birth weight. Obstet Gynecol. 2009;114(4):770-6.
5. Hangartner TN. Osteoporosis due to disuse. In: V. Matkovic (Ed). Physical Medicine and Rehabilitation Clinics of North America: Osteoporosis. Philadelphia:W.B.Saunders Company;1995.pp. 579-94.
6. Jacobson PC, Beaver W, Grubb SA, et al. Bone density in women: college athletes and older athletic women. J Orthop Res. 1984;2(4):328-32.
7. Australian Institute of Health and Welfare, National Perinatal Statistics Unit. Australia's mothers and babies 2000. Canberra; 2003.
8. Kramer MS, McDonald SW. Aerobic exercise for women during pregnancy. Cochrane Database of Syst Rev. 2006;(3): CD000180.
9. Burnett CW. The value of antenatal exercises. J Obstet Gynaecol Br Emp. 1956;63(1):40-57.
10. Artal R, Gardin S. Historical perspectives. In: Artal Mittlemark R, Wiswell RA, Drinkwater BL, editors. Exercise in Pregnancy, 2nd edition. Baltimore: Williams and Wilkins; 1991.
11. Williams M. Keeping fit for Pregnancy and Labour. London: National Childbirth Trust; 1970.
12. Rhodes P. Antenatal and postnatal physiotherapy. Practioner. 1971;206(236):758-64.
13. Bing E. Six Practical Lessons for an Easier Childbirth. New York: Bantam; 1994.
14. Noble E. Essential Exercises for the Childbearing Years. Boston: Houghton Miffin; 1995.
15. Artal R, Wiswell R. Exercise in Pregnancy. Baltlmore: Williams and Wilkins; 1986.
16. American College of Obstetrics and Gynecology (ACOG). Guidelines for Prenatal Exercises. Washington, DC: ACOG; 1986.
17. Bell RJ, Palma SM, Lumley JM. The effects of vigorous exercise during pregnancy on birth weight. Aust N Z J Obstet Gynaecol. 1995;35(1):46-51.
18. Cooper K, Cooper M. The New Aerobics for Women. New York: Bantam Books; 1988.
19. Dale E, Mullinax K. Physiological adaptations and considerations of exercise during pregnancy. In: Wilder E, editor. Obstetrics

and Gynecologie Physical Therapy. London,New York: Churchill Livingstone; 1988.

20. Drinkwater BL. Artal R. Heat stress and pregnancy. In: Artal Mittlemark R, Wiswell RA, Drinkwater BL, editors. Exercise in Pregnancy, 2nd edition. Baltimore: Williams and Wikins; 1991.
21. Clapp JF. The effects of maternal exercise on early pregnancy outcome. Am J Obstet Gynecol. 1989;161(6 Pt 1):1453-7.
22. Weissgerber TL, Wolfe LA, Davies GA.The Role of Regular Physical Activity in Preeclampsia Prevention Med Sci Sports Exerc. 2004;36(12):2024-31.
23. Clapp JF 3rd. The effects of maternal exercise on fetal oxygenation and feto-placental growth. Eur J Obstet Gynecol Reprod Biol. 2003;110(Suppl. 1):S80-5.
24. Chambers JC, Fusi L, Malik IS, et al. Association of maternal endothelial dysfunction with preeclampsia. JAMA. 2001;285(12):1607-12.
25. Jackson MR, Gott P, Lye SL, et al. The effects of maternal aerobic exercise on human placental development: placental volumetric composition and surface areas. Placenta. 1995;16:179-91.
26. Powers SK, Ji LL, Leeuwenburgh C. Exercise training-induced alterations in skeletal muscle antioxidant capacity: a brief review. Med Sci Sports Exerc. 1999;31(7):987-97.
27. Desouza CA, Shapiro LF, Clevenger CM, et al. Regular aerobic exercise prevents and restores age-related declines in endothelium-dependent vasodilation in healthy men. Circulation. 2000;102(12):1351-7.
28. Weight management before, during and after pregnancy. NICE Public Health Guidance. July 2010. Available from URL: http://www.nice.org.uk/nicemedia/live/13056/49926/49926.pdf.
29. Exercise in Pregnancy (RCOG Statement 4). January 2006. Available from URL: http://www.rcog.org.uk/womens-health/clinical-guidance/exercise-pregnancy.

Pain Abdomen

15

CHAPTER

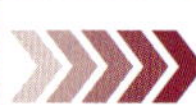

Nalini Mahajan, Shivani Singh

INTRODUCTION

Pain abdomen in early pregnancy is a frequent presenting complaint of an expecting mother. Depending on the severity of pain and the level of anxiety, patients may present to the emergency or to routine outpatient clinics. Medical and surgical causes of acute abdomen further complicate diagnosis and management. Any delay in the treatment can be disastrous for both mother and the fetus. It is important, therefore, that the obstetrician be conversant with the various causes of pain abdomen in early pregnancy to offer the appropriate treatment.

CAUSES

Causes of first trimester pain abdomen can be divided into the following groups as discussed below (Table 1).

TABLE 1: **Causes of pain abdomen in first trimester**

Physiological causes	• Round ligament pain • Ovarian pain
Pathological causes	
Obstetric	• Urinary retention • Hyperemesis gravidarum • Ectopic and heterotopic pregnancy • Threatened/incomplete/inevitable abortion • Hydatidiform mole
Gyneco-logical	• Ovarian cyst • Adnexal torsion • Fibroid Degeneration • Pelvic inflammatory disease
Medical	• Urinary tract infection • Gastric reflux • Irritable bowel syndrome • Worm infestation • Chronic constipation • Sickle cell crisis • Porphyria
Surgical	• Appendicitis • Ureteric calculus • Peptic ulceration • Cholecystitis • Diverticulitis • Pancreatitis • Inflammatory bowel disease • Obstruction/volvulus • Subrectus hematoma • Trauma • Aneurysm rupture

PRESENTATION

Based on the clinical presentation, pain abdomen in early pregnancy can be grouped under 2 major headings.

Acute Pain

Acute pain results in the patient presenting to the emergency. The incidence of acute abdomen during pregnancy is 1 in 500–635 pregnancies.

Subacute/Chronic Pain

These patients present to the out patient department (OPD) with varying degrees of abdominal discomfort.

Acute abdomen occurring with early pregnancy presents a management challenge since investigations and procedures have to be such that they safeguard an ongoing pregnancy without compromising the health of the mother and one has to be well versed with the physiological changes of pregnancy. A multidisciplinary approach must be adopted when dealing with this challenging situation.

DIFFERENTIAL DIAGNOSIS

A wide range of possible differential diagnosis should be considered when a patient presents with acute abdomen, because of conditions, that are pregnancy specific, coincidental, or more likely to occur in pregnancy (Table 2).

Precaution: Care must be taken to minimize manipulation of the uterus during surgery.

DIAGNOSIS

The diagnosis of abdominal pain in early pregnancy can be tricky. Clinical evaluation is confounded by the normal anatomical and physiological changes occurring in pregnancy. Diagnostic accuracy can be achieved by keeping the following key points in mind.

Accurate History

Critically review the history of pain—location, onset, nature, duration, and radiation. Detail the relationship of pain to eating, activity, urination, defecation, and bleeding per vaginum. It is also important to take a menstrual history with date of the last menstrual period, past obstetric, surgical, and medical history. A well taken history will more often than not give a lead to the diagnosis.

Physical Examination

Assessing the general status of the patient is imperative to ascertain the degree of emergency.

TABLE 2: Differential diagnosis of acute pain abdomen in pregnancy

Incidental to pregnancy	*Conditions associated with pregnancy*	*Due to pregnancy*
Gastrointestinal • Acute appendicitis • Acute pancreatitis • Peptic ulcer • Gastroenteritis • Hepatitis • Bowel obstruction • Bowel perforation • Herniation • Meckel diverticulitis • Toxic megacolon • Pancreatic pseudocyst	• Acute pyelonephritis • Acute cystitis • Acute cholecystitis • Acute fatty liver of pregnancy • Rupture of rectus abdominis muscle • Torsion of the pregnant uterus	**Early pregnancy** • Ruptured ectopic pregnancy • Septic abortion with peritonitis • Acute urinary retention due to retroverted gravid uterus

Contd...

Contd...

Incidental to pregnancy	*Conditions associated with pregnancy*	*Due to pregnancy*
Genitourinary • Ovarian cyst rupture • Adnexal torsion • Ureteral calculus • Rupture of renal pelvis • Ureteral obstruction **Vascular** • Superior mesenteric artery syndrome • Thrombosis/infarction-specifically mesenteric venous thrombosis • Ruptured visceral artery aneurysm • Splenic artery aneurysm **Respiratory** • Pneumonia • Pulmonary embolism **Others** • Intraperitoneal hemorrhage • Splenic rupture • Abdominal trauma • Acute intermittent porphyria • Diabetic ketoacidosis • Sickle cell disease		**Later pregnancy (to complete the list)** • Red degeneration of myoma • Torsion of pedunculated myoma • Placental abruption • Placenta percreta • HELLP (hemolysis, elevated liver function, and low platelets) syndrome-spontaneous rupture of the liver • Uterine rupture • Chorioamnionitis

- *Abdominal examination* is done to localize any areas of tenderness, to look for palpable masses, and rule out any guarding rigidity and rebound tenderness
- *Pelvic examination* can pick out polyps, erosions lacerations, bleeding through the os, tenderness in fornices, cervical excitation pain, etc. which can be completely missed on an ultrasound.

Investigations

- *Hematological and biochemical investigations* along with *urinalysis* and *stool examination* should be carried out as required
- *Ultrasound* plays a key role as a diagnostic modality
- *Magnetic resonance imaging (MRI)* provides excellent anatomic resolution and tissue characterization. Not all MRI contrast agents are approved for use in pregnancy. Intravenous gadolinium crosses the placenta, and the effects on the fetus are not understood. Although, no adverse fetal effects have been documented, the National Radiological Protection Board advises against the use of MRI in the first trimester[1]
- *Laparoscopy* has been used as a diagnostic tool in acute abdomen. The Society of American Gastrointestinal Endoscopic Surgeons have concluded that the laparoscopic approach is safe and effective in the diagnosis and treatment of acute abdominal pathology during pregnancy, and offers many advantages over open surgery.

MANAGEMENT

For reasons of simplicity, the various causes, their diagnosis, and treatment have been dealt with individually.

Physiological Causes

Some degree of mid-line abdominal or pelvic pain occurs normally in pregnancy due to the stretching of the uterine wall with its peritoneal coat, stretching of the supportive ligaments of the uterus, gas, or constipation.

Round Ligament Pain

Round ligament pain may result in short cramp like or a stabbing, sharp ache in one or both sides of the abdomen, extending till groin. It is more often on the right side, presumably because the uterus is twisted to the right during pregnancy. It increases on prolonged standing or sudden movements. Fortunately, this pain is relieved relatively quickly simply by resting, changing positions, or taking an analgesic.

Ovarian Pain

This pain results from a corpus luteal cyst of pregnancy and is usually localized on one side. It is more frequently seen in women who have received ovarian stimulation especially polycystic ovary syndrome patients. A transvaginal ultrasound (TVS) shows a large sized corpus luteal cyst along with an intrauterine gestation sac. Conservative management with mild analgesics forms the basis of management.

Pathological Causes

Some of these are rare but do find mention in literature.

Obstetric Causes

- *Acute urinary retention*: It occurs often in association with a retroverted uterus in the late first trimester. The pain increases progressively and is more midline, as time progresses there is pain in the lumbar region, as well due to back pressure effects on the kidney. The telltale midline bulge disappears on catheterization. Short term catheterization is the answer and the condition resolves as the uterus grows out of the pelvis. Urinary infection should be excluded. Occasionally, the uterus may become incarcerated in the pelvis and requires physical manipulation for correction
- *Hyperemesis gravidarum*: It may lead to pain either in the epigastric region due to hyperacidity and reflux esophagitis, or a lower abdominal pain, musculoskeletal in nature, due to repeated retching. Treatment of hyperemesis resolves the situation
- *Ectopic pregnancy*: It is the most common obstetric cause of acute abdomen. The classic triad of symptoms of ectopic pregnancy consists of amenorrhea, vaginal bleeding, and lower abdominal pain which may be acute or chronic in nature.[2] On examination, there may be abdominal distension, guarding, rigidity and rebound tenderness, cervical motion tenderness with a slightly enlarged, and globular uterus. A significantly raised beta human chorionic gonadotropin (HCG) and a sonography revealing an empty uterine cavity with free fluid/blood in pelvis or a adnexal mass with mixed echogenicity, clinches the diagnosis.[3] After emergency resuscitative measures, the patient is taken up for salpingectomy or linear salpingostomy by performing a laparotomy or laparoscopy, if she is hemodynamically stable. Medical management with injection of methotrexate at the dose of 50 mg/m^2 may be given in early unruptured ectopic.[4] (*See* Chapter 16: Ectopic Pregnancy).
- *Threatened/incomplete/septic abortion*: Patient has a variable period of amenorrhea, lower abdomen pain or cramps, backache, and bleeding/abnormal discharge per vaginum with or without history of passage

of products of conception (POC). On examination the uterus is soft and bulky; the internal and external os may be open. Per speculum examination may show products extruding through the os. Sepsis may present with signs of peritonitis (abdominal rigidity, guarding and rebound tenderness, and high fever). Investigations would include a urine pregnancy test, total leukocyte count (TLC) and a TVS. Treatment is conservative in threatened abortion. Evacuation of POC is done if there is an incomplete abortion. High dose antibiotics will be required in septic abortion

- *Hydatidiform mole*: Women with hydatidiform mole have a history of amenorrhea with cramp like pain, associated with spotting or bleeding per vaginum. This may be associated with passage of grape-like vesicles through vagina in late stages. Per vaginum examination reveals a very soft bulky uterus. Extremely high β-HCG levels may be present. TVS shows snow storm appearance with absence of fetal parts (in case of complete mole). Suction evacuation followed by methotrexate therapy form the mainstay of the treatment.

Gynecological Causes

- *Pelvic inflammatory disease*: Symptoms of pelvic inflammatory disease include pain in lower abdomen along with vaginal discharge which may be associated with fever, tachycardia, malaise, or backache. There is adnexal tenderness or mass on pelvic examination. TLC, C-reactive protein and erythrocyte sedimentation rate are raised. Triple swab test should be performed in all suspected cases which includes:
    - High vaginal swab to identify bacterial vaginosis, candidal infections, and *Trichomonas vaginalis*
    - Endocervical swab in transport medium (charcoal or noncharcoal) to diagnose gonorrhea
    - Endocervical swab for a chlamydial DNA amplification test to diagnose *Chlamydia trachomatis.*

  Ultrasound shows an intrauterine gestational sac with free fluid in pelvis, adnexal mass, and probe tenderness.
- *Ovarian cysts*: Ovarian cysts occur in pregnancy with a frequency ranging from 1 in 81 to 1 in 1000. Severity of presenting symptoms depend on if there is hemorrhage, torsion, or rupture of the cyst. The patient may have mild chronic lower abdominal discomfort that suddenly intensifies with tenderness and guarding with an adnexal mass. TVS shows ovarian cyst and a separate corpus luteum of pregnancy. Invasive treatment will depend on severity of symptoms

Note: CA 125, CEA and AFP, are not considered reliable tumor markers in pregnancy. Morphological and Doppler scoring systems should be used to differentiate benign from malignant masses and to assess the blood supply

- *Fibroid torsion or degeneration*: Fibroids occur in 0.5–1.0% of pregnancies and increase in size in early pregnancy. Pedunculated fibroids carry a risk of torsion. Red degeneration occurs in 5–10% of pregnant women with myomas. Patients present with an acute onset of significant localized abdominal pain with vomiting, low-grade fever, and tenderness over a mass in the uterus. Ultrasonography shows a degenerating myoma which has a mixed echodense or echolucent appearance. Treatment includes analgesia with narcotic or anti-inflammatory agents
- *Adnexal torsion*: Pregnancy predisposes to adnexal torsion, with 1 in 5 adnexal torsions occurring during pregnancy.[5] The condition is associated with an ovarian mass in 50–60% of patients, mostly a dermoid. It occurs more frequently on the right side and in the first trimester, occasionally in the second, and rarely in the third. Patients present with acute, severe, colicky, unilateral, lower abdominal

or pelvic pain, nausea, vomiting, fever, and a tender adnexal mass. Ultrasonography with color Doppler can be useful in diagnosing the condition. Treatment is surgical, and consists of untwisting of the pedicle with cystectomy and fixation. Salpingo-oopherectomy is warranted if necrosis has occurred. Pregnancy outcome associated with adnexal torsion generally is good.

Surgical and Medical Causes

- *Appendicitis*: It is the most common general surgical emergency in pregnancy with an incidence of 1 in 2,000. The incidence of perforation is 25% in pregnancy, increasing to 66% if surgery is delayed for more than 24 hours. Maternal and fetal morbidity and mortality rates increase once perforation occurs. There is fever, tachycardia, abdominal pain, and tenderness located in right lower quadrant in the first trimester with nausea and vomiting. Rebound tenderness, rigidity, and Rovsing's sign can be demonstrated in 50–65% of patients. Rectal tenderness is usually present, particularly in the first trimester. Appendectomy preferably using laparoscopic approach is done (*See* Chapters 27 and 28: Surgery and Anesthesia and Laparoscopy).

Note:
- Though pregnancy does not affect the overall incidence of appendicitis, the severity may be increased
- The importance of a raised TLC in appendicitis is undermined by the fact that TLC can be as high as 15,000/mm^3 in normal pregnancy. Also severe disease can occur with a normal count.

- *Ureteric calculus/urinary tract infection*: Patient comes with complaint of pain, usually in the flank, dysuria, gross hematuria, urgency, and nausea. Ultrasound may pick up a ureteric calculus and indicate the status of the pelvicalyceal system. Urine should be sent for culture. In case of recurrent pyelonephritis, urological evaluation including ultrasonography of kidney, ureter, bladder is recommended along with chronic suppressive therapy using nitrofurantoin 100 mg each night. Urine is sent for culture every month.[6] Treatment depends on the size and location of the stone, the degree of obstruction, the severity of symptoms, and the presence of infection. Most stones pass with hydration. Minimally invasive procedures can be considered

Precaution: Extracorporeal shock-wave lithotripsy has not been approved for use in pregnancy.

- *Gastric reflux/peptic ulceration*: Gastric reflux is common and peptic ulceration is rare. These conditions may be difficult to diagnose, as upper gastrointestinal symptoms are common in pregnancy
- *Constipation/irritable bowel syndrome*: Bowel colic improves and constipation worsens with the raised progesterone levels of pregnancy
- *Cholecystitis*: Pregnant women have asymptomatic cholelithiasis in 4.5% and acute cholecystitis in 0.05%. Right upper quadrant pain radiating to the back with vomiting, fever, and tenderness in the right upper quadrant may be the presenting symptom. Up to 40% of these patients will require surgery during gestation. Laparoscopic approach is suitable if intervention is required in early pregnancy

Caution: Surgery should not be delayed as patients experience increase in hospitalization, spontaneous abortion, preterm labor, and preterm delivery if not operated.

- *Pancreatitis*: Pancreatitis is a rare, though potentially devastating disease. The case to delivery ratio ranges from 1:1,289 to 1:3,333. Epigastric pain and tenderness is the main finding. Treatment is conservative. The maternal mortality rate ranges from 0 to 37%

Note: Serum amylase testing is diagnostic though a slight, rise occurs in normal pregnancy too.

- *Inflammatory bowel disease*: Inflammatory bowel disease may present with passage of blood and mucus rectally, altered bowel habits, and colicky pain. Treatment is conservative

- *Obstruction/volvulus*: Obstruction or volvulus is rare during the first trimester. Increased mobility of the bowel and displacement of the bowel into the upper abdomen by the growing uterus are implicated in these cases. Pain may be constant or periodic. This condition may require an upright plain X-ray of abdomen for diagnosis. Treatment is surgical with correction of fluid and electrolyte imbalance
- *Meckel's diverticulitis*: May mimic acute appendicitis
- *Subrectus hematoma*: It can occur spontaneously with severe, localized superficial pain. Mass is not always evident
- *Worm infestation*: Often, pain is more chronic and colicky
- *Sickle cell crisis*: It is usually diagnosed prepregnancy and homozygous state may result in severe crisis precipitated by infection
- *Porphyria*: Although rare, may present for the first time during pregnancy. It is associated with hypertension, disorientation, and dark urine. Management is conservative with aggressive rehydration and analgesia.

Very Rare Causes of Acute Abdomen during Pregnancy

- *Mesenteric venous thrombosis*: This is an extremely rare but potentially lethal event. Treatment is resection of the involved segment with institution of chronic anticoagulation
- *Rupture of visceral artery aneurysm*: Splenic artery aneurysms are probably the most common.

CONCLUSION

The diagnostic work up of an acute abdomen may be more difficult in pregnant women due to the normal anatomical and physiological changes of pregnancy. Ultrasound is the main diagnostic tool. Prompt clinical diagnosis and surgical intervention when indicated is necessary to minimize maternal and fetal mortality. General anesthesia is considered safe in pregnancy and a laparoscopic approach (except in a hemodynamically unstable patient) is gaining popularity.

REFERENCES

1. Garden AS, Griffiths RD, Weindling AM, et al. Fast-scan magnetic resonance imaging in fetal visualization. Am J Obstet Gynecol. 1991;164(5 Pt 1):1190-6.
2. Clayton HB, Schieve LA, Peterson HB, et al. Ectopic pregnancy risk with assisted reproductive technology procedures. Obstet Gynecol. 2006;107(3):595-604.
3. Ko PC, Liang CC, Lo TS, et al. Six cases of tubal stump pregnancy: complication of assisted reproductive technology? Fertil Steril. 2011;95(7):2432.
4. Kadar N, Caldwell BV, Romero R. A method of screening for ectopic pregnancy and its indications. Obstet Gynecol. 1981;58(2):162-6.
5. Origoni M, Cavoretto P, Conti E, et al. Isolated tubal torsion in pregnancy. Eur J Obstet Gynecol Reprod Biol. 2009;146(2): 116-20.
6. Cunningham FG, Lucas MJ. Urinary tract infection complicating pregnancy. Baillieres Clin Obstet Gynaecol. 1994;8(2): 353-73.

Ectopic Pregnancy

16

CHAPTER

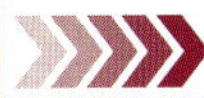

Ameet Patki, Alok Sharma

INTRODUCTION

An ectopic pregnancy (EP) is a complication of pregnancy in which the pregnancy implants outside the uterine cavity. With rare exceptions, EPs are not viable. Furthermore, they are dangerous for the mother, internal bleeding being a common complication. Most EPs occur in the fallopian tubes but implantation can also occur in the cervix, ovaries, and abdomen. An EP is a potential medical emergency, and, if not treated properly, can lead to death.

DIAGNOSIS AND LABORATORY STUDIES

In order to reduce the morbidity and mortality associated with EP, a high index of suspicion is necessary to make a prompt and early diagnosis. Hence, screening every female patient in the reproductive years presenting with abdominal pain, cramping, or vaginal bleeding for EP should be a norm.

Blood (ABO and Rh Type)

Blood typing (ABO and Rh) and antibody screening should be done in all pregnant patients with bleeding to identify Rh negative pregnant patients in whom bleeding would be associated with an increased risk of Rh isoimmunization. Such patients require to be injected with 50 µg of anti-D immunoglobulin to prevent the occurrence of hemolytic disease of the newborn. Blood must be typed and cross matched in order to ensure the availability of blood products in case of excessive blood loss. Hemoglobin or hematocrit levels must be measured serially in order to quantify blood loss.

Beta-human Chorionic Gonadotropin

In early healthy intrauterine pregnancies, serum levels of beta-human chorionic gonadotropin (β-hCG) doubles approximately every 2 days (1.4–2.1 days). Kadar et al. established that the lower limit of the reference range to which serum β-hCG should increase during a 2-day period is 66%.[1] An increase in β-hCG of less than 66% is associated with an abnormal intrauterine pregnancy or an extra uterine pregnancy.

Note:

Fifteen percent of healthy intrauterine pregnancies do not increase by 66% and that 13% of all EPs have normally rising β-hCG levels of at least 66% in 2 days.

No single serum β-hCG level is diagnostic of an EP and serial serum β-hCG levels are necessary to differentiate between normal and abnormal pregnancies.

Serial β-hCG estimations are required, the major disadvantage of which is the potential for delay in reaching the diagnosis and subsequent management. Furthermore, serial β-hCG titers do not indicate the location of the pregnancy. Hence, additional diagnostic modalities, including ultrasound and other biochemical markers are needed.

Prognostic Evaluation of Serial Beta-human Chorionic Gonadotropin Assay

Serial β-hCG assay offer four different possibilities:
1. β-hCG above discriminatory zone with empty uterus always suggests EP
2. β-hCG below the discriminatory zone limits; the diagnostic capability of transvaginal scan (TVS) since intrauterine gestational sac won't be evident. They need serial scans correlating with serum hormone level
3. Subnormal rise indicates degenerating trophoblasts, likely to resolve spontaneously and could be either extrauterine or intra-uterine
4. Rapidly growing β-hCG level signals danger and suggests functionally active rupture.

Progesterone

A single serum progesterone level is another tool that is useful in differentiating abnormal gestations from healthy intrauterine pregnancies. Because in most EPs, progesterone levels range between 10 ng/mL and 25 ng/mL, the clinical utility is limited.

Other Novel Serum Markers

There are some other markers like increased serum creatine kinase levels, decrease pregnancy specific β(1)-glycoprotein SP1, human placental lactogen, or pregnancy-associated plasma protein A (PAPP-A) but none can differentiate an ectopic from early pregnancy. Serum interleukin-8 (IL-8), IL-6, and tumor necrosis factor (TNF) concentrations also increased in women with ectopic. Several other serum and urine markers are currently under investigation to help distinguish normal and abnormal pregnancies. These include serum estradiol, inhibin, pregnanediol glucuronide, placental proteins, and a quadruple screen of serum progesterone, estriol, and alpha-fetoprotein. At present, the use each of these markers is only as a research tool until substantial clinical evidence proves their role in clinical medicine.

Imaging Studies

Ultrasonography

Visualization of an intrauterine sac, with or without fetal cardiac activity, often is adequate to exclude EP.[2] The exception to this is in the case of heterotopic pregnancies, which are more common in patients undergoing ovarian stimulation and assisted reproduction as they have a ten-fold increased risk of heterotopic pregnancy. TVS, with its greater resolution, can be used to visualize an intrauterine pregnancy by 24 days postovulation, or 38 days after last menstrual period, which is about 1 week earlier than transabdominal ultrasonography. The gestational sac is the first structure that is recognizable on TVS. A pseudosac may be mistaken for a gestational sac and it is a collection of fluid within the endometrial cavity created by bleeding from the decidualized endometrium often, associated with an extrauterine pregnancy. The true gestational sac is located eccentrically within the uterus beneath the endometrial surface and has an echogenic choriodecidual reaction around it, whereas the pseudosac fills the endometrial cavity and does not show an echogenic rim. The criteria for TVS diagnosis of ectopic pregnancy is given in table 1.

Note: The effectiveness of using ultrasonography with discriminatory zone of hCG levels and demonstration of free fluid in the cul-de-sac, which may represent hemoperitoneum, has been well established as a diagnostic criterion for EP.

TABLE 1: Criteria for diagnosis of ectopic pregnancy by transvaginal scan

Stage	*Transvaginal scan findings*
Type 1A	Well-defined tubal ring displaying fetal heart
Type 1B	Well-defined tubal ring displaying no fetal heart
Type 2	Ill-defined fetal heart
Type 3	Free pelvic fluid, empty uterus, and displaying no adnexal mass

Adapted from Rottem et al. Editors Transviginal Sonography, New York 1991, Elsevier.

Transvaginal Color Doppler Sonography

Color-flow Doppler ultrasonography has been demonstrated to improve the diagnostic sensitivity and specificity of transvaginal ultrasonography, especially in cases where a gestational sac is questionable or absent. Furthermore, color-flow Doppler ultrasonography can potentially be used to identify involuting EPs which can be treated with expectant management. Its introduction added another tool to display the increased vascular areas randomly dispersed in the adnexal complex mass and assess the trophoblastic activities, which correlate well with the β-hCG titer.

DIAGNOSTIC PROCEDURES

Dilatation and Curettage

A simple way to rule out an EP is to establish an intrauterine pregnancy by dilatation and curettage. Where tissue obtained is positive for villi floating in saline or by histological diagnosis on frozen or permanent section

Culdocentesis

It is performed by inserting a needle through the posterior fornix of the vagina into the cul-de-sac and attempting to aspirate blood. When nonclotted blood is found in conjunction with a suspected EP, operative intervention is indicated because the likelihood of a ruptured EP is high. Culdocentesis is of historical interest because its use today is obsolete. Improved technology with sonography and hormonal assays are far superior in sensitivity and specificity in reaching the correct diagnosis.

Laparoscopy/Laparotomy

Patients in pain and/or those who are hemodynamically unstable should proceed to laparoscopy/laparotomy. Laparoscopy allows assessment of the pelvic structures, size and exact location of EP, presence of hemoperitoneum, and presence of other conditions, such as ovarian cysts and endometriosis, which, when present with an intrauterine pregnancy, can mimic an EP. Furthermore, laparoscopy provides the option to treat once the diagnosis is established. Laparoscopy can miss up to 4% of early EPs.

SCREENING FOR ECTOPIC PREGNANCY

Transvaginal ultrasonography and serum β-hCG determinations have proven diagnostic value in the evaluation of symptomatic women with suspected EP. Some have advocated applying the same diagnostic tools to screen asymptomatic women at increased risk for EP. In practice, women at risk might be instructed to contact their clinician as soon as pregnancy is suspected and, if confirmed, receive careful monitoring with serial β-hCG determinations and timely ultrasonography. The alternative is to evaluate only those in whom clinical symptoms of pain or vaginal bleeding emerge. The rationale for screening at risk women is that early diagnosis of EP allows early intervention and noninvasive treatment that may help to minimize tubal damage and to reduce costs.[3,4]

Results of a decision analysis suggest that screening probably is justified when the risk of EP is approximately 8% or higher. At that risk level, screening may be expected to prevent one to two ruptured EPs and to yield less than one false positive diagnosis for every 100 women screened.[5] Accepting a 2% background rate of EP and considering the increased incidence associated with certain risk factors, screening seems justified for women with previous tubal surgery or EP and those with known tubal pathology or who conceive with an intrauterine device *in situ* or after a sterilization procedure. Screening is more difficult to justify for women in whom a history of infertility or pelvic infection is the only risk factor.

RISK FACTORS

Although women with EP frequently have no identifiable risk factors, a prospective case-controlled study has shown that increased awareness of EP and a knowledge of the associated risk factors helps identify women at higher risk in order to facilitate early and more accurate diagnosis.[6] Most risk factors are associated with risks of prior damage to the fallopian tube. These factors include:

TABLE 2: Risk factors for ectopic pregnancy

Fallopian tube damage	• Previous tubal surgery (female sterilization) • Previous pelvic surgery (caesarean section and ovarian cystectomy) • Previous abdominal surgery (appendicectomy and bowel surgery) • Confirmed genital infection[7] • Pelvic inflammatory disease, commonly caused by chlamydial infection
Infertility[8]	• Documented tubal disease • Assisted reproductive technology[8] • Endometriosis • Unexplained infertility[8]
Contra-ceptives[9]	• Failure • Progestogen-only contraception • Intrauterine contraceptive device
Others	• Cigarette smoking[10] • Age more than 35 years • Previous ectopic pregnancy • Previous miscarriage (spontaneous or induced)

DIFFERENTIAL DIAGNOSIS

Obstetric Causes

- Threatened or incomplete miscarriage
- Early pregnancy with pelvic tumors
- Septic abortion.

Gynecological Causes

- Pelvic inflammatory disease
- Ruptured or hemorrhagic corpus luteum
- Salpingitis
- Adnexal torsion
- Degenerating fibroids
- Dysfunctional uterine bleeding
- Endometriosis
- Ovarian torsion
- Tubo-ovarian abscess.

Nongynecological Diseases

- Appendicitis
- Urinary calculi
- Gastroenteritis
- Intraperitoneal hemorrhage
- Perforated peptic ulcer.

MANAGEMENT CHOICES

Over the past decade, the management of EP has evolved from a radical operative approach (salpingectomy) to a more conservative surgical or medical treatment. This has been possible due to early diagnosis, advanced laparoscopic techniques, and ability to monitor the patient after conservative surgical or medical treatment. However, the type of treatment must be individualized and depends more on clinical presentation.

Catastrophic Presentation

Ectopic pregnancies frequently present as life-threatening emergencies. The patient presenting in shock with an acute abdomen should be stabilized and taken up for surgery immediately.

- Fluid resuscitation and placement of Foleys catheter must be carried out immediately
- Blood should be drawn for hematocrit and cross-matched for 4 units of blood
- Surgical approach: The patient should be taken for surgery as quickly as possible. Either a low midline vertical incision or a transverse suprapubic incision can be used. Upward traction on the uterus coupled with digital pressure on the involved tube will stop the bleeding so that fluid resuscitation, including transfusion if needed, can be completed. Only then should the hemoperitoneum be cleared and the involved adnexa stabilized in the operative field. Usually salpingectomy is done. There is no need to remove the ipsilateral ovary. Hysterectomy is not indicated unless the EP is interstitial or cornual, and the uterine rupture is so severe that it cannot be repaired.

Subacute Presentation

In the hemodynamically stable patient once the diagnosis of EP has been made, options include surgical, medical, or expectant management (Fig. 1). The goal of treatment is to minimize disease and treatment related morbidity, while maximizing reproductive potential. Anti D immunoglobulin should be given to all Rh-negative women.

Clinical Prediction Tools

Clinical prediction tools have been developed to aid management decision making. Fernandez et al. developed a score based on gestational age, β-hCG level, progesterone level, abdominal pain, hemoperitoneum volume, and hematosalpinx diameter[11] (Table 3). A score of more than 12 predicts a more than 80% success with expectant or nonsurgical management.

Similarly, to predict response to a single-dose of methotrexate, Elito et al. developed a score based on β-hCG level, ultrasound findings, size of the mass (cm), and color Doppler image aspects[12] (Table 4). A score of greater than or equal to 5 ensures a success rate of 97% with a single dose of methotrexate.

Expectant Management

Expectant management may be offered to asymptomatic women with small adnexal masses (<4 cm), lower β-hCG levels (<1000 mIU/mL), and evidence of spontaneous resolution (e.g., falling β-hCG levels) who are willing to accept the risk of tubal rupture. Rising β-hCG levels, pain, hemodynamic instability, or hemoperitoneum on ultrasound dictate switching to active management.

Note: Eighty percent of women with initial β-hCG levels <1000 mIU/mL experience spontaneous resolution.

Medical Management

Methotrexate, a folic acid antagonist, is a well-studied medical therapy. Methotrexate may be used for primary treatment of EP, for persistent EP following tubal sparing surgery, as prophylaxis to reduce persistent EP following salpingostomy, and in cornual and cervical pregnancies. Eligibility criterion is shown in box 1.[13] Other therapeutic agents include hyperosmolar glucose, potassium chloride, prostaglandins, and mifepristone.

Systemic Therapy

Methotrexate Therapy

Protocols for methotrexate therapy include single-dose and multiple-dose regimens. Methotrexate, regardless of the protocol, had an overall 89% crude success rate. Side effects of methotrexate include bone marrow suppression, elevated liver enzymes, rash, alopecia, stomatitis, nausea, and diarrhea. The time to resolution of the EP is 3–7 weeks after methotrexate therapy.

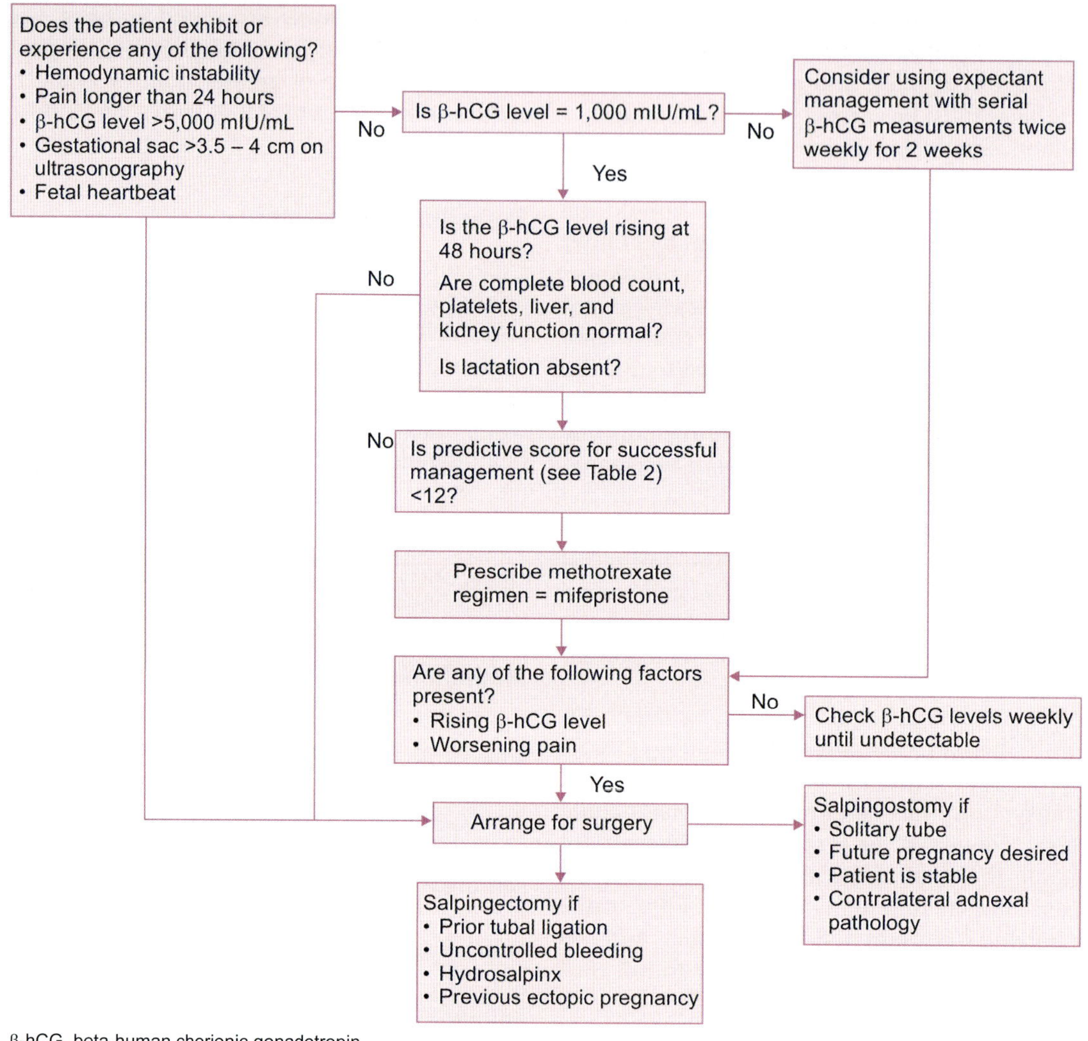

FIGURE 1 Management options in ectopic pregnancy.

TABLE 3: Predictive score for expectant management or nonsurgical treatments[11]

Criterion	*1 point*	*2 points*	*3 points*
β-hCG (mIU/mL)	<1,000	1,000–5,000	>5,000
Progesterone (ng/mL)	<5	5–10	>10
Abdominal pain	Absent	Induced	Spontaneous
Hematosalpinx (cm)	<1	1–3	>3
Hemoperitoneum (mL)	0	1–100	>100

Score <12: 80% success with various nonsurgical treatments, including expectant management. β-hCG, beta-human chorionic gonadotropin.

TABLE 4: Predictive score for single dose methotrexate (50 mg/m² intramuscularly)[12]

Parameters	*0 point*	*1 point*	*2 points*
β-hCG (mIU/mL)	>5,000	1,500 – 5,000	<1,500
Aspects of the image	Live embryo	Tubal ring	Hematosalpinx
Size of the mass	>3.0–3.5	2.6–3.0	<2.5
Color Doppler	High risk	Medium risk	Low risk

Score ≥5: 97% success with single-dose methotrexate. β-hCG, beta-human chorionic gonadotropin.

Box 1: Patients eligible for methotrexate

- No rupture
- Hemodynamically stable
- Gestational sac <3.5 cm
- β-hCG <5,000 mIU/mL
- No fetal cardiac activity on ultrasonography

β-hCG, beta-human chorionic gonadotropin.

Contraindications: Some women are not appropriate candidates for medical therapy and should be managed surgically (Box 2)

Direct Injection in Sac

Methotrexate: The advantages cited for the direct instillation of methotrexate, laparoscopically or transvaginally under ultrasound guidance include higher local drug concentrations, less systemic distribution, a smaller therapeutic dose, and less toxicity. Despite the theoretical advantages of direct injection of methotrexate, success rates in practice appear unacceptably low.[14]

Prostaglandin: Unruptured tubal pregnancies may be treated with an injection with 0.5–1.5 mg of prostaglandin F2 into the affected tube which has similar effects to methotrexate but has lead to cardiac arrhythmia, cardiopulmonary edema, and gastrointestinal symptoms.

Box 2: Contraindications to medical therapy

Absolute contraindications

- Hemodynamically unstable
- Signs of impending or ongoing ectopic mass rupture (i.e., severe or persistent abdominal pain or >300 mL of free peritoneal fluid outside the pelvic cavity)
- Clinically important abnormalities in baseline hematologic, renal, or hepatic laboratory values
- Immunodeficiency, active pulmonary disease, and peptic ulcer disease
- Hypersensitivity to methotrexate
- Coexistent viable intrauterine pregnancy
- Breastfeeding
- Unwilling or unable to be compliant with post-therapeutic monitoring
- Do not have timely access to a medical institution

Relative contraindications

- Gestation sac >3.5 cm in dimension
- Embryonic cardiac activity present
- High β-hCG concentration

β-hCG, beta-human chorionic gonadotropin.

Surgical Therapy

Surgical therapy may be either open laparotomy or laparoscopy. Ideally, all EPs requiring surgery should be treated laparoscopically. A recent Cochrane review indicated that laparoscopic surgery for EP was a cost-effective approach.[14]

Indications for Surgical Therapy

- Candidate not suitable for medical therapy
- Failed medical therapy
- Heterotopic pregnancy with a viable intrauterine pregnancy
- Patient is hemodynamically unstable and requires immediate treatment.

Advantages of Laparoscopic Surgery

- Less postoperative pain
- Faster recovery
- Short hospital stay
- Lower rate of postoperative complications like wound infection
- Cost-effectiveness
- Reduced postoperative analgesic requirement
- Reduced adhesion formation.

Complications due to Laparoscopic Surgery

- Missed diagnosis
- Bleeding
- Incomplete removal of EP
- Visceral injury
- Leakage of purulent exudates
- Intra-abdominal abscess
- Hernia at the port site.

Indications for Laparotomy

- Patient is hemodynamically unstable
- Cervical, interstitial, or abdominal EP
- Patients having large hematoma due to large ruptured EP
- Presence of more than 1,500 cc hemo-peritoneum
- Patients with underlying cardiac diseases and chronic obstructive pulmonary disease
- History of abdominal surgery in the past
- Patients at increased risk of complications with general anesthesia.

Salpingectomy

Regardless of the route of approach, salpingectomy is indicated in the following situations:

- The tube is severely damaged
- There is uncontrolled bleeding
- There is a recurrent EP in the same tube
- There is a large tubal pregnancy of size >5 cm
- The EP has ruptured
- The woman has completed her family and future fertility is not desire
- Ectopic pregnancy has resulted due to sterilization failure
- Ectopic pregnancy has occurred in a previously reconstructed tube
- Patient requests sterilization
- Hemorrhage continues to occur even after salpingostomy
- Cases of chronic tubal pregnancy.

Salpingostomy

In the absence of any of the above indications for salpingectomy, salpingostomy may be performed like if it is a solitary tube, or contralateral tube is diseased provided patient is stable and desirous of future pregnancy. Salpingostomy removes the EP while preserving the fallopian tube. Weekly quantitative β-hCG testing is required to rule out persistent EP, which occurs in 5–8% of patients following salpingostomy.[15] The likelihood of persistent EP following salpingostomy increases with:

- An EP <2 cm in diameter
- Salpingostomy performed <6 weeks from the last menstrual period
- A β-hCG level >3,000 mIU/mL
- Progesterone level over 35 nmol/L combined with a daily change in β-hCG over 100 mIU/mL.

Fimbrial Evacuation

If the EP is at the fimbria, then fimbrial evacuation is feasible, in the absence of indications for salpingectomy.

Partial Salpingectomy

Partial salpingectomy may be indicated if the pregnancy is in the mid portion of the tube, none of the indications for salpingectomy are present, and the patient may be a candidate for tubal reanastomosis later.

Follow-up

All patients who have not had the entire EP removed by salpingectomy need to have their weekly hCG levels observed until these levels return to nonpregnant values. If, during this time span the hCG level either plateaus or rises, treat the patient with methotrexate.

Contraception

Patients should all be on some form of effective contraception until such time as their hCG levels have returned to nonpregnant levels.

UNUSUAL LOCATIONS

More than 95% of EPs occur in the fallopian tube, usually in the distal half. However, pregnancies can implant in a wide variety of sites, including the ovary, intramyometrial portion of the tube or uterine cornua, lower uterine segment or cervix, prior caesarean section scar, and peritoneal cavity. These pregnancies are usually diagnosed later than tubal pregnancies, and catastrophic rupture with hemorrhage and shock is more likely to occur in these non-tubal pregnancies.

Cervical Pregnancy

Cervical pregnancy arises from implantation in the cervical epithelium instead of the endometrium. The patient usually presents with heavy vaginal bleeding and a cervical mass. The cervix may be effaced and dilated. It is sometimes difficult to distinguish a cervical implantation from an incomplete abortion with products of conception passing through the cervix. Medical management is preferred if patient is not bleeding. The pregnancy may be removed with suction curettage, but bleeding from the implantation site is often very heavy. Paracervical injection with dilute vasopressin may aid hemostasis. Hemostatic techniques like uterine packing, use of an intracervical Foley catheter balloon, deep lateral cervical stitches, or cerclage with either the MacDonald or Shirodkar techniques have been tried. Hysterectomy may be necessary if hemorrhage is severe.

Abdominal Pregnancy

Abdominal pregnancy accounts for approximately 0.003% of all pregnancies. It arises either from primary implantation in the abdominal cavity or secondary implantation after tubal abortion. Women with abdominal pregnancy may present with abdominal pain, unusual fetal lie, or unusually prominent fetal parts. If partial placental separation has occurred, the patient may present in shock with intra-abdominal hemorrhage. Maternal mortality rates have been reported to be ranging from 2% to 18%. The fetus should be removed, the umbilical cord tied as close as possible to the placenta, and the placenta left *in situ*. If left in place, the placenta may remain functional for up to 50 days. Any attempt to separate the placenta from abdominal organs or the abdominal wall may result in severe blood loss and, therefore, should be avoided. Methotrexate has been used to hasten the resorption. When massive bleeding is encountered, abdominal packs can be used to control bleeding and left in place with removal at a second procedure. Arterial embolization has also been used successfully.

Ovarian Pregnancy

Ovarian pregnancy implants on the ovarian stroma. The incidence has been estimated to range from 1 in 7,000 to 1 in 40,000 deliveries. Management is cystectomy with repair of the ovary or oophorectomy if cystectomy cannot be accomplished.

Caesarean Scar Pregnancy

Implantation of an otherwise normal pregnancy into a prior caesarean delivery uterine scar is seen with increased frequency as the caesarean delivery rate has increased.[16] Pain and bleeding are most common, but up to 40% of women are asymptomatic, and the diagnosis is made during routine sonographic examination. Management is gestational-age dependent and includes methotrexate treatment, curettage, hysteroscopic resection, uterine-preserving resection by laparotomy or laparoscopy, a combination of these, or hysterectomy.

Other Rare Sites of Ectopic Pregnancy

A number of intra-abdominal placental implantations have been cited in case reports. Most are variation of abdominal pregnancy. Splenic, hepatic retroperitoneal, and omental pregnancy are reported in literature. In most patients, laparotomy is preferred by many for these ectopic abdominal pregnancies.

Prognosis

One measure of long-term morbidity in the patient treated for EP is future reproductive potential. Fertility following EP depends upon several factors, the most important of which is a prior history of infertility. The treatment choice, whether surgical or nonsurgical, also plays a role. For example, the rate of intrauterine pregnancy may be higher following methotrexate compared to surgical treatment. Rate of fertility may be better following salpingostomy than salpingectomy. A review of published reports on laparoscopic salpingostomy revealed a tubal patency rate of 86%, a pregnancy rate of 66%, and a repeat EP rate of 23%.[17] Although fewer data are available on methotrexate use, reported outcomes are similar, with a tubal patency rate of 81% and a pregnancy rate of 70%, but with a repeat EP rate of 11%, which is less than that seen with laparoscopy.[18]

Ectopic pregnancy is a common first trimester emergency. High-resolution ultrasonography and sensitive hCG determinations permit earlier diagnosis. Therapeutic laparoscopy has resulted in a reduction in operative morbidity, hospital stay, cost and recovery time.

REFERENCES

1. Kadar N, Bohrer M, Kemmann E, et al. The discriminatory human chorionic gonadotropin zone for endovaginal sonography: aprospective, randomized study. Fertil Steril. 1994;61(6): 1016-20.
2. Stein JC, Wang R, Adler N, et al. Emergency physician ultrasonography for evaluating patients at risk for ectopic pregnancy: a meta-analysis. Ann Emerg Med. 2010;56(6):674-83.
3. Cacciatore B, Stenman UH, Ylöstalo P. Early screening for ectopic pregnancy in high-risk symptom free women. Lancet. 1994;343(8896):517-8.
4. Mol BW, Hajenius PJ, Ankum WM, et al. Screening for ectopic pregnancy in symptom-free women at increased risk. Obstet Gynecol. 1997;89(5 Pt 1):704-7.
5. Mol BW, van der Veen F, Bossuyt PM. Symptom-free women at increased risk of ectopic pregnancy: should we screen? Acta Obstet Gynecol Scand. 2002;81(7):661-72.
6. Karaer A, Avsar FA, Batioglu S. Risk factors for ectopic pregnancy: a case-control study. Aust N Z J Obstet Gynaecol. 2006;46(6):521-7.
7. Akande V, Turner C, Horner P, et al. British Fertility Society Impact of *Chlamydia trachomatis* in the reproductive setting: British Fertility Society Guidelines for practice. Hum Fertil (Camb). 2010;13(3):115-25.
8. Clayton HB, Schieve LA, Peterson HB, et al. Ectopic pregnancy risk with assisted reproductive technology procedures. Obstet Gynecol. 2006;107(3):595-604.
9. Furlong LA. Ectopic pregnancy risk when contraception fails. A review. J Reprod Med. 2002;47(11):881-5.
10. Talbot P, Riveles K. Smoking and reproduction: the oviduct as a target of cigarette smoke. Reprod Biol Endocrinol. 2005;3:52.
11. Fernandez H, Lelaidier C, Thouvenez V, et al. The use of a pretherapeutic, predictive score to determine inclusion criteria for the non-surgical management of ectopic pregnancy. Hum Reprod. 1991;6(7):995-8.
12. Elito J Jr, Reichmann AP, Uchiyama MN, et al. Predictive score for the systemic treatment of unruptured ectopic pregnancy with a single dose of methotrexate. Int J Gynaecol Obstet. 1999;67(2):75-9.
13. Practice Committee of the American Society for Reproductive Medicine. Medical treatment of ectopic pregnancy. Fertil Steril. 2006;86(5 Suppl 1):S96-102.
14. Hajenius PJ, Mol F, Mol BW, et al. Interventions for tubal ectopic pregnancy. Cochrane Database Syst Rev. 2007;(1):CD000324.
15. Mol F, Mol BW, Ankum WM, et al. Current evidence on surgery, systemic methotrexate and expectant management in the treatment of tubal ectopic pregnancy: a systematic review and meta-analysis. Hum Reprod Update. 2008;14(4):309-19.
16. Rotas MA, Haberman S, Levgur M. Cesarean scar ectopic pregnancies: etiology, diagnosis, and management. Obstet Gynecol. 2006;107(6):1373-81.
17. Ichinoe K, Wake N, Shinkai N, et al. Nonsurgical therapy to preserve oviduct function in patients with tubal pregnancies. Am J Obstet Gynecol. 1987;156(2):484-7.
18. Stovall TG, Ling FW. Single-dose systemic methotrexate: an expanded clinical trial. Am J Obstet Gynecol. 1993;168 (6 Pt 1):1759-62.

Gestational Trophoblastic Disease

17

CHAPTER

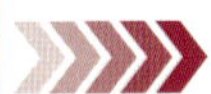

Harshad Parasnis

INTRODUCTION

Gestational trophoblastic disease (GTD) is a term that describes a continuum of tumors that arise in the fetal chorion with a wide range of biologic behavior and potential for metastases. These tumors are fetal allograft in maternal tissues and share some characteristics, such as chemosensitivity and chemocurability, production of human chorionic gonadotropin (hCG), and origin in fetal chorion, a genetically different tissue from the host.[1-3] In order to allay confusion regarding the terminology of GTD, the World Health Organization (WHO) study group on GTD has recognized four clinicopathological entities for GTD to include the conditions of:

1. Complete and partial hydatidiform mole (HM)
2. Invasive mole
3. Choriocarcinoma
4. Placental site trophoblastic tumor (PSTT).

The latter three conditions constitute gestational trophoblastic tumors, all of which may metastasize and are potentially fatal if untreated.

HYDATIDIFORM MOLE

Hydatidiform mole is a pregnancy characterized by vesicular swelling of placental villi and varying degrees of trophoblastic proliferation, involving both the cytotrophoblast and syncytiotrophoblast. It includes two distinct entities, complete hydatidiform mole (CHM) and partial hydatidiform mole (PHM).

Complete Hydatidiform Mole

It is an abnormal conceptus without any embryo or fetus, with gross hydropic swelling of the placental villi and usually pronounced trophoblastic hyperplasia involving both the cytotrophoblast and syncytiotrophoblast.

Partial Hydatidiform Mole

It is an abnormal conceptus with an embryo or fetus that tends to die early, and a placenta subject to focal villous swelling leading to cistern formation and focal trophoblastic hyperplasia, usually involving the syncytiotrophoblast only. The unaffected villi appear normal and vascularity of the villi disappears following fetal death.

Bilateral theca lutein cysts are seen in the ovary and are multilocular cysts lined by lutein cells, containing amber colored or serosanguinous fluid are formed due to overstimulation of lutein elements by excess amounts of hCG from the proliferating trophoblasts.

INVASIVE MOLE

Invasive mole is a tumor or tumor-like process arising from the HM invading the myometrium by direct extension or by venous channels, and characterized by trophoblastic hyperplasia and persistence of placental villous structures.

CHORIOCARCINOMA

Choriocarcinoma is a carcinoma arising from the trophoblastic epithelium that shows both cytotrophoblastic and syncytiotrophoblastic elements. It is characterized by abnormal trophoblastic hyperplasia and anaplasia with absence of villi and presence of extensive hemorrhage and necrosis.

PLACENTAL SITE TROPHOBLASTIC TUMOR

Placental site trophoblastic tumor is a tumor that arises from the trophoblast of the placental bed and is composed of mainly intermediate trophoblastic cells. It is very rare.

INCIDENCE

The incidence of HM varies in different parts of the world, but has been falling. The incidence of HM ranges from 0.5 cases to 8.3 cases per 1,000 live births. Review of literature shows that the incidence of molar pregnancy is 7–10 times greater in Asian countries as compared to North America or Europe. In India and Middle East, the incidence is approximately 1 in 160 pregnancies.

The incidence of invasive mole and choriocarcinoma are 1 per 15,000 pregnancies and 1 per 40,000 pregnancies, respectively. In Asia, the reported incidence of choriocarcinoma is 1 in 250 to 1 in 6,000 pregnancies. Complete mole has 9–20% risk of developing gestational trophoblastic neoplasia (GTN) while the risk in partial mole is about 3–5%. Up to 50% cases of choriocarcinoma develop from HM, while 25% cases each follow abortion or tubal pregnancy and normal term pregnancy.

CYTOGENETICS OF HYDATIDIFORM MOLE

Cytogenetic studies show that HM is the result of abnormal gametogenesis and fertilization. The complete and partial moles are separate entities with different genetic background. CHM commonly results from fertilization of an empty egg from which nuclear materials has been lost or inactivated, by a single or more sperm, with one of the mechanism discussed below.

Monospermic Homozygous

Here, maternal haploid set of 23 chromosomes is lost before fertilization by an unknown mechanism. The empty egg is fertilized by a sperm containing haploid set of 23X chromosomes. The duplication of this 23X chromosomes to 46XX without cell division results later in the formation of CHM.

Dispermic Diploidy Heterozygous

Occasionally, an empty ovum is fertilized by two sperms carrying X and X or X and Y chromosomes resulting in 46XX or 46XY chromosomal pattern in CHM.

Partial mole are most commonly due to a fertilization error in which a normal ovum is fertilized by two sperms resulting in a triploid karyotype (69XXY). The fertilization error may arise by diandry (one maternal and two paternal set of chromosomes) and less frequently by digyny (two maternal and one paternal set of chromosomes). This triploid conceptus has multiple congenital malformations. As the result of this there are differences in complete and partial mole (Table 1).

TABLE 1: Characteristics of partial hydatidiform mole and complete hydatidiform mole

	PHM	CHM
Embryonic/fetal tissue	Present	Absent
Karyotype	Triploid (diandrous) 69,XXY or 69, XYY	Paternal (androgenetic) 46 XX (96%) 46 XY (4%)
Hydatidiform swelling of villi	Focal/ patchymaze like cisterns	Diffuse
Stromal inclusions	Present	Absent
Villous scalloping	Present	Absent
Trophoblastic hyperplasia	Focal	Diffuse
Trophoblastic neoplsia	5%	20%

PHM, partial hydatidiform mole; CHM, complete hydatidiform mole.

PRESENTATION OF MOLAR PREGNANCY

Classic Features of Molar Pregnancy

- Irregular vaginal bleeding
- Spontaneous expulsion of grape like vesicles occurs mostly around 16 weeks of gestation
- Hyperemesis
- Excessive uterine enlargement
- Early failed pregnancy
- Anemia is often out of proportion to the amount of blood lost due to rapid growth of the tumor, hypervolemia, and concealed bleeding inside the uterus.

Rarer Presentations

- Hyperthyroidism
- Early onset preeclampsia
- Abdominal distension due to theca lutein cysts.

Very Rare Presentation

- Acute respiratory failure (due to metastatic disease)
- Neurological symptoms such as seizures (due to metastatic disease)
- Acute abdomen due to torsion, infarction, internal hemorrhage, or rupture of the theca lutein cysts.

Note: In contrast to CHM, partial moles are frequently misdiagnosed as threatened or missed abortion, have small for date uterus, and low hCG levels.

DIAGNOSIS OF HYDATIDIFORM MOLE

Ultrasonography

Ultrasonography is an accurate and sensitive method for the diagnosis.

- Complete mole: Characteristic vesicular or snowstorm pattern due to generalized swelling of the chorionic villi with absence of fetus (except partial mole)
- Partial molar pregnancy; the finding of multiple soft markers, including both cystic spaces in the placenta and a ratio of transverse to anterioposterior dimension of the gestation sac of greater than 1.5, is required for the reliable diagnosis of a partial molar pregnancy.

Human Chorionic Gonadotropin

- Estimation of hCG levels is a very reliable method for diagnosis, response to treatment, remission, and recurrence in trophoblastic disease. In molar pregnancy, hCG levels greater than 2 multiples of the median may help in diagnosis.

INVESTIGATIONS

After diagnosis, the workup of molar pregnancy includes:

- Complete blood count
- Chest X ray: To rule out pulmonary metastasis. Four forms of pulmonary metastatic lesions seen:
  1. Snowstorm or miliary pattern
  2. Single or multiple discrete rounded opacities

3. Embolic pattern due to pulmonary artery occlusion with resultant unilateral or multisegmental loss of vascular marking and right ventricular hypertrophy
4. Pleural effusion.

- Coagulation profile: It would also help to diagnose disseminated intravascular coagulation in clinically suspicious cases.

COMPLICATIONS

- Uterine perforation with attendant hemorrhage and intraperitoneal bleeding
- Pre-eclampsia
- Acute cor pulmonale from pulmonary embolization
- Disseminated intravascular coagulation
- Anemia
- Thyrotoxicosis: Thyroid storm can be precipitated if beta-adrenergic blockers are not given prior to induction of anesthesia for molar evacuation
- Recurrence of molar pregnancy: It occurs in 0.5–2.6% cases
- Malignant change: It is seen in 20% of CHM and 5% of PHM
- Maternal mortality: It has decreased from 10% in the past to 1% due to the modern management of molar pregnancy.

TREATMENT

Evacuation of Molar Pregnancy

Time of Evacuation

Once the diagnosis of HM is established, the uterus should be evacuated without waiting for spontaneous expulsion of the mole. In twin pregnancy with a viable fetus and a molar pregnancy, after counseling, the pregnancy may be allowed to continue.

Before Evacuation

- Evaluate patient for the presence of associated medical complications including:
  - Hyperthyroidism
  - Anemia
  - Preeclampsia.
- Blood should be typed and cross matched
- Baseline hCG levels should be determined.

Method

Suction evacuation: Suction evacuation is the preferred method of evacuation, independent of the uterine size. Oxytocin infusion may be started at the end of the evacuation to minimize the bleeding. There is theoretical concern over the routine use of potent oxytocic agents because of the potential to embolize and disseminate trophoblastic tissue through the venous system. Anti-D should be given to Rh negative women.

Incomplete evacuation: If incomplete evacuation is suspected, an ultrasonography after 1 week of evacuation is done. If there is evidence of residual tissue, a repeat curettage has to be performed to ensure complete removal of all molar tissue so that the further bleeding and elevation or persistence of the hCG is a pointer for the diagnosis of GTN.

Note: Routine repeat curettage after evacuation of the mole is not warranted.

Medical induction of labor: Presently, there is no place for medical induction of labor in the management of molar pregnancy. Data from the management of molar pregnancies with mifepristone and misoprostol are limited. Suction curettage is the method of choice for evacuation of partial molar pregnancies except when the size of the fetal parts deters the use of suction curettage. In these cases, medical evacuation can be used. In twin pregnancy with a viable fetus and a molar pregnancy, after counseling, the pregnancy may be allowed to continue.

Hysterectomy: In elderly multiparous patients who are not desirous of further reproductive function, hysterectomy with mole-*in-situ* may be an option. Though, hysterectomy will not *prevent* the risk of subsequent development of GTN, it *reduces* the risk. These patients are also advised to come for follow-up.

Prognosis

Local uterine invasion occurs in 15% of cases and distant metastasis occurs in 4% of cases following molar evacuation. For rest of the patients, evacuation is curative.

Note: Histology in molar pregnancy has no influence on subsequent prognosis. Hence, the need for follow-up after molar evacuation.

FOLLOW-UP AFTER MOLAR PREGNANCY

After molar evacuation, meticulous follow-up is done to detect any continued trophoblastic activity. The follow-up visit should include physical examination, serial hCG estimation, USG, and chest X ray.

Serum hCG Assay

After a normal pregnancy, hCG levels require up to 20 days to become undetectable, hence hCG estimation is started after 3 weeks post-evacuation

- First estimation: At 3 weeks
- Every 2 weeks: Till hCG becomes undetectable. There is no distinct benefit from doing weekly estimations as has been advocated by some authority
- If undetectable at 8 weeks: Monthly urine hCG assay for 6 months. Most patients achieve normal values by 8 weeks after evacuation
- If hCG levels abnormal at 8 weeks: Risk of progression to choriocarcinoma is 1%. Assays done
    - Monthly for 1 year
    - Three monthly for the second year.

Chest X ray

It should be done at 1 and 2 months post-evacuation.

Pelvic Examination

Pelvic examination should be performed to detect theca lutein cyst which usually regress spontaneously in 2–4 months (mean 8 weeks).

Contraception

Contraception should be advised:

- For 6 months if hCG levels become undetectable within 8 weeks after evacuation
- For 2 years in patients whose hCG levels become undetectable after 8 weeks
    - *Barrier contraception*: Though less effective, it is the most preferred method (condoms or diaphragm with the use of spermicides)
    - *Oral contraceptive pills*: The controversy of using combined *oral contraceptive* (OC) pills persists. However, low dose OC pills can be safely prescribed without increasing the risk of persistent disease, once the hCG levels become undetectable
    - *Intrauterine devices*: They are not recommended due to fear of perforation and irregular bleeding that simulates persistent trophoblastic activity on follow-up
    - *Permanent methods*: For couples that do not wish for further pregnancy, sterilization is the most appropriate method.

Note: A high index of suspicion for progression of molar pregnancy to choriocarcinoma, early diagnosis with meticulous follow-up and early referral for initiating specific therapy are the key to reducing the morbidity and mortality associated with choriocarcinoma.

CHEMOPROPHYLAXIS

Although routine use of chemoprophylaxis at time of evacuation may reduce the incidence of GTN in high-risk patients, there is no benefit in low-risk patients and it is not recommended. If any of them develop GTN in spite of the prophylactic chemotherapy, they will have a more resistant disease requiring multiagent chemotherapy.

Note: The routine use of prophylactic chemotherapy at the time of evacuation of the mole is not recommended.

INDICATIONS FOR THERAPY

Widely accepted indications for therapy after evacuation of a mole are:

- An abnormal hCG regression pattern (a 10% or greater rise in hCG levels or a plateauing hCG of three stable values over 2 weeks)
- An hCG rebound
- Histologic diagnosis of choriocarcinoma or placental site trophoblastic tumor
- The presence of metastases
- High hCG levels (>20,000 mIU/mL more than 4 weeks postevacuation)
- Persistently elevated hCG levels 6 months postevacuation.

POST-MOLAR GESTATIONAL TROPHOBLASTIC NEOPLASIA

Approximately 10–17% of HM develop invasive mole while 2–3% of HM progress to choriocarcinoma. The incidence of GTN after complete and partial mole is 8% and 0.5%, respectively.

Criteria for Diagnosis of Post-Molar Gestational Trophoblastic Neoplasia

The diagnosis of GTN is made on the basis of elevated hCG levels supported, but not necessarily, by histologic or radiologic evidence.

- Histological evidence of choriocarcinoma
- Plateau of hCG for more than 4 measurements over a period of 3 weeks or longer
- Rise in hCG on three consecutive weekly measurements over a period of 2 weeks or longer
- hCG level more than 20,000 IU/L 4 weeks after evacuation
- hCG remaining positive after 16 weeks after evacuation.

Metastatic Work-up in Gestational Trophoblastic Neoplasia

Metastatic work-up should include:

- Chest X-ray for diagnosis of lung metastasis
- Computed tomography (CT) scan or ultrasonography to diagnose liver metastasis
- Magnetic resonance imaging (MRI) or CT scan to diagnose brain metastasis.

FIGO STAGING OF GESTATIONAL TROPHOBLASTIC NEOPLASIA

After diagnosing GTN, staging International Federation of Gynecology and Obstetrics (FIGO) is required to determine the extent of the disease and the factors affecting the prognosis.

Stage I: Disease confined to the uterus.

Stage II: GTN extends outside the uterus, but limited to genital organs.

Stage III: GTN extends to the lungs with or without known genital involvement.

Stage IV: All other metastatic sites.

RISK SCORING

The modified WHO scoring system is used to decide management. In the new risk scoring system, ABO blood groups are omitted and liver metastasis is given a score of 4 (Table 2).

- Low risk: 6 or less
- High risk: 7 and above.

TREATMENT OF LOW RISK GESTATIONAL TROPHOBLASTIC NEOPLASIA

Patients of FIGO stage I, II, and III with WHO score of 6 or less or of duration less than 4 months or hCG value is less than 40,000 IU/L are low-risk GTN and treated with single agent chemotherapy.

TABLE 2: Risk factor scoring system treatment of low-risk GTN patients of FIGO stage I

	0	*1*	*2*	*4*
Age (years)	<40	>40		
Antecedent pregnancy	Mole	Abortion	Term	
Pregnancy event to chemotherapy	<4 months	4–6 months	7–12 months	>12 months
hCG (IU/mL)	<1,000	1,000–10,000	10,000–1,00,000	>1,00,000
Largest tumor including uterine	<3	3–5 cm	>5 cm	
Site of Metastases	Lung	Spleen, kidney	GI tract	Liver, brain
Number of metastases identified		1–4	5–8	>8
Prior chemotherapy			Single drug	two or more drugs

GTN, gestational trophoblastic neoplasia; FIGO, International Federation of Gynecology and Obstetrics; hCG, human-chorionic gonadotropin.

Single Agent Chemotherapy Schedules

- Methotrexate with leucovorin rescue: Methotrexate 1 mg/kg intramuscularly on days 1, 3, 5, and 7 with folinic acid 0.1 mg/kg on days 2, 4, 6, and 8. It is given 24 hours after each dose of methotrexate. Course could be repeated every 2 weeks depending on the response[4]
- Actinomycin-D: 9–12 mg/kg intravenousy daily for 5 days repeated every 2 weeks.

Monitoring During Chemotherapy

Monitoring is done to detect drug toxicity and to assess response to treatment prior to each course a complete blood count, renal functional test, liver functional test, serum hCG measurements, and chest X-ray is done. Brain CT/MRI should be done when there is suspicion of metastasis.

Length of Therapy

Usually 2–3 courses of chemotherapy should be given beyond first negative hCG level, especially if the fall of hCG was slow.

Response: With single agent chemotherapy, most trophoblastic centers report a near 100% cure rate for nonmetastatic GTN.

TREATMENT OF HIGH RISK GESTATIONAL TROPHOBLASTIC NEOPLASIA

Patients with FIGO stage I, II, III with WHO risk score of 7 or greater, or FIGO stage IV are high risk GTN and are treated with etoposide, methotrexate, and dactinomycin alternating with cyclophosphamide and vincristine (EMA-CO) as the primary combination therapy.[5] Due to risk of chemotherapy complications, like leucopenia, this schedule must be given in a well equipped institution.

MANAGEMENT OF PLACENTAL SITE TROPHOBLASTIC TUMOR

Surgery remains the treatment of choice for disease localized to the uterus, while metastatic PSTT is treated with hysterectomy followed by multiagent chemotherapy at well equipped institutions.

POST-THERAPY PREGNANCY

Patients must be advised to wait for 12 months after completion of chemotherapy before undertaking pregnancy. There is an increased risk of developing recurrent molar pregnancy in patients with past history of GTD. Artificial reproductive technology opens up new vistas for patients with GTD. Some studies have reported increased incidence of spontaneous abortion, but there is no increase in incidence of congenital malformation inspite of potentially mutagenic chemotherapy. In the subsequent pregnancy, early ultrasonography must be done to confirm normal gestation.

Note:
- There is no evidence of activation of GTD due to subsequent pregnancy event
- After the delivery hCG assay must be done at 3 weeks and at 3 months to rule out persistent trophoblastic disease.

RECURRENT MOLAR PREGNANCIES

This is also known as familial recurrent hydatidiform mole and is a rare condition. It is an autosomal recessive condition that presents with CHM of biparental rather than androgenetic origin. The mutated gene NALP7 is carried on the long arm of chromosome 19.[6] Such women are incapable of having normal pregnancies and should be advised *in vitro* fertilization with donor oocytes.

Gestational trophoblastic disease presents primarily in the first trimester. Clinical suspicion and USG are the mainstay of diagnosis. Suction evacuation is treatment of choice. Close follow-up is necessary. Monitoring in subsequent pregnancy is also required

REFERENCES

1. Fleming ID. Gestational trophoblastic tumors. In: American Joint Committee on Cancer. AJCC Cancer Staging Manual, 5th edition. Philadelphia: Lippincott-Raven Publishers; 1997. pp. 211-14.
2. Parasnis HB, Parulekar SV. Clinical Manual of Gynecologic Oncology, 1st edition. Bhalani Publishing House; 1994.
3. Ernest I Kohorn. The FIGO 2000 staging and risk factor scoring system for gestational trophoblastic neoplasia. In: Hancock BW, Newlands ES, Berkowitz RS, Cole LA, editors. Gestational Trophoblastic Disease. 2nd ed. 2003. pp. 175-81.
4. Tumors of the placental trophoblast. In: Morrow CP, Curtin JP, editors. Synopsis of Gynecologic Oncology. 5th ed. New York, NY: Churchill Livingstone; 1998. pp. 315-53.
5. Newlands ES, Bagshawe KD, Begent RH, et al. Results with the EMA/CO (etoposide, methotrexate, actinomycin D, cyclophosphamide, vincristine) regimen in high risk gestational trophoblastic tumors, 1979 to 1989. Br J Obstet Gynecol. 1991;98(6):550-7.
6. Fisher RA, Sebire NJ. Recurrent molar pregnancies. In: Arora M, editor. Recurrent Pregnancy Loss. India: New Delhi. Jaypee Medical Publishers; 2007. p. 46-53.

HIV Positive Mother

18

CHAPTER

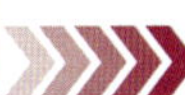

Sarita Agarwal

INTRODUCTION

Human immunodeficiency virus (HIV) epidemic is nearly 26 years old. Since the beginning of HIV epidemic more than 60 million people have been infected globally and as on November 2009, total 33.4 million people are living with HIV/AIDS (acquired immunodeficiency syndrome) worldwide. HIV presently accounts for the highest number of deaths attributable to any single infective agent. Globally, coverage for services to prevent mother-to-child HIV transmission rose from 10% in 2004 to 45% in 2008 [World Health Organization (WHO), United Nations Children's Fund (UNICEF), and Joint United Nations Programme on HIV and AIDS (UNAIDS), 2009]. The drop in new HIV infections among children in 2008 suggests that these efforts are saving lives.

HIV AND PREGNANCY

There is no evidence to suggest that pregnancy enhances progression of disease. However, HIV infection during pregnancy has been found to be associated with increased risk of abortion, preterm labor, and intrauterine growth restriction (IUGR). Perinatal transmission of HIV and childhood infection is major cause for concern. Twenty-five to thirty-five percent of transmission occurs in the antenatal period, mainly in the later part of pregnancy. Seventy to seventy-five percent of vertical transmission occurs during labor and delivery. The proportion of transmission attributable to breast feeding worldwide from HIV is 14%.[1]

Factors Affecting Mother to Child Transmission

Numerous factors influence HIV perinatal transmission and these are often responsible for the observed variability in transmission rates (Table 1).

Maternal Viral Load

The strongest predictor of transmission is the maternal viral load. Garcia et al. showed that there are no factors affecting mother to child transmission (MTCT) when maternal viral load is below 1,000 copies/mL.[2] However, there is insufficient evidence for existence of a plasma load threshold below which MTCT never occurs.

Maternal Immune Depletion

An increased risk of vertical transmission is noted with lowered CD4 T cell counts in mother.[3]

TABLE 1: Factors affecting mother to child transmission

Viral	*Maternal*	*Obstetric procedures enhancing transmission*	*Neonatal*
• Viral load-no MTCT if viral load <1,000 copies/mL • Viral genotype and phenotype: transmission in low HIV-2 • Viral resistance	**More if** • Low CD4 • AIDS • Opportunistic infection. • Sexually transmitted disease • Nutritional deficiency • Behavioral factors-tobacco, alcohol, drug addiction and smoking **Less if** • ART given	• CVS • Amniocentesis • Cordocentesis • ARM • PROM >4 hours • Invasive fetal monitoring • Intrapartum hemorrhage • Vaginal delivery	• Breast feeding • Mixed feed • Mastitis • Prematurity • Genetic • Multiple pregnancy

MTCT, mother to child transmission; HIV, human immunodeficiency virus; AIDS, acquired immunodeficiency syndrome; ART, antiretroviral therapy; CVS, chorionic villous sampling; ARM, artificial rupture of the membranes; PROM, premature rupture of membranes.

Genital Tract Infection

Irrespective of whether genital lesions are present, genital tract infections increase the risk of MTCT. Clinical vaginitis or vaginosis of any etiology at the last antenatal visit was associated with MTCT.

Nutritional Deficiencies

Some studies have shown that transmission rates are higher when nutritional deficiencies coexist. This possibly is an important factor responsible for the geographical differences in transmission rates. An example of this is, the reduction of perinatal transmission by vitamin A supplementation as demonstrated by Semba et al. in a rural African population.[4]

Drug Use

Use of drugs (cocaine, heroin, opiates, methadone, and injecting drugs) by HIV positive women in pregnancy has shown to increase perinatal transmission.

Cigarette Smoking

An association has been documented between cigarette smoking in pregnancy and an increased risk of mother to child transmission.

Unprotected Sexual Intercourse

It probably leads to a higher chance of genital infection and has also been found to increase perinatal transmission.

Opportunistic and Coexisting Infection

Presence of opportunistic and coexisting infection, viz., tuberculosis, malaria, etc. further increases the risk of transmission.

Intrapartum Events

Intrapartum events are crucial factors governing MTCT since this is the period where the risk is highest. The following events have all been associated with an increased risk of perinatal transmission:

- Duration of membrane rupture more than 4 hours

- Preterm births
- Chorioamnionitis
- Invasive procedures during labor and delivery.

Note: An elective cesarean section (before the onset of labor) prevents perinatal transmission but an emergency cesarean section performed in labor for prolonged or difficult labor has been associated with increased transmission rates.[1]

Breast Feeding

Breast feeding increases the risk of MTCT, more so with recently acquired HIV infection in the mother and presence of mastitis (clinical and subclinical).

Recommendation for Screening of HIV in Pregnant Women

Every pregnant woman should be offered HIV screening universally as early as possible, in each new pregnancy because, appropriate intervention can reduce the risk of MTCT of HIV. However, testing is not compulsory. As a substantial proportion of pregnant women present to health facilities at the time of labor, HIV testing and counseling should be recommended to all women of unknown HIV status in labor, or as soon as possible after delivery.

Indication of Repeat Testing

Repeat testing late in pregnancy should also be recommended to HIV negative women in high prevalence area and women with high risk of acquiring the infection.

Confirmatory Tests

If screening test by rapid enzyme-linked immunosorbent assay (ELISA) is positive the diagnosis is to be confirmed with two more ELISA/rapid simple tests with different antigenic test principle. When a patient presents in labor without HIV report, a rapid test using single ELISA may be appropriate but needs to be confirmed subsequently with the three test principle. The three tests done are chemiluminescence, immunohistochemistry, and a western blot test which is confirmatory. Single test positive is sufficient to discard blood, semen, or organ donation

GENERAL PRINCIPLES REGARDING USE OF ANTIRETROVIRAL THERAPY IN PREGNANCY

Initial Evaluation

Initial evaluation of an infected pregnant woman should include an assessment of HIV disease status by CD4 count and WHO staging.

Indication for Treatment

The women in pregnancy require antiretroviral (ARV) drugs for two goals.

Antiretroviral Therapy

For their own health: Those with CD4 count less than 350/mm^3 irrespective of WHO staging and those in WHO stage III or IV irrespective of CD4 count need antiretroviral therapy (ART) and should receive it life-long.

Antiretroviral Prophylaxis

Prevention of MTCT: Those who do not require it for their own health but for prevention of MTCT (ARV prophylaxis) should receive effective antenatal, peripartum, and postnatal ARV based interventions.

Drugs and Duration of Antiretroviral Prophylaxis

Recent data indicate greater benefits of starting ARV prophylaxis for prevention of parent to child transmission (PPTCT) earlier during pregnancy and support extended ARV prophylaxis to mothers or infants during the breastfeeding period preventing transmission through breastfeeding (Pepi Malawi trial, Swen trial).[5,6]

Antiretroviral drugs are classified as follows:

- Nucleoside reverse transcriptase inhibitors (NRTI)
  - Lamivudine (XTC)
  - Zidovudine (ZDV/AZT)
  - Emtricitabine (FTC)
  - Abacavir (ABC)
  - Tenofovir (TDF)
  - Didanosine (DDI)
  - Stavudine (d4T)
- Non-nucleoside reverse transcriptase inhibitors (NNRTI)
  - Efavirenz (EFV)
  - Nevirapine (NVP)
- Protease inhibitors
  - Indinavir (IDV)
  - Lopinavir (LVP)
  - Ritonavir
- Fusion inhibitors
  - Enfuvirtide (T-20)
- Entry inhibitors CCR5 co-receptor antagonist
  - Maraviroc
- HIV integrase strand transfer inhibitors
  - Raltegravir
  - Dolutegravir
- Combination Drugs
  - Atripla (efavirenz + emtricitabine + tenofovir).

Drug with Transplacental Passage Indicated

Zidovudine (ZDV/AZT) should be included in the antenatal ARV regimen as it has shown maximum efficacy in prevention of mother-to-child transmission (PMTCT), unless there is severe toxicity, contraindications, or documented resistance. If antenatal ZDV is not possible, at least one agent with known transplacental passage (ABC, DDI, FTC, D4T, TDF, NVP), lopinavir/ritonavir (LVP/r) should be part of ARV regimen.[7,8]

Contraindicated Drugs

Avoid use of EFV or other potentially teratogenic drugs in the first trimester and drugs with known adverse potential for mother. Since the neural tube closes at approximately 28 days gestation, if a woman receiving EFV is recognized as pregnant before 28 days gestation, EFV should be stopped and substituted with NVP or a protease inhibitor. If a woman is diagnosed as pregnant after 28 days gestation, EFV should be continued. There is no indication for abortion in women exposed to EFV in the first trimester of pregnancy as there is very low quality, conflicting evidence on the risks of EFV causing neural tube defects. Although, women who become pregnant while receiving EFV may consider temporarily suspending treatment, this is not recommended. The ART regimen may be changed if necessary, but should continue without interruption. Discontinuation of ART could lead to an increase in viral load, which could result in a decline in immune status and an acceleration of disease progression, thereby increasing the risk of HIV transmission to the fetus.[9]

ANTIRETROVIRAL PROTOCOLS

The ART protocols are defined according to clinical situations which are specific to whether the woman is on ART or not, her requirement for ART, and if she has needed and received prophylaxis. For the baby treatment differs according to whether the baby is breast fed or not[7,8] (Table 2).

ANTENATAL CARE FOR HIV POSITIVE WOMEN

The first task in caring for an HIV infected woman who is pregnant or considering pregnancy is to provide counseling that will allow her to make informed reproductive choices. For this, the patient needs education and information about the risk of perinatal transmission of HIV, potential complications of pregnancy, continuation or modification (or possibly, initiation) of ART, and the support she will need to optimize maternal and fetal outcomes.

TABLE 2: ART protocols

Clinical situations	*For mother*	*For newborn*
HIV-infected woman who is already receiving ART and becomes pregnant	Continue current HAART regimen if successfully suppressing viremia. Except avoid use of EFV or other potentially teratogenic drugs in the first trimester and drugs with known adverse potential for mother (combination D4T/DDI). Continue ART during labor, after delivery and life-long	Daily AZT or NVP from birth until 6 weeks of age
HIV-infected pregnant woman who is not on antiretroviral but, has indications for antiretroviral therapy for own health	*Time to start*: Should start ART irrespective of gestational ageand continue throughout pregnancy, delivery, and thereafter *Regimen*: The preferred first-line ART regimen should include an AZT + 3TC backbone: • AZT + 3TC + NVP or • AZT + 3TC + EFV *Alternative regimens*: Alternative regimens that are recommended include: • TDF + 3TC (or FTC) + NVP • DF + 3TC (or FTC) + EFV Avoid use of EFV or other potentially teratogenic drugs in the first trimester and drugs with known adverse potential for mother (combination D4T/DDI).	*For breastfeeding infants*: Daily NVP from birth until 6 weeks of age *For nonbreastfeeding infants*: Daily AZT or NVP from birth until 6 weeks of age
HIV-infected pregnant woman who is not on antiretroviral therapy and does not require ART for her own health	*Time to start*: ARV prophylaxis should be started from as early as14 weeks gestation (second trimester) or as soon as possible when women present late in pregnancy and labor and it is to be continued till 1 week after all exposure to breast feeding has ended *Regimen*: The preferred first-line ARV Prophylaxis regimen should include: • Antepartum daily AZT • Sd-NVP at onset of labor* • AZT + 3TC during labor and delivery • AZT + 3TC for 7 days postpartum *Alternative regimens*: Alternative regimens that are recommended include an AZT + 3TC backbone: • AZT + 3TC + LVP/r • AZT + 3TC + EFV • AZT + 3TC + ABC • TDF + XTC+ EFV	*In breastfeeding infants:* Maternal ARV prophylaxis should be coupled with daily administration of NVP to the infant from birth until one week after all exposure to breastmilk has ended *In nonbreastfeeding infants*: Maternal ARV prophylaxis should be coupled with daily administration of AZT or NVP from birth until 6 weeks of age

Contd...

Contd...

Clinical situations	*For mother*	*For newborn*
HIV-infected woman who has received no antiretroviral therapy or prophylaxis prior to labor (during labor protocol)	Administration of single dose NVP has shown to develop resistance limiting subsequent use of NVP and other NNRTI also. Hence, consideration should be given to adding 3TC and AZT with single dose NVP during labor and maternal AZT/3TC for 7 days postpartum, which may reduce development of NVP resistance. If above protocol is not feasible then administer at least single dose NVP during labor to mother (A 200 mg NVP tablet is given at the onset of labor. Give at least 2 hours before birth for best efficacy)	*In breastfeeding infants*: Single-doseNVP plus AZT for 6 weeks *In nonbreastfeeding infants*: Single dose NVP within 72 hours of birth to infant (2 mg/kg of body weight)
Women who did not receive any ARV prophylaxis for PPTCT	Evaluate by CD4 count and WHO staging for need for initiation of postpartum antiretroviral therapy	AZT given for 6 weeks to the infant, started as soon as possible after birth. Consultation with a pediatric HIV specialist is recommended

*sd-NVP and AZT+3TC intra-and post-partum can be omitted if mother receives more than 4 weeks of AZT during pregnancy.

HIV, human immunodeficiency virus; ART, antiretroviral therapy; ARV, antiretroviral; PPTCT, prevention of parent to child transmission; HAART, highly active antiretroviral therapy; EFV, Efavirenz; D4T/DDI, stavudine/ didanosine; AZT, zidovudine; 3TC, lamivudine, epivir; NVP, nevirapine; TDF, tenofovir; LVP, lopinavir; ABC, abacavir; XTC, lamivudine; NNRTI, non-nucleoside reverse transcriptase inhibitors; WHO, World Health Organization.

Along with standard antenatal care, the following must be included:

- Assessment of severity of disease: Assess and follow up immune status (CD count)
- Detecting opportunistic infection: Identify illnesses resulting from compromised immune status such as tuberculosis, pneumocystis carinii pneumonia, and treat as appropriate
- Sexually transmitted diseases screen: Screen for other sexually transmitted infections, surface antigen of the hepatitis B virus (HBsAg), and hepatitis C virus (HCV) at first visit and repeat at 28 weeks. Treat them, if any
- Pap smear: Do Pap smear screening for cervical dysplasia
- Nutrition: Importance of balanced diet with adequate calories should be stressed and implemented
- Anemia prophylaxis: Prevention of anemia by prophylactic iron, folic acid, and high protein diet is a must
- Discouraging addictions: Discourage smoking, alcohol, illicit drugs, and unsafe sex
- Psychological support: Psychological support and counseling is a must
- Support services: Linkage of woman to HIV related care, treatment, and support services.

Investigations

- Antenatal care investigation should include urine examination, complete blood count, blood group and typing, venereal disease research laboratory test (VDRL), HBsAg, and HCV
- Initial CD4 count to be done and repeated every 3 month
- Tests for quantitative viral load and CD8 counts if feasible
- When patient are on either ARV therapy or prophylaxis, appropriate investigations for drug toxicity like anemia, lactic acidosis,

hyperglycemia, hepatitis, pancreatitis, renal dysfunction, and electrolyte imbalance may be needed
- Fetal anomaly scan has to be done if there is first trimester exposure to highly active anti-retroviral therapy (HAART) or co-trimoxazole.

SPECIAL CONSIDERATIONS FOR OPPORTUNISTIC INFECTION PROPHYLAXIS DURING PREGNANCY

If CD4 count declines and viral load increases it invites opportunistic infection and prophylaxis for prevention of these infections is important. The prophylaxis is specific to the disease (Box 1). For women who require prophylaxis, trimethoprim-sulfamethoxazole is the preferred agent, although some specialists advice against giving pyrimethamine during pregnancy due to an increased risk of folate deficiency. Folate supplementation should be given to reduce the risk of neural tube defects

The care of HIV pregnant patient requires attention to many aspects like control of the disease, prevention of transmission to the baby, prophylaxis of opportunistic infections, and care of the baby.

Box 1: Opportunistic infections prophylaxis in HIV positive pregnant woman

- *Pneumocystis carinii pneumonia*: CD4 count <200 cell/cmm trimethoprim + sulfamethoxazole (septran) double strength 2 tab BD three times a week + folic acid
- *Toxoplasma*: CD4 count <100 cells/cmm trimethoprim + sulfamethoxazole
- *Tuberculosis*: CD4 count <50 cells/cmm, *mycobacterium avium* complex isoniazid + pyridoxine
- *Genital herpes*: Suppression therapy is indicated if recurrent

REFERENCES

1. Dunn D, Newell ML, Ades AE, et al. Risk of HIV-1 transmission through breastfeeding. Lancet. 1992;340(8819):585-8.
2. Garcia PM, Kalish LA, Pitt J, et al. Maternal Levels of plasma human immunodeficiency virus type 1 RNA and the risk of perinatal transmission. Women and Infants Transmission Study Group. N Engl J Med. 1999;341(6): 394-402.
3. Natural history of vertically acquired Human Immunodeficiency Virus-1.Infection. Pediatrics. 1994;94(6 Pt 1):815-9.
4. Semba KD, Miotti PG, Chilhangwi, et al. Maternal Vitamin A Deficiency and Mother to Child Transmission of HIV-1. Lancet. 1994;339:1593-7.
5. Kumwenda NI, Hoover DR, Mofenson LM, et al. Extended antiretroviral prophylaxis to reduce breast-milk HIV-1 transmission. N Engl J Med. 2008;359(2):119-29.
6. SWEN Study Team. Extended -dose nevirapine to 6 weeks of age for infants to prevent HIV transmission via breastfeeding in Ethiopia, India, and Uganda: an analysis of three randomized controlled trials. Lancet. 2008;372(9635):300-13.
7. WHO. Rapid advice: antiretroviral therapy for HIV infection in adult and adolescent. [online] available from www.who.int/hiv/pub/arv/advice/en/index.html [accessed october, 2013].
8. Guidelines for the management of occupational exposure to HIV and recommendations for post exposure prophylaxis, U.S. Department of Health and Human Services May 24, 2010.
9. U.S. Department of Health and Human Services. Guidelines for the Use of Antiretroviral Agents in HIV-1-Infected Adults and Adolescents. January 10, 2011.

TORCH Infection

19
CHAPTER

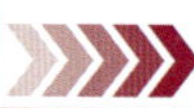

Subhash C Biswas, Ram P Dey

INTRODUCTION

TORCH is an acronym for a special group of infections which may be acquired by a woman before or during pregnancy with disastrous consequences for the fetus. All are grouped together because they can cause a cluster of symptomatic birth defects in newborns, collectively called the TORCH syndrome.

"TORCH" group of infections includes

- Toxoplasma infection
- Other infections, such as syphilis, varicella-herpes zoster (VZV), and hepatitis B
- Rubella
- Cytomegalovirus (CMV)
- Herpes simplex virus (HSV).

Klein and Remington[1] have suggested that this classification is too limiting and that several additional infectious agents should be considered in the "other" category, such as enteroviruses, *Borrelia burgdorferi* (the cause of Lyme disease) and, of course, human immunodeficiency virus (HIV). However, this review includes the traditional TORCH infection only.

INCIDENCE

Incidence of these infections has a wide variability with regards to endemicity, geographical distribution, and socioeconomic groups (Table 1).

PATHOGENESIS

The placenta constitutes a protective immunologic barrier that shields the fetus, a graft of foreign tissue, from the mother's humoral and cell-mediated immune responses. This makes the fetus especially susceptible to infection during the first trimester before full development of placenta. Early in pregnancy, the most complex events in embryogenesis take place, exposing sensory organs, such as the eyes and ears at risk. The organisms being of relatively low virulence, seldom lead to fetal death beyond the earliest stages of embryogenesis but result in persistence of organisms leading to post-natal sequelae in life (see below). The fetus is infected mainly by transplacental spread except in HSV where infective secretion is the vehicle of spread. In most cases, the maternal illness is mild but the impact on the developing fetus is more severe. It is difficult to determine the percentage of fetal loss due to infection during early pregnancy.

Note: The degree of severity of effect is dependent on the gestational age of the fetus when infected, the causative agent and their virulence, the damage to the placenta, and the severity of maternal disease.

However, certain agents are preferentially transmitted during different trimester of pregnancy (Table 2).

TABLE 1: Incidence and fetal affection in TORCH infections

Infective agent	*Global incidence*	*Seroprevalence (India)*	*Fetal affection*
Syphilis[2]	2.2/10,000	1.4–2.4%	Primary: 50–75% (in active lesion) Secondary: 50% Latent: 10–30%
Toxoplasmosis[3]	1 in 10,000 live births	4–57%	<5 weeks— no fetal affection Third trimester: 60%
Cytomegalo-virus[4]	1–2% of all pregnancies	0–6%	First trimester: up to 2% Second trimester: 6–10% Third trimester: 11–28% Symptomatic at birth:10% Late sequelae: 5–25%
Rubella[5]	Eliminated in developed countries	55–95%	<10 weeks: 80–90% 10–12 weeks: 50% >12 weeks: 33%
Herpes simplex[6]	Variable	22% seropositive for HSV2	33% transmission rate (HSV1) and 2.7% (HSV2)
Varicella[7]	1–5/10,000	95–100%	Embryopathy: 2–10% Congenital varicella syndrome (8–20 weeks): 1.3%

HSV, herpes simplex virus.

TABLE 2: Time of transmission of TORCH infection

Toxoplasmosis	*Mainly third trimester*
CMV	All three trimesters, more severe in second trimester
HSV	All three trimesters with different outcomes
Syphilis	After 16 weeks gestation
Varicella	<9 weeks ≥36 weeks gestation
Rubella	<12 weeks of gestation

CMV, cytomegalovirus; HSV, herpes simplex virus.

SPECTRUM OF FETAL AFFECTION WITH TORCH INFECTIONS DURING PREGNANCY

Many systems in the fetus are affected by TORCH infections. Some effects are listed below:

- Resorption of embryo or miscarriage
- Small-for-gestational-age or intrauterine growth restriction
- Congenital heart disease
- Cataract or significant visual impairment
- Hearing impairment
- Microcephaly
- Mental retardation
- Hepatosplenomegaly, anemia, and hyperbilirubinemia
- Pneumonia
- Skin rash
- Central nervous system (encephalitis, calcification in brain tissue and seizures)
- Stillborn/perinatal death.

In addition to these symptoms, each of the TORCH infections has its own characteristic differentiating symptom cluster in newborns.

SCREENING

Recommendations by Infections and pregnancy Study Group (UK):

- Sporadic miscarriage is so common that detailed infective screening cannot be justified economically (Grade C)

- TORCH screening is unhelpful and should be abandoned in the investigation of recurrent miscarriage (Grade C).

As per the Royal College of Obstetricians and Gynaecologists (RCOG) Guideline (2011),[8] any severe infection that leads to bacteremia or viremia can cause sporadic miscarriage. The role of infection in recurrent miscarriage is unclear. For an infective agent to be implicated in the etiology of repeated pregnancy loss, it must be capable of persisting in the genital tract and avoiding detection, or must cause insufficient symptoms to disturb the woman. Toxoplasmosis, rubella, cytomegalovirus, and herpes infections do not fulfill these criteria and routine TORCH screening should be abandoned. However, universal antenatal screening for syphilis is recommended for communities where prevalence is high or patients are at high risk. Serological testing in addition to routine early screening should be performed twice during the third trimester, i.e. in between 28 weeks and delivery.

DIAGNOSIS

All women with history of exanthematous rash, fever and genital lesions in pregnancy are high-risk groups and should undergo evaluation for TORCH infections. There are two components for establishing TORCH infection: maternal affection and fetal affection. These can be carried out by serology and imaging (Table 3).

Serology

Serologic tests are used to diagnose acute infection in pregnant women, which must be confirmed at reference laboratory before abortion or treatment with potentially toxic drugs. In general, immunoglobulin M (IgM) production is the acute reaction followed by IgG in 1–3 weeks. Ideally two samples should be taken 3 weeks apart. Diagnosis of acute maternal infection is made by one of the following:

- Seroconversion (IgG negative mother, to IgG positive)
- Fourfold increase in IgG serial titer over 2–3 weeks
- Demonstration of pathogen specific IgM.

"Avidity" or "functional affinity" defines the net antigen binding force of populations of antibodies, and has highly diagnostic value in timing the maternal infection in positive serology cases. IgG antibodies of low avidity suggests recent infection, although it is not an absolute indicator. Whereas, high avidity rules out recent infection of less than 4 months duration, even if IgM is positive.[9]

The IgM is not necessarily indicative of recent infection and can persist for years. Hence, further investigation is only required in mothers who seroconvert during pregnancy or have an initially high antibody titer. For example, the IgM can persist for up to 4 months after the acute episode and thus the infection could have been acquired before pregnancy, which is associated with negligible risk to the fetus.[10]

Isolation of the Parasite

The isolation of the parasite by means of mouse inoculation may be done but results are available only after 4–5 weeks. Polymerase chain reaction (PCR) can be done. The combination of amniocentesis and placental tissue culture from chorion villous sampling (CVS) (which has a positive predictive value of 90%) may reduce the waiting period to 5 days, but there is risk of overwhelming fatal infection.[11]

Note: For establishment of fetal infection amniocentesis rather than CVS is recommended for PCR. Cordocentesis is no longer recommended.

Tests to Establish Specificity

Each disease has a specific test to establish diagnosis:

- Toxoplasmosis: Sabin-Feldman dye test (old), enzyme linked immunosorbent assay (ELISA), immunofluorescence assay (IFA), and modified direct agglutination

TABLE 3: TORCH infections in pregnancy

Virus	*Manifestations of maternal infection*	*Transmission to fetus/neonate*	*Clinical manifestation in fetus/neonate*	*Long-term sequelae*	*Preventive measures against maternal or neonatal infection*
Toxoplasmosis	Asymptomatic (90%) resemble infectious mononucleosis cervical lymphadenopathy	Transplacentally in acute infection	85% subclinical	Later surface as chorioretinitis, hearing loss and developmental delay	Avoid cats, under cooked meat and awareness of hygiene Confirm fetal affection by amniocentesis with PCR and institute drug treatment with spiramycin
Varicella-zoster	Chickenpox, pneumonia, and respiratory insufficiency	Maternal viremia	Fetal varicella syndrome Neonatal varicella Zoster in infancy	Limb hypoplasia cutaneous scarring (cicatrices) Microcephaly psychomotor retardation	Vaccination (before pregnancy) VZIG to ameliorate or prevent maternal and neonatal infection
Syphilis	Manifestation vary from primary, secondary, and tertiary state	Transplacentally in acute infection	Quite variable, rhinitis, maculopapular rash, chondritis hepatosplenomegaly, etc.	Keratitis, deafness frontal bossing sabershins, and notched teeth	Sex education of parents primary treatment with penicillin of infective mother
Rubella	Subclinical rash, adenopathy, and arthralgias	Maternal viremia	Congenital rubella syndrome (cataracts, heart disease, deafness) Purpura	Cataracts, heart defects deafness, and other nerve damage	Vaccination (before pregnancy)
Cytomegalovirus	Subclinical, fever mononucleosis-like	Maternal viremia contact with infected genital secretions at birth, breast milk	Cytomegalic inclusion disease (hepatosplenomegaly, jaundice, petechial rash, microcephaly, chorioretinitis, cerebral calcifications)	Deafness neurologic damage	Good hygiene, seronegative or filtered blood products
Herpes simplex	Subclinical genital herpes	Maternal viremia (rare) contact with genital or skin lesion or infected secretions	Microcephaly, vesicular skin lesions, localized or disseminated infection; encephalitis	Neurologic damage and recurrent skin lesions	Cesarean sections within 4–6 hours of ruptured membranes Acyclovir for mother in pregnancy and prophylactic to exposed neonate at birth

VZIG, varicella zoster immune globulin.

- Syphilis: Direct microscopic examination of wet mount, immunofluorescent staining, fluorescent treponemal antibody-absorption (FTA-ABS), treponema pallidum immobilization (TPI), treponema pallidum hemagglutination assay (TPHA), microhemagglutination (MHA)-TP, and treponema pallidum particle agglutination assay (TPPA)
- CMV: Direct IFA, enzyme immunoassays (EIA), and PCR of amniotic fluid
- HSV: Viral culture, ELISA, and PCR assay for HBV DNA
- Rubella: Reverse transcriptase (RT)-PCR for viral DNA.

Ultrasonographic Parameters of Fetal Infection

The following ultrasound markers may be found:

- Intrauterine growth restriction
- Ventricular dilation (most common finding in toxoplasma infections)
- Intracranial calcification
- Hepatomegaly
- Increased placental thickness
- Ascites
- Microcephaly
- Hydrops fetalis
- Echogenic bowel (seen in 22% patients with CMV infections)
- Limb abnormalities (in VZV infections)
- Increase in middle cerebral artery peak systolic velocity (MCA-PSV) resulting from fetal anemia
- Heart defects: atrial septal defect (ASD), ventricular septal defect (VSD), and patent ductus arteriosus (PDA) in rubella infections.

Note: These sequelae identified by ultrasound, are characteristically seen in severe CMV, toxoplasma, and syphilis infections while in HSV and varicella infections the ultrasound may be normal.

MANAGEMENT

- Adolescents and nonpregnant seronegative women for rubella IgG and varicella zoster to be offered vaccination and refrain from pregnancy for 1 month from vaccination
- Counseling of pregnant women and infected family members about the risk of affection and long-term neurological sequelae to the baby and maternal complications especially in patients with chicken pox and syphilis
- Counseling of partner to get himself investigated and treated for other sexually transmitted diseases if a woman has syphilis or HSV
- Offer termination of pregnancy, if fetal affection is severe
- Transfer patient to a tertiary care institute
- Preventative measures for patients at high risk for toxoplasmosis and CMV. Avoidance of intercourse in third trimester for HSV infection
- Institute therapy if seroconversion is recent to minimize fetal infection
  - *Toxoplasmosis*: Spiramycin 3 IU/day for 3 weeks every month if maternal infection is established. Pyrimethamine and sulfadiazine combination for fetal infection
  - *Syphilis*: Centers for Disease Control and Prevention recommendation for treatment of patients with syphilis in pregnancy
    - Primary disease or early latent (<1year): Benzathine penicillin G 2.4 million units intramuscularly (IM) in a single dose
    - Late Latent (>1 year) or unknown duration: Benzathine penicillin G 7.2 million units administered in three doses of 2.4 million units each week at 1 week interval
    - *Neurosyphilis*: Procaine penicillin 2.4 million units IM once daily plus probenecid, 500 mg orally QDS, for 10–14 days. In patients sensitive to penicillin desensitization in 3–4 days is recommended

- *Herpes simplex virus*: Acyclovir is given orally 200 mg five times a day for 7–14 days. Severe HSV: intravenously (IV) acyclovir 5–10 mg/kg/8 hourly for 2–7 days is administered
- *Cytomegalovirus*: Eradication of virus is beyond the scope of modern medicine. If the host is severely immunocompromized, ganciclovir will provide relief from chorioretinitis. It is given after 27-week gestation through umbilical vein 10 mg/day for 5 days followed by 15 mg/day for 3 days followed by 20 mg/day for 4 days
- *Rubella*: Patients developing thrombocytopenia or encephalitis may benefit from glucocorticoids or platelet transfusion
- *Varicella Zoster Virus*: Varicella zoster immunoglobulin (VZIG) to be administered to susceptible women within 48 hours of exposure to infection. Oral acyclovir may be given to reduce severity of maternal affection. Neonates to be given VZIG at birth

• Prior intimation to neonatologist of nature of TORCH infection so that prompt neonatal care can be instituted
• Mode of delivery should be vaginal unless obstetric indications arise for all infections, except in cases of HSV with active genital lesions.[12,13] In these cases, caesarean section at the onset of labor irrespective of the condition of membranes is advocated. Also, fetal HSV infection has been attributed to use of fetal scalp electrodes even in absence of active lesions. Hence, scalp electrodes should be avoided in HSV cases.

CONCLUSION

Pregnancy is associated with decreased maternal cell-mediated immunity. TORCH infections can pose a serious threat to the fetus and the newborn. Depending on gestational age, transplacental infection may give rise to asymptomatic to severe long-term sequelae in the children. The lack of specific treatment options against most of the infections imply, that prevention is the most important approach to disease containment. The development of vaccines and newer drugs hold the promise of reducing the incidence of fetal infection and disability in future.

REFERENCES

1. Klein J, Remington J. Current concepts in infections of the fetus and newborn. In: Infectious Diseases of the Fetus and Newborn Infant. Remington J, Klein J, editors. Saunders: Philadelphia, PA;2001. pp.1-24.
2. Rawston S. Treponema pallidum (Syphilis). In: Principles and Practice of Pediatric Infectious Diseases. Long S, Pickering L and Prober C, editors. Churchill-Livingston: New York; 2003. pp. 954-65.
3. Boyer KM. Toxoplasmosis: Current status of diagnosis, treatment and prevention. Semin Pediatr Infect Dis. 2000;11:165-71.
4. Griffiths PD. Strategies to prevent CMV infection in the neonate. Semin Neonatol. 2002;7(4):293-9.
5. Mellinger AK, Cragan JD, Atkinson WL, et al. High incidence of congenital rubella syndrome after a rubella outbreak. Pediatr Infect Dis J. 1995;14(7):573-8.
6. Brown ZA, Selke S, Zeh J, et al. The acquisition of herpes simplex virus during pregnancy. Its frequency and impact on pregnancy outcome. N Engl J Med. 1997;337(8):509-15.
7. Van der Zwer WC, Vandenbroucke-Grauls CM, van Elburg RM, et al. Neonatal antibody titers against varicella-zoster virus in relation to gestational age, birth weight, and maternal titer. Pediatrics. 2002:109(1):79-85.
8. RCOG Greentop Guideline No 17 Recurrent Miscarriage, Investigation and Treatment of Couples, May 2011
9. Candolfi E, Pastor RR, Filisetti D, et al. IgG avidity firms up the diagnosis of acute toxoplasmosis on the first serum sample in immunocompetent pregnant women. Diagn Microbial Infect Dis. 2007;58(1):83-88.
10. Foulon W, Naessens A, de Catte L, et al. Detection of congenital toxoplasmosis by chorionic villus sampling and early amniocentesis. Am J Obstet Gynecol. 1990;163(5 Pt 1):1511-3.
11. Morris DJ. Congenital cytomegalovirus infection. BMJ. 1987;295(6592):269-70.
12. Watts DH, Brown ZA, Noney D, et al. A double-blind randomized, placebo-controlled trial of acyclovir in late pregnancy for the reduction of herpes simplex virus shedding and cesarean delivery. Am J Obster Gynecol. 2003:188:836.
13. Moris DJ. Genital cytomegalovirus infection. BMJ. 1987;295: 269-70.

Medical Disorders

20

CHAPTER

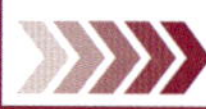

Sujata Misra, Sudhanshu Nanda

INTRODUCTION

Medical disorders in pregnancy encompasses a myriad of disorders, each with variable subtypes and symptoms, which is indeed very challenging. In an era poised to reduce maternal mortality, diagnosis and treatment of these disorders is mandatory. The disorders may be metabolic or infectious and include cardiovascular, respiratory, genitourinary, gastrointestinal, and hematopoietic system.

DIABETES MELLITUS

Gestational diabetes mellitus (DM) affects 3–15% of pregnancies and is associated with risks to both, the woman and the developing fetus. Miscarriage, preeclampsia, and preterm labor are more common in women with pregestational diabetes. In addition, diabetic retinopathy can worsen rapidly during pregnancy. Stillbirth, congenital malformations, macrosomia, birth injury, perinatal mortality, and postnatal adaptation problems (such as hypoglycemia) are some problems seen in the newborn.

Management

The management of diabetes in pregnancy includes a careful combination of diet, exercise, and insulin therapy.[1]

Preconception Care

Preconception care and tight glycemic control during the first trimester is beneficial both, to the mother and the fetus (Table 1).

TABLE 1: Preconception care in diabetes mellitus

Counseling	*Goal for glycemic management*	*Self-management skills are essential for attaining good glycemic control*
The importance of avoiding unplanned pregnancy should be an essential component of diabetes education from adolescence for women with diabetes	To obtain the lowest glycosylated hemoglobin test level possible without undue risk of hypoglycemia in expecting mothers, both in the preconception period and the first trimester	• Use of appropriate meal plan • Self-monitoring of blood glucose • Self-administration of insulin and adjustment of insulin doses • Treatment of hypoglycemia • Incorporate safe physical activity • Development of techniques to reduce stress and cope with the denial

Note: To prevent congenital malformations it is important to have a strict glycemic control prepregnancy and during the first trimester.

Insulin Requirement in Patients with Pregestational Diabetes

If near euglycemia had been achieved before conception and the prepregnancy insulin regimen incorporates two or more insulin injections a day, it may be suitable to achieve the near euglycemia necessary for a successful outcome of the pregnancy by:

- Using three injections of regular human insulin or rapid acting insulin analogs with each meal giving the patient more flexibility with regard to eating and exercise
- Preprandial regular or rapid-acting insulin analogs can be particularly helpful during the first trimester, when nausea and anorexia are common
- Controlling the fasting plasma glucose concentration requires predinner or bedtime neutral protamine Hagedorn (NPH) insulin.

Note: Short-acting human insulin should be administered 30 minute prior to meal to counter the slowness at the onset of action of human insulin. On the other hand, the new rapid-acting insulin analogs, when administered with meals start acting within 10–15 min. Therefore, short-acting insulin analogs are effective in controlling the postprandial peak.

Adjusting insulin doses is simpler with self monitoring of blood glucose (SMBG) four times a day because each component of the insulin regimen affects only one SMBG value. Monitoring before meals and 2 hours after a meal is recommended (Table 2).

TABLE 2: Management of diabetes

Medical nutrition therapy (MNT)	*Insulin treatment*	*Target blood glucose levels*
For women with • With normal body weight the diet is 30–35 kcal/kg of actual weight • With less than 90% of desirable body weight it is 35–40 kcal/kg • With more than 120% of desirable body weight it is 24 kcal/kg *Caloric composition* • 40–50%: Complex and high-fiber carbohydrates • 20%: Protein • 30–40%: Unsaturated fats *Calorie distribution* • 10–20% at breakfast • 20–30% at lunch • 30–40% at dinner • 30% with snacks, especially a bedtime snack to reduce nocturnal hypoglycemia	*Indication for insulin* • Insulin is essential if diet control and exercise fail to achieve euglycemia[3] • If the fasting plasma glucose concentration on the OGTT is >120 mg/dL *Dose* The initial dose of NPH insulin could be as low as 4 units and the dose of insulin can be adjusted on follow-up Combination of short-acting insulin and intermediate-acting insulin in the morning and evening • If prelunch blood sugar is high: Regular insulin is usually necessary in the morning to handle the postbreakfast hyperglycemia, as there is a lag period before the intermediate-acting insulin begins to work. The above regimen of regular and intermediate acting insulin in the morning controls hyperglycemia in most cases • If the postdinner blood sugar is high: A small dose of regular insulin is necessary before dinner in addition to the regular and intermediate acting insulin given in the morning	Maintenance of mean blood glucose level <105 mg/dL is ideal for good fetal outcome.[4] Perinatal mortality is proportional to maternal blood glucose level during the last weeks of pregnancy.[5]

Contd...

Contd...

Medical nutrition therapy (MNT)	*Insulin treatment*	*Target blood glucose levels*
	• If FBS is high: Combination of regular-and intermediate-acting insulin before dinner may be necessary • If the patient continues to have fasting hyperglycemia: The intermediate-acting insulin has to be given at bedtime instead of pre-dinner and the dose has to be individualized. Split-mixed dosage: This is referring to the combination of short and intermediate acting insulin being split • Two-thirds of total dose: In the morning • One-third: In the evening (for each combination) • One-third dose should be regular insulin • Two-thirds should be intermediate-acting	

OGTT, oral glucose tolerance test; NPH, neutral protamine Hagedorn; FBS, fasting blood sugar.

Note:
- In pregnant women with type I diabetes, the requirement of insulin may fall during the early part of the first trimester due to increased insulin sensitivity
- Preprandial regular or rapid-acting insulin analogs can be particularly helpful during the first trimester, when nausea and anorexia are common.

During the first trimester, there is no difference in the insulin requirement between type 1 and type 2 subjects. However, the insulin requirement significantly increases during the second trimester and third trimester (10% increase for patients with type 1 DM as compared to 33–40% in those with type 2 DM) owing to the increased concentration of circulating placental hormones.[2]

Newer Insulin Analogs in Pregnancy

The rapid-acting analog insulins are useful in pregnancy complicated by diabetes, since they are more able to reduce postprandial hyperglycemia with respect to regular insulin. Studies in pregnancy are limited to lispro and aspart (category "B"), both demonstrating clinical effectiveness, with no evidence of teratogenesis, low antigenicity, and placental transport of autoantibodies similar to human regular insulin. Use of long-acting glargine insulin (category "C") in pregnancy awaits randomized controlled trials to confirm its safety and efficacy in pregnancy.[6]

Oral Hypoglycemic Agents

The oral hypoglycemic agents—glibenclamide and metformin are currently classified by the Food and Drug Administration (FDA) as Category B drugs for use in pregnancy.[7,8] No adverse neonatal outcome has been reported with these drugs and effects were comparable to insulin.[9-12]

CHRONIC HYPERTENSION

Chronic hypertension is defined as blood pressure exceeding 140/90 mmHg before pregnancy or prior to 20 weeks' gestation. It complicates at least 5% of all pregnancies. Although the primary risk of chronic hypertension in pregnancy is development of superimposed preeclampsia later in pregnancy, there is no evidence to suggest that pharmacologic treatment of mild hypertension reduces the incidence of pre-eclampsia in this population.

Goal of Treatment: The goal of pharmacologic treatment should be a diastolic blood pressure (DBP) of less than 100–105 mmHg and an systolic blood pressure (SBP) less than 160 mmHg. Women with pre-existing end-organ damage from chronic hypertension should have a lower threshold for starting antihypertensive medication (i.e., >139/89) and a lower target blood pressure (<140/90).

Three treatment options are available in cases of mild chronic hypertension once pregnancy is detected.

1. Antihypertensive medication may be withheld or discontinued, with subsequent close observation of blood pressure. As blood pressure drops during normal pregnancy and no data support the use of medication in patients with blood pressures less than 160/100 mmHg, the authors recommend this option most often write.
2. If a woman is on pharmacologic treatment with an agent not recommended for use in pregnancy, she may be switched to an alternative antihypertensive agent preferred for use in pregnancy.
3. If a woman is on pharmacologic treatment with an agent acceptable for use in pregnancy, she may continue her current antihypertensive therapy.

Note: Methyldopa or nifedipine are the preferred antihypertensive medications in the first trimester of pregnancy.

Women with hypertension in pregnancy should be monitored for the development of worsening hypertension and/or the development of superimposed preeclampsia (the risk being approximately 25%)

THYROID DISORDERS

Thyroid disorders, both hypothyroidism and hyperthyroidism have been listed in table 3.

Note: Propylthiouracil should be used when antithyroid drug therapy is started during the first trimester.

TABLE 3: Hypothyroidism and hyperthyroidism in pregnancy

	Hyperthyroidism	*Hypothyroidism*
Common cause	Graves' disease, 80–85%	• Hashimoto's thyroiditis-autoimmune disorder • Inadequate treatment of a pre-existing hypothyroidism • Over treatment of a hyperthyroid woman with antithyroid medications
Incidence	1 in 1,500 pregnant patients	Approximately, 2.5% of women will have a slightly elevated thyroid stimulating hormone (TSH) of greater than 6 and 0.4% will have a TSH greater than 10 during pregnancy
Fetal/ neonatal issues	• Fetal tachycardia • Small for gestational age babies • Prematurity • Stillbirths • Congenital malformations	• Severe cognitive abnormalities • Neurological abnormalities Developmental abnormalities
Drug therapy	• *Propylthiouracil* should be used when antithyroid drug therapy is started during the first trimester • *Methimazole* should be used when antithyroid drug therapy is started after the first trimester	*Levothyroxine* Thyroid function tests should be checked approximately every 6–8 weeks during pregnancy to ensure that the woman has normal thyroid function throughout pregnancy

Propylthiouracil (PTU) generally has been preferred in pregnancy because of concerns about rare but well-documented teratogenicity associated with methimazole, namely, aplasia cutis and choanal or esophageal atresia. However, recent concerns about rare but potentially fatal PTU hepatotoxicity have led to a re-examination of the role of PTU in the management of hyperthyroidism in pregnancy, and it is recommended that PTU be reserved for patients who are in their first trimester of pregnancy, or who are allergic to or intolerant of methimazole.

ANEMIA

Anemia increases the maternal morbidity, fetal and neonatal mortality, and morbidity significantly.

Maternal Risks

They include poor weight gain, preterm labor, pregnancy induced hypertension (PIH), placenta previa, accidental hemorrhage, eclampsia, premature rupture of membrane (PROM), etc.

Fetal and Neonatal Complications

They include prematurity, low birth weight, poor Apgar score, fetal distress, and neonatal distress.

Any woman with anemia must be given folic acid to prevent neural tube defects. Nutritional anemia should be corrected by oral/parenteral replaced of iron and vitamin B12.

Note: Babies whose mothers had anemia during their first trimester experienced higher rates of cardiovascular morbidities and mortalities in their adult lives.

SICKLE CELL ANEMIA

Prenatal Care

The prenatal assessment visit allows counseling and an outline of care for the duration of the pregnancy. If conception accidentally occurs when women is taking hydroxyurea, the couple should be told that a paucity of information exists on which to determine the effect of hydroxyurea on the fetus. The primary focus is to identify maternal risks for low birth weight, preterm delivery, and genetic risks for fetal abnormalities. A baseline hemoglobin concentration of 6–8 g/dL is typical for patients with sickle cell disease (SCD) along with a high reticulocyte count and sickle cells on the peripheral smear.

Note: Return visits are recommended 2 weeks after the initial visit. Pregnant women with SCD should be observed closely if blood pressure rises above 125/75 mmHg.

Indications for Blood Transfusion during Pregnancy with Sickle Cell Disease

The role of prophylactic transfusions in pregnancy is controversial.[13,14] Avoid routine prophylactic transfusions for uncomplicated pregnancies but consider transfusions for women who have complications, such as preeclampsia, severe anemia, or increasing frequency of pain crisis. Women who have had previous pregnancy losses or who have multiple gestation may benefit from the early use of transfusions to maintain the hemoglobin level, above 9 g/dL.

THALASSEMIA

Thalassemia is due to quantitative disorders of globin chain production that affects α-chain or the β-chain of the hemoglobin molecule. Heterozygous individuals carry the thalassemia trait and present with anemia. Women who have thalassemia trait should be identified before pregnancy so that they can be alerted to the one in four chance of having a hydropic fetus if their partner carries the same trait. Techniques of antenatal diagnosis should be discussed. In hemoglobin H disease (deletion of 3 α-globin gene) daily folate supplementation is required and transfusion may be needed.

β-Thalassemia

Partners of women with β-thalassemia need antenatal screening to determine the risk of major hemoglobinopathy. The transfusion regimen must be monitored carefully. Iron chelation therapy must be reviewed. Oral and intravenous iron supplementation is contraindicated. Assessment of liver, heart, and endocrine system should be carried out on follow-up.

Recommendation: With thalassemia ideally, iron status is optimized prepregnancy and chelation is discontinued periconceptionaly, at least for the first trimester.

THROMBOCYTOPENIA

Thrombocytopenia is encountered in 7–8% of all pregnancies.

Immune Thrombocytopenic Purpura

It is the most common cause of thrombocytopenia in first trimester. Five characteristics of immune thrombocytopenic purpura (ITP) make the diagnosis likely:

1. Moderate thrombocytopenia (50,000–100,000/μL).
2. A preconception or early gestation platelet count that is less than 100,000/μL.
3. Normal to increased megakaryocyte levels as determined by bone marrow biopsy.
4. Exclusion of other systemic disorders or use of drugs that might be associated with decreasing platelet counts.
5. An absence of splenomegaly.

The mother is at risk for spontaneous hemorrhage, particularly if the platelet count drops to less than 20,000/μL. The maternal immunoglobulin G (IgG) will cross the placenta and could cause fetal thrombocytopenia.

Note: A mother in the first or early second trimester who has thrombocytopenia will have either ITP or gestational thrombocytopenia although the latter is much more common in later gestation.

Patients with ITP require special considerations during their prenatal care. Patients should avoid nonsteroidal anti-inflammatory agents, aspirin, and trauma.

Patients with platelet counts greater than 30,000/μL and no bleeding generally do not require treatment. First line of therapy for ITP in pregnant patients should be corticosteroids. However, increased incidence of PIH, gestational diabetes, and premature rupture of the fetal membranes has been seen with steroids. High-dose (2 g/kg) intravenous immunoglobulin (IVIg) is suggested as an alternative first-line therapy for pregnancy-associated ITP. Since responses to IVIg are often transient, multiple courses of therapy during gestation may be required, at significant expense and patient inconvenience. IVIg should be strongly considered only when more than 10 mg/day of prednisone is required to maintain the maternal platelet count above 30,000/μL. Intravenous anti-D has also been used with success. Cytotoxic agents are avoided in pregnancy.

HEART DISEASES

Frequency of detection of heart disease among pregnant women fluctuates from 0,4% to 4.7%. The rheumatic heart diseases compound 75–90% of all lesions of the heart in pregnant women, most common being mitral insufficiency or stenosis. Cardiocirculatory changes which can significantly impact underlying cardiac disease begin early in pregnancy (within the first 5–8 weeks).

Regardless of the cardiac lesion, maternal outcome generally depends on the functional class of the patient. Most patients with pregnancy and valvular heart disease can be managed medically. Recommendations for patients with volume overload lesions include restricted physical activity, salt restriction, and diuretics. Diuretics are given cautiously avoiding rigorous volume depletion and uteroplacental hypoperfusion. Reassurance and the use of tranquilizers and sedatives are appropriate. Anemia, infections and arrhythmias should be addressed promptly as they can be very detrimental to the cardiac patient. Digoxin, beta blockers, adenosine, sotalol, lidocaine, and procainamide can be safely used for the treatment of supraventricular arrhythmias during pregnancy. Amiodarone is best avoided because of the risk of fetal hypothyroidism. Angiotensin converting enzyme inhibitors and angiotensin receptor blockers are contraindicated during pregnancy because of the risks of urogenital defects, intrauterine growth retardation, and fetal death.

Open Heart Surgery

The current recommendation for open heart surgery during pregnancy includes:

- Avoidance of open heart surgery, if at all possible, during the first trimester. The risk of teratogenesis due to drug administration and possibly cardiopulmonary bypass during the first trimester of pregnancy is always present, and any surgical procedure should be avoided during this time
- Use of high-flow, high-pressure, and normothermic bypass during the procedure
- Fetal heart and uterine monitoring to allow adjustments to the blood flow and pharmacological manipulations to ensure adequate placental perfusion
- If the fetus is more than 28 weeks of gestational age, to opt for cesarean section concurrently just prior to the cardiac operation.

ASTHMA

Asthma treatment is organized around assessment and monitoring of asthma, including objective measures of pulmonary function, control of factors contributing to asthma severity, patient education, and a stepwise approach to pharmacologic therapy.

Mild Intermittent Asthma

Short-acting bronchodilators, particularly short-acting inhaled beta 2-agonists, are recommended as quick relief medication for treating symptoms as needed in patients with intermittent asthma.

Note: Albuterol is the preferred short-acting inhaled beta 2-agonist because it has an excellent safety profile during pregnancy.

Persistent Asthma

The preferred treatment for persistent asthma is daily low dose inhaled corticosteroid which is considered safe in pregnancy.[15] Published data are minimal on using leukotriene receptor antagonists during pregnancy.

Note: Budesonide is the preferred inhaled corticosteroid

If asthma still persists two preferred treatment options are noted: either a combination of low dose inhaled corticosteroid and a long-acting inhaled beta 2-agonist, or increasing the dose of inhaled corticosteroid to the medium dose range. If increasing the inhaled corticosteroid dose to a high-dose range is insufficient to manage asthma symptoms, then the addition of systemic corticosteroid is warranted; although the data are uncertain about some risks of oral corticosteroids during pregnancy, severe uncontrolled asthma poses a definite risk to the mother and fetus.

Asthma Exacerbations during Pregnancy

High-dose short-acting inhaled beta 2-agonist by nebulization every 20 minutes or continuously for 1 hour along with inhaled ipratropium bromide, oxygen (O) to achieve O_2 saturation more than 95% and oral/systemic corticosteroid.

SYSTEMIC LUPUS ERYTHEMATOSUS

Systemic lupus erythematosus (SLE) is one of the most common autoimmune disorders that affect women during their childbearing years. None of the medications used in the treatment of SLE is absolutely safe during pregnancy. Hence, use of medications should be decided after careful assessment of the risks and benefits in consultation with the patient. During the first trimester, most of the drugs should be avoided. In the absence of any historical features of antiphospholipid syndrome (recurrent pregnancy loss, venous, or arterial thromboembolism), patients with lupus anticoagulant and/or high levels of anticardiolipin antibodies should receive low-dose aspirin and heparin.

TUBERCULOSIS

The commonly used medicines for tuberculosis are perfectly safe in pregnancy for the mother and the baby. Although anti-TB drugs can cross the placenta and reach the baby, these drugs do not have an adverse effect on the fetus.[16] The treatment for pregnant women is the same as for nonpregnant women. This is usually a combination of four drugs: (1) Isoniazid, (2) Rifampicin, (3) Pyrazinamide, and (4) Ethambutol later tapered to two drugs. Streptomycin should be avoided in pregnancy.

Precautions

- An adequate intake of pyridoxine with isoniazid during the entire period of therapy
- Prophylactic vitamin K administration to baby at birth for preventing hemorrhagic disease of the newborn.

Medical disorders in pregnancy, especially in first trimester need to be dealt with carefully so as to prevent effects on the developing fetus, either through drugs given to treat the condition or because of the condition itself.

REFERENCES

1. Franz MJ, Bantle JP, Beebe CA, et al. Evidence-based nutrition principles and recommendations for the treatment and prevention of diabetes and related complications. Diabetes Care. 2003;26 (Suppl 1):S51-61.
2. Langer O, Anyaegbunam A, Brustman L, et al. Pregestational diabetes: insulin requirements throughout pregnancy. Am J Obstet Gynecol. 1988;159(3):616-21.
3. Jovanovic-Peterson L. The diagnosis and management of gestational diabetes mellitus. Clin Diabetes. 1995;13:32.
4. Langer O, Levy J, Brustman L, et al. Glycemic control in gestational diabetes mellitus: how tight is tight enough: small for gestational age versus large for gestational age? Am J Obstet Gynecol. 1989;161(3):646-53.
5. Karlsson K, Kjellmer I. The outcome of diabetic pregnancies in relationship to the mother's blood sugar level. Am J Obstet Gynecol. 1972;112(2):213-20.
6. Torlone E, Di Cianni G, Mannino D, et al. Insulin analogs and pregnancy: an update. Acta Diabetol. 2009;46(3):163-72.
7. Notelovitz M. Sulphonylurea therapy in the treatment of the pregnant diabetic. S Afr Med J. 1971;45(9):226-9.
8. Zucker P, Simon G. Prolonged symptomatic neonatal hypoglycemia associated with maternal chlorpropamide therapy. Pediatrics. 1968;42(5):824-5.
9. Langer O, Conway DL, Berkus MD, et al. A comparison of glyburide and insulin in women with gestational diabetes mellitus. N Engl J Med. 2000;343(16):1134-8.
10. Kremer CJ, Duff P. Glyburide for the treatment of gestational diabetes. Am J Obstet Gynecol. 2004;190(5):1438-9.
11. Glueck CJ, Goldenberg N, Wang P, et al. Metformin during pregnancy reduces insulin, insulin resistance, insulin secretion, weight, testosterone and development of gestational diabetes: prospective longitudinal assessment of women with polycystic ovary syndrome from preconception throughout pregnancy. Hum Reprod. 2004;19:510-21.
12. Glueck CJ, Goldenberg N, Pranikoff J, et al. Height, weight, and motor-social development during the first 18 months of life in 126 infants born to 109 mothers with polycystic ovary syndrome who conceived on and continued metformin through pregnancy. Hum Reprod. 2004;19:1323-30.
13. Koshy M, Burd L, Wallace D, et al. Prophylactic red cell transfusion in pregnant patients with sickle cell disease. A randomized cooperative study. N Engl J Med. 1988;319(22):1447-52.
14. Tuck SM, James CE, Brewster EM, et al. Prophylactic blood transfusion in maternal sickle cell syndromes. Br J Obstet Gynaecol. 1987;94(2):121-5.
15. EPR-2.NAEPP Expert Panel Report 2. Guidelines for the Diagnosis and Treatment of Asthma. NIH Publication No.97-4051. Bethesda, MD: U.S. Department of Health and Human Services; National Institutes of Health; National Heart, Lung, and Blood Institute, 1997. [online] Available from: http://www.nhlbi.nih.gov/guidelines/ asthma/asthgdln.htm. [Accessed November, 2013].
16. Anderson G.D. Tuberculosis in pregnancy. Semin Perinatol. 1997;21(4):328-35.

Vaginal Discharge

21

CHAPTER

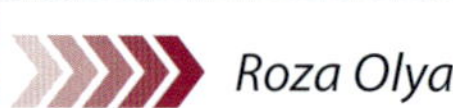

Roza Olyai

INTRODUCTION

Vaginal discharge can be normal in pregnancy and is physiological. However, vaginal thrush is common in pregnancy and bacterial vaginosis may lead to adverse pregnancy outcome. It is imperative that normal vaginal discharge is differentiated from abnormal vaginal discharge.

PHYSIOLOGICAL DISCHARGE

Physiologic vaginal discharge in pregnancy is colorless or white, non irritating, and odorless or has mild odor and is noninfective in nature with no sequelae. This physiologic discharge is formed by mucoid endocervical secretions in combination with sloughing epithelial cells, normal bacteria, and vaginal transudate. It can sometimes, be malodorous and accompanied by irritative symptoms.

The pH of the normal vaginal secretions is 4.0–4.5. The acidic environment is hostile to growth of pathogens and inhibits adherence of bacteria to vaginal squamous epithelial cells. Microscopic examination reveals a predominance of squamous cells and rare polymorphonuclear leukocytes.

Under the influence of estrogen, the normal vaginal epithelium cornifies and produces glycogen. This acts as a substrate for lactobacilli, thereby protecting women against infection from a number of pathogens. On the other hand, the endocervix is lined with columnar epithelium and is more susceptible to infection with certain pathogenic organisms. These differences explain, in part, why cervicitis occurs in the absence of vaginitis and vice versa.

There is hypertrophy of the vaginal epithelium, during pregnancy leading to an increased number of glycogen-containing cells, and these cells are shed into the vagina. Pregnancy may also predispose women to infective conditions, such as candida vulvovaginitis.

NORMAL FLORA

The number of bacteria recoverable from the lower female genital tract is relatively staggering. The isolation of a given bacteria does not necessarily confer functional significance to it. Table 1 shows the list of aerobic and anaerobic bacteria isolated from the lower female genital tract.[1]

Note: The microbial load of a given bacteria appears to govern the relative risk of asymptomatic versus symptomatic infection.

TABLE 1: Bacteria in female lower genital tract

Aerobes	*Anaerobes*
Gram-positive	• *Bacteroides* species
• Gram-positive rods	• *B. bivius*
○ Diphtheroids	• *B. fragilis*
○ Lactobacilli	• *B. melaninogenicus*
• Gram-positive cocci	• *Clostridium* species
○ *Staphylococcus aureus*	○ *C. perfringens*
○ *Staphylococcus epidermidis*	• *Eubacterium* species
○ Streptococcus species	• *Fusobacterium* species
– Alpha-hemolytic	• *Gaffkya* species
– Beta-hemolytic	• *Lactobacillus* species
– Nonhemolytic	• *Peptococcus* species
– Group D	
Gram-negative rods	
• *Escherichia coli*	
• *Klebsiella* and *Enterobacter* species	
• *Proteus* species	
• *Pseudomonas* species	

ABNORMAL DISCHARGE

Abnormal vaginal discharge may be green, yellow, brown, or red in color with foul smelling odor, pruritus, irritation, dysuria, or dyspareunia depending on the type of infection.[2] Infective vaginal discharge in a pregnant lady poses greater risk in the transmission of human immune deficient virus (HIV), and other complications, such as abortion, prematurity, and premature rupture of membranes.[3]

CAUSES

The causes of vaginal discharge in pregnancy are similar to those in nonpregnant state (Box 1).

Box 1: Causes of vaginal discharge in pregnancy

- Physiological discharge of pregnancy
- Sexually transmitted infections
  - *Trichomonas vaginalis*
  - *Chlamydia trachomatis*
  - *Neisseria gonorrhoeae*
  - Herpes simplex infection
  - Human papilloma virus
  - Human immunodeficiency virus
- Other infections
  - *Candida* species vulvovaginitis
  - Bacterial vaginosis
  - Toxic shock syndrome
- Neoplasms
  - Cervical polyps
  - Cervical ectropian
- Iatrogenic
  - Drug induced
  - Foreign bodies

DIFFERENTIAL DIAGNOSIS

It is important to note the type of discharge and the possible diagnosis, so that the appropriate treatment is given. Frequently when the discharge is physiologic, all the patient needs is reassurance. Table 2 lists the clinical features of the three common infections and their clinical manifestations, commonly encountered in clinical practice.[4]

INVESTIGATIONS

The main approach to a patient with vaginal discharge in pregnancy is by clinical history and examination. Laboratory investigations are the most useful way of diagnosing infective causes of vaginal discharge, as many a times, classical clinical presentation may not be there, and these infections are asymptomatic. Table 3 shows the laboratory tests done for the diagnosis of the infections commonly encountered.[4]

TABLE 2: Clinical features of vaginal infections

	Bacterial vaginosis	*Candidiasis*	*Trichomoniasis*
Symptoms	• Thin discharge • Offensive or fishy odor • No itching	• Thick and yellow • Nonoffensive • Vulval itch or soreness • Superficial dyspareunia • External dysuria	• Scanty to profuse or frothy yellow discharge • Offensive • Vulval itch • External dysuria • Low abdominal pain
Signs	Discharge coating vagina and vestibule	Normal findings or vulval erythema, edema, fissuring satellite lesions	Vulvitis and vaginitis, so-called strawberry cervix satellite lesions (uncommon 2%)

TABLE 3: Laboratory tests for vaginal discharge

Specimen	*Investigation*	*Infection detected*
High vaginal swab from lateral wall	Microscopy and Gram staining	Bacterial vaginosis Amsel's criteria (3/4) • White discharge • pH > 4.5 • Fishy odor on addition of potassium hydrooxide (KOH) to the discharge • Clue cells (vaginal epithelial)
	Wet mount with 10% KOH and saline	*Candida* spores and pseudohyphae cells surrounded by bacteria
	Saline wet microscopy	*Trichomonas vaginalis* (direct visualization of flagellate protozoa)
	Culture	*Neisseria gonorrhoeae* (chocolate agar) *Candida* (Sabouraud's medium) if microscopy inconclusive

Implications of These Infections and Their Management

There is increasing evidence that *Trichomonas vaginalis* (TV) infection may be associated with preterm delivery and low birth weight.[5-7] There is no indication for routine screening for TV in pregnancy. Bacterial vaginosis is associated with late miscarriage, chorioamnionitis, preterm labor, premature rupture of membranes, low birth weight, and postpartum endometritis. Bacterial vaginosis and vaginal trichomoniasis have been implicated with an increased risk of transmission of HIV. The presence of vulvovaginal candidiasis may be suggestive of diabetes (overt or gestational). Table 4 shows the implications and the treatment of the three commonly encountered infections.

Note: Treatment with topical azoles is recommended in pregnancy for candidiasis, as stated above, but longer duration of treatment (7 days) may be required. Oral regimens are avoided due to potential teratogenicity.[7,8]

TABLE 4: Complications and treatment of vaginitis

	Bacterial vaginosis	*Candidiasis*	*Trichomoniasis*
Clinical implication and complications	• Chorioamnionitis • Preterm labor • Premature rupture of membranes • Low birth weight • Postpartum endometritis • Increased risk of transmission of HIV	May be suggestive of overt or gestational diabetes mellitus	Increased risk of transmission of HIV
Treatment	• Oral metronidazole 400 mg three times a day for 5 days • Metronidazole vaginal gel 5 g every night for 5 nights • Metronidazole vaginal gel 5 g every night for 5 nights • Oral clindamycin 300 mg twice daily for 7 days • Clindamycin cream for 3 days	Clotrimazole pessary: • Single dose 500 mg • 200 mg every night for 3 days or • 100 mg every night for 6 days	• Metronidazole: 400 mg three times a day for 5–7 days • Tinidazole: 500 mg BD for 5–7 days

HIV, human immunodeficiency virus; BD, twice a day.

PRACTICE POINTS

- Candidiasis, bacterial vaginosis, and trichomoniasis are the three commonly encountered infections in pregnancy
- Important to differentiate physiological discharge from pathological discharge, simply by checking the pH of the discharge. If it is less than 4, consider it a physiologic discharge which only needs reassurance
- Impact of bacterial vaginosis in pregnancy may lead to—chorioamnionitis, preterm labor, premature rupture of membranes, low birth weight, postpartum endometritis, and increased risk of transmission of HIV
- Trichomoniasis and bacterial vaginosis—increased risk of transmission of HIV
- Candidiasis in pregnancy should be given vaginal azole regimens and may require up to 7 days treatment
- Pregnant women with bacterial vaginosis should be treated as nonpregnant women.

Vaginal discharge in pregnancy is a common complaint and must be diagnosed accurately for correct treatment.

REFERENCES

1. Larsen B. Microbiology of the female genital tract. In: Pastorck J editor. Obstetric and Gynecologic Infectious Disease. New York: Raven Press;1994. pp.11-25.
2. Osoba AO, Onifade O. Venereal disease among pregnant women in Nigeria. W Afr Med J. 1993;22:23-25.
3. Joint United Nations Program on HIV/AIDS (2003).AIDS epidemic update. Geneva.
4. Royal College of Obstetricians & Gynaecologists; British Association for Sexual Health and HIV. The management of women of reproductive age attending non-genitourinary medicine settings complaining of vaginal Discharge. J Fam Plann Reprod Health Care. 2006;32(1):33-42.
5. Saurina GR, McCormack WM. Trichomoniasis in pregnancy. Sex Transm Dis. 1997;24(6):361-2.
6. Cotch MF, Pastorek JG 2nd, Nugent RP, et al. Trichomonas vaginalis associated with low birth weight and preterm delivery. The Vaginal Infections and Prematurity Study Group. Sex Transm Dis. 1997;24(6):353-60.
7. Clinical Effectiveness Group (Association for Genitourinary Medicine and the Medical Society for the Study of Venereal Diseases). (2001). National Guideline for the management of Bacterial Vaginosis. [online] Available from: www.bashh.org/guidelines/2002/bv_0601. [Accessed November, 2013].
8. Department of Health. (2004). PRODIGY Guidance–Candida–femalegenital. [online] Available from www.prodigy.nhs.uk/guidance.asp. [Accessed November, 2013].

Breast Diseases

22

CHAPTER

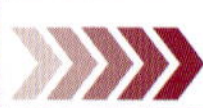

Madhuri Patel, Rahul Chauhan

INTRODUCTION

Pregnancy causes unique physiological changes in the mammary glands in response to hormonal stimulation. Most of the benign lesions seen in breast during pregnancy are usually same as those in nonpregnant women. However, some breast disorders are unique to pregnancy. Although most disorders related to pregnancy are benign, pregnancy associated breast carcinoma (PABC) represents up to 3% of all breast malignancies.

PHYSIOLOGICAL CHANGES OF BREAST DURING FIRST TRIMESTER OF PREGNANCY

Early in the second month of the first trimester of pregnancy, increase in size of breasts begins due to increase in circulating hormones estrogen, progesterone, and prolactin. This initial period of change occurs under estrogenic influence and is characterized by marked ductular sprouting with some branching and discrete lobular growth, simultaneous involution of the fibro fatty stroma and an increase in glandular vascularity, often accompanied by infiltration by mononuclear cells (Fig 1). Early in pregnancy, the colostrum is usually thick and yellow. As delivery approaches, it turns pale and nearly colorless.[1]

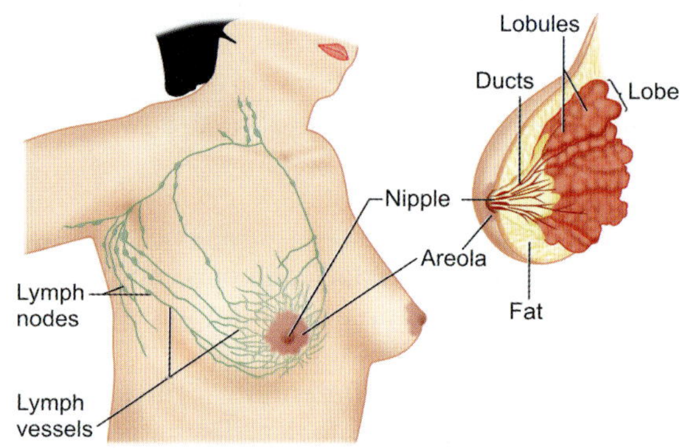

FIGURE 1 Changes in breast during pregnancy.

IMAGING OF BREAST IN PREGNANCY

Ultrasound

Ultrasound is used before mammography to evaluate a palpable mass. Ultrasound can accurately diagnose a lump with cyst or a solid mass, but is much less accurate at distinguishing between benign and cancerous lesions.[2]

Mammograms

Mammography during pregnancy may be considered for women with signs or symptoms, or ultrasound suspicious of a breast cancer. The gland appears very dense, heterogeneously coarse, nodular, and confluent with a marked decrease in adipose tissue and a prominent ductal pattern. Small studies have found that mammography poses little to no harm to the fetus during pregnancy if a lead shield is placed on the abdomen to block any possible radiation scatter.[3]

Note: The sensitivity of mammography in pregnant and lactating women is decreased due to increased parenchymal density. Instead, ultrasonography becomes the most appropriate radiologic method for evaluating breast masses.

Magnetic Resonance Imaging

Magnetic resonance imaging (MRI) is indicated in breast lumps in pregnant women having a suspicion of cancer on mammography. MRI could play an important role in the differential diagnosis of pregnancy-related breast lumps, particularly during puerperium, thus avoiding unnecessary surgical biopsies. Until more data are available, the use of MRI during pregnancy should be carefully planned in selected case.[2-4]

EFFECT OF PREGNANCY ON DISEASES PRE-EXISTING IN BREAST

Most of the breast tumors diagnosed during pregnancy are pre-existing but are manifested during this time due to changes or growth of the tumor.

Fibroadenoma

Fibroadenoma is one of the most common tumors of pregnancy and pregnancy may cause growth, infarction, and secretory hyperplasia in these tumors. The changes are discussed below.

Growth of Fibroadenoma

Fibroadenoma is a hormone sensitive tumor most commonly found during pregnancy or lactation. The increased hormone levels associated with pregnancy and lactation can induce tumor growth. Hence, existing or unknown fibroadenomas may be discovered during pregnancy. The benign radiologic appearance of the fibroadenoma during pregnancy is similar to its appearance in a nonpregnant women. However, in some of the pregnant women, ultrasound reveals a fibroadenoma with a prominent ductal pattern and proliferative changes under hormonal stimulation, leading to manifestations resembling those of complex fibroadenomas (Fig. 2A) and cyst formation (Fig. 2B). Cytological analysis and results may be suspicious because of several normal physiologic changes in cellularity during pregnancy and lactation. Suspicious finding on cytology should be confirmed on core biopsy.

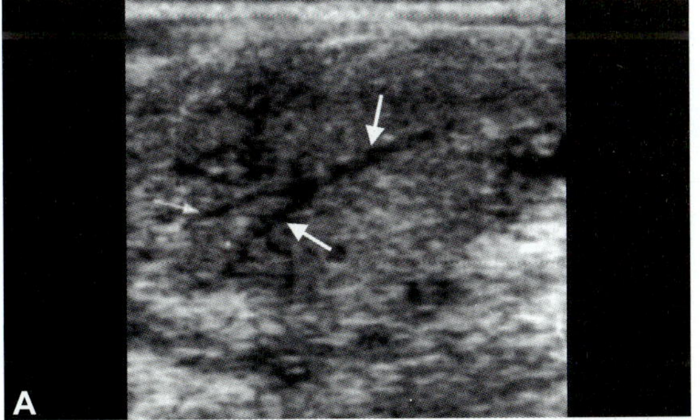

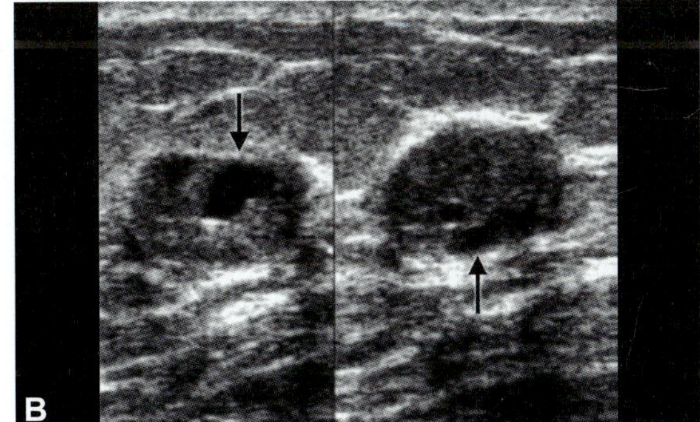

FIGURE 2 **A,** Complex fibroadenoma; **B,** Cyst formation in fibroadenoma.

Infarction in Fibroadenoma

Fibroadenomas and lactating adenomas can develop foci of infarction during pregnancy. This phenomenon is usually detected in the third trimester or after delivery, and is rare earlier. It can be clinically suspected if sudden pain occurs in a previously painless fibroadenoma. Intravascular thrombosis has been suggested as a causative factor. The radiological features of fibroadenomas with infarction show more lobulated margins, a heterogeneous echotexture, and acoustic shadowing. If large infarcts occur, the tumor may show suspicious findings requiring histological analysis on core biopsy.

Secretory Hyperplasia or Lactational Change in Fibroadenoma

Secretory hyperplasia sometimes develops in fibroadenomas during pregnancy due to the epithelial hormone-sensitive component of the tumor responding to the gravid hormonal stimulation in a similar way as occurs in the mammary parenchyma. If the tumor is allowed to remain in the breast or is not detected until after delivery, it will be classified as a fibroadenoma with lactational change. Milk may be extracted at fine needle aspiration when fibroadenomas demonstrate lactational changes. These fibroadenomas with secretory hyperplasia may change in appearance on ultrasound, showing discrete heterogeneity in their echotexture with hyperechogenic areas, dilated ducts, and cysts, thereby, resembling complex fibroadenomas. Microcalcifications may be found at mammography, making fibroadenomas with secretory hyperplasia more conspicuous.[5-7]

BENIGN DISEASES CLOSELY RELATED TO PHYSIOLOGICAL CHANGE

Gestational and Secretory Hyperplasia

Usually gestational hyperplasia is related to pregnancy and secretory hyperplasia is related to lactation. Two different mammographic manifestations can coexist, round punctate calcifications represent hyperplasia in the lobular acini, whereas linear calcifications correspond to ductal hyperplasia. Microcalcifications secondary to gestational or secretory hyperplasia must be distinguished clinically from a different entity known as pregnancy like hyperplasia or pseudo-lactational hyperplasia, which manifests with the same radiological and pathological findings in nonpregnant and nonlactating women (Fig. 3A), Malignant potentiality has not been described in secretory or lactational hyperplasia.

Spontaneous Bloody Nipple Discharge

Spontaneous bloody nipple discharge is an uncommon clinical condition during pregnancy and lactation. During the third trimester of pregnancy, proliferative changes within the ducts of the breasts may lead to bloody discharge from the nipple. This occurs when proliferative spurs of epithelium that extend into the ducts are traumatized, resulting in bleeding. Clinical follow-up is advised if no pathologic results are found and physical and ultrasound examinations are normal. Galactography is recommended if bloody secretion is limited to one duct because spontaneous secretion usually involves more than one duct (Fig. 3B). It must be remembered that nipple discharge represents an uncommon manifestation of PABC.[5]

Gigantomastia

Gigantomastia is a very rare condition that complicates about one of every 100,000 pregnancies.[1,5] It is characterized by massive enlargement of the breasts, resulting in tissue necrosis, ulceration, infection, hemorrhage, and complications that can be life threatening in certain cases. Although, its etiology is unknown, gigantomastia is believed to represent an abnormal response to hormonal stimulation during pregnancy. Both glands grow dramatically, and increased weight of 4–6 kg per

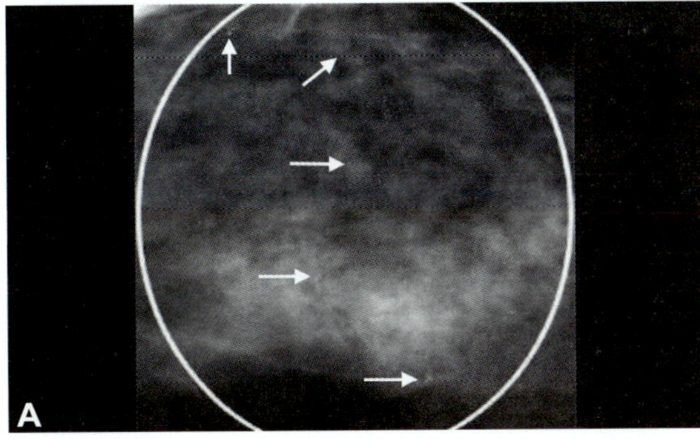

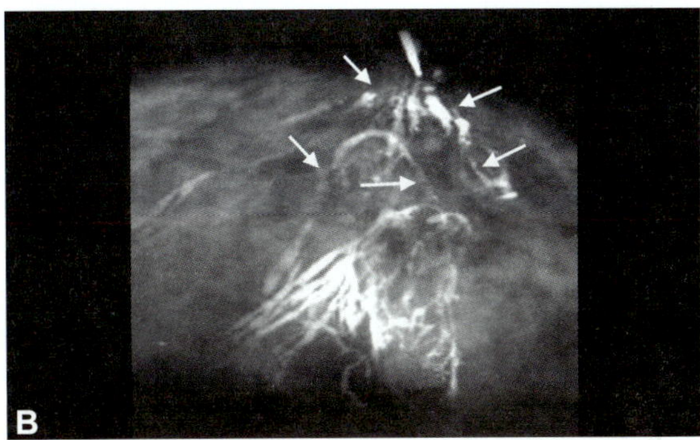

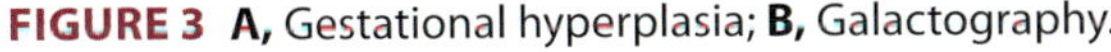
FIGURE 3 **A,** Gestational hyperplasia; **B,** Galactography.

breast has been reported, resulting in dyspnea. The diagnosis of gigantomastia is based on clinical findings. Radiological and pathological studies are not required if no associated disorders are present. Treatment is based on bromocriptine administration, but surgical intervention (reduction mammoplasty or simple mastectomy with posterior reconstruction) is required if the disorder progresses.

Granulomatous Mastitis

Granulomatous mastitis is a very rare inflammatory disease of unknown cause that has been closely related to pregnancy, lactation and within 5 years of pregnancy. Inflammatory factors have been reported as a possible cause but a recent study isolated corynebacterium in up to 75% of cases. Generally, manifests as a distinct firm to hard mass that may involve any part of the breast but tends to spare the subareolar regions. The US appearance of multiple clustered, often contiguous tubular hypoechoic lesions has been considered suggestive of granulomatous mastitis. Unfortunately, this is an uncommon manifestation whose imaging features most often resemble those of carcinoma (Fig. 4A).The diagnosis of granulomatous mastitis is based on exclusion, since it depends on the demonstration of a particular histologic pattern: a noncaseating, nonvasculitic granulomatous inflammatory reaction centered on lobules, combined with the exclusion of other granulomatous reactions, especially tuberculosis and fungal infections as well as sarcoidosis (Fig. 4B). The prognosis is often good, but local recurrence has been reported. Corticotherapy has proved effective. Primary treatment has classically been based on excisional biopsy, but close surveillance without surgery has also proved adequate in the management of cases involving spontaneous resolution. If corynebacterium is isolated with microbiologic or pathologic studies, antibiotic therapy based on the administration of penicillin should be effective.

Benign Neoplasia of the Breast

Benign tumors of the breast include lactating adenoma and fibroadenoma. Fibroadenoma has already been discussed.

Lactating Adenoma

Despite the name, lactating adenomas are more common during pregnancy than during lactation. Lactating adenomas typically present as painless palpable masses. The histology is characteristic, lobulated masses of acini or lobules, densely packed together with little intervening stroma and

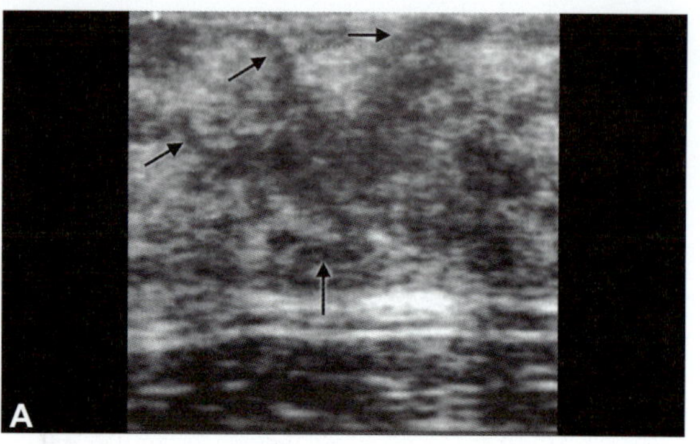

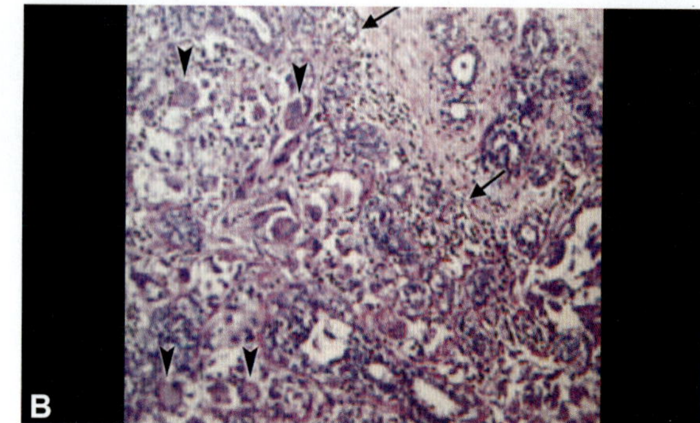

FIGURE 4 Granulomatous mastitis. **A,** Ultrasound; **B,** Histopathological.

intact basement membrane. Despite abundant proliferative changes, there are no atypia. Pregnancy associated changes usually are noted, including intracytoplasmic or supranuclear vacuolation and secretions in gland lumens. The major task is to differentiate this benign mass from breast cancer. Diagnostic fine-needle aspiration cytology is an acceptable method of diagnosis. Large numbers of very similar cells are present, with some nuclear enlargement, prominent nucleoli, cellular dispersion against a background suggestive of necrosis, prominent cytoplasmic vacuoles, and a foamy/wispy appearance of the cytoplasm.[4,6]

MALIGNANT TUMORS

Malignant diseases include PABC, and pregnancy-related Burkitt lymphoma of the breast

Pregnancy Associated Breast Carcinoma

Pregnancy associated breast carcinoma is defined as breast cancer that occurs during pregnancy or within 1 year of delivery with the incidence of 0.3/1,000 pregnancies.[2,3] It occurs between the age group of 32 years and 38 years of age. With many women choosing to delay childbearing, it is likely that the incidence of breast cancer during pregnancy will increase. Most common presentation is a palpable mass. Swelling, erythema, and diffuse breast enlargement are less common. No damaging effects on the fetus from maternal breast cancer have been demonstrated, and there are no reported cases of maternal-fetal transfer of breast cancer cells.[8]

Diagnosis: The physiological changes of the breasts of pregnant and lactating women may hinder detection of small masses so early diagnosis of breast cancer may not occur. An average delay in diagnosis of 5–15 months from onset of symptoms is common and is a major factor responsible for the advanced stage and poor prognosis associated with PABC. Therefore, cancers are typically detected at a later stage than in a nonpregnant, age-matched population. To detect breast cancer, pregnant and lactating women should practice self-examination and undergo a breast examination as part of the routine prenatal examination by a doctor. If an abnormality is found, diagnostic approaches, such as ultrasound and mammography may be used (Fig. 5). Diagnosis may be safely accomplished with a fine-needle aspiration, core biopsy, or excisional biopsy.[8,9] Core biopsy is the standard procedure for assessing breast masses during pregnancy. It is a safe, cost-effective, and easy method for making a precise diagnosis. The risk of bleeding is slightly increased due to the increased vascularity associated with pregnancy and lactation. The risk of infection and milk fistula

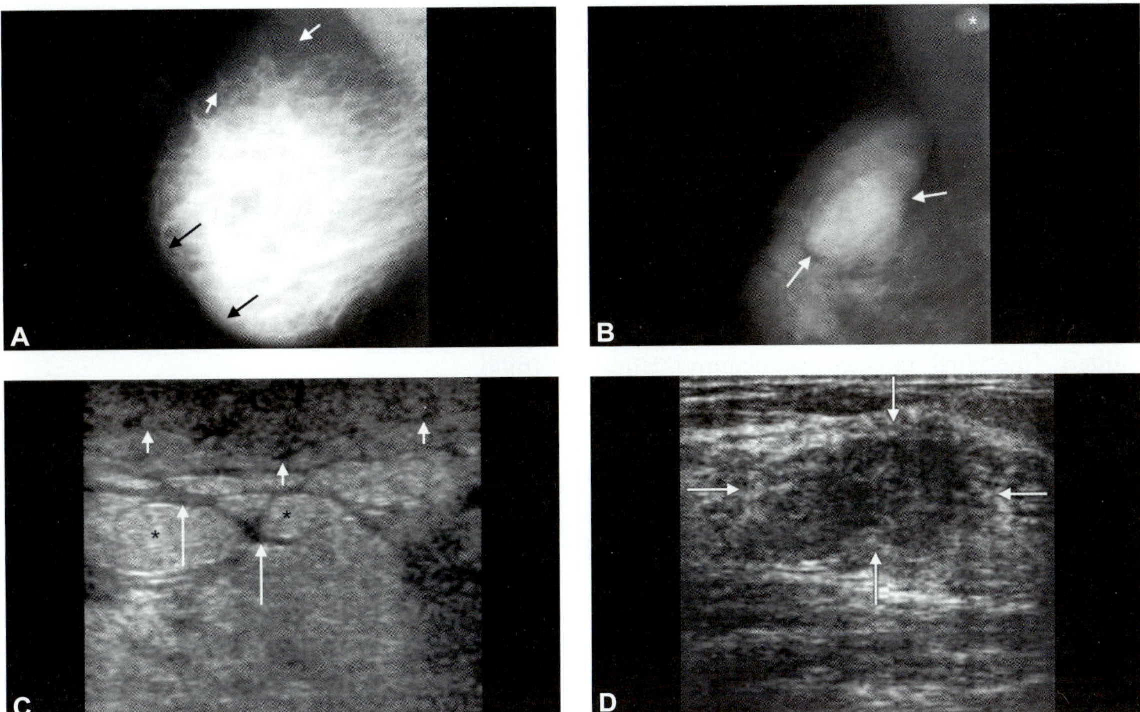

FIGURE 5 Inflammatory carcinoma. **A,** Mammogram shows a marked diffuse increase in parenchymal density with skin thickening and thickened trabeculae due to dilated lymphatic vessel; **B,** Ultrasound image shows skin thickening, a network of hypoechoic and anechoic tubular structures representing enlarged lymphatic vessels. PABC; **C,** Mammogram reveals a large lobular mass with obscured margins; and **D,** Ultrasound image shows an irregular heterogeneous hypoechoic mass with indistinct margin.

formation are also increased. Obviously, these complications are more prone to develop with core biopsy than with fine-needle aspiration, but they occur infrequently.

Caution:

- Since 25% of mammograms in pregnancy may be negative in the presence of cancer, a biopsy is essential for the diagnosis
- Any palpable mass and all masses found during pregnancy should be evaluated carefully
- Several cellular changes normally occur in the epithelium of the breasts of pregnant women leading to a false-positive results
- Diagnosis of carcinoma with cytological analysis must be interpreted with caution. Core biopsy is mandatory if malignancy is suspected.

Staging: Nuclear scans cause fetal radiation exposure. If such scans are essential for evaluation, hydration and foley catheter drainage of the bladder can be used to prevent retention of radioactivity. Timing of the exposure to radiation relative to the gestational age of the fetus may be more critical than the actual dose of radiation delivered. Radiation exposure during the first trimester can lead to congenital malformations, especially microcephaly. A chest X-ray with abdominal shielding is relatively safe but it should be used only when it is essential for making treatment decisions. Evaluation of the liver can be performed with ultrasound, and brain metastases can be diagnosed with a MRI scan, both of which avoid fetal radiation exposure. However, no data evaluating the safety of MRI during pregnancy are available.

Note:

For the diagnosis of bone metastases, a bone scan is preferable to a skeletal series because the bone scan delivers a smaller amount of radiation and is more sensitive

Hormone receptor assays are usually negative in pregnant breast cancer patients, because of receptor binding by high serum estrogen levels associated with pregnancy.[8,9]

Treatment of early stage cancer (stages I and II): Surgery (modified radical mastectomy) is the treatment of choice. Conservative surgery with postpartum radiation therapy has been used for breast preservation. Data on the immediate and long-term effects of chemotherapy on the fetus are limited.[8] Studies using adjuvant hormonal therapy alone or in combination with chemotherapy for breast cancer in pregnant women are also limited. Therefore, no conclusion has been reached regarding these options.

Precaution:

- If adjuvant chemotherapy is necessary, it should not be given during the first trimester to avoid the risk of teratogenicity
- Radiation therapy, if indicated, should be withheld until after delivery since it may be harmful to the fetus at any stage of development.

Treatment of late stage disease (stages III and IV): First-trimester radiation therapy should be avoided. Chemotherapy may be given after the first trimester as discussed above. As the mother may have a limited life span and there is a risk of fetal damage with treatment during the first trimester, issues regarding continuation of the pregnancy should be discussed with the patient and her family.

Note: Termination of pregnancy may be considered based on the age of the fetus if maternal treatment options such as chemotherapy and radiation therapy are significantly limited by the continuation of the pregnancy.[5]

PABC in BRCA germline mutation carriers: BRCA 1 or BRCA 2 mutation carriers are at high risk for breast cancer, making strict surveillance mandatory. Therefore, before pregnancy and after delivery a complete clinical and radiologic evaluation is necessary to exclude any pathologic process. Ultrasound and MRI evaluation are of great value.

Pregnancy-related Burkitt Lymphoma of the Breast

Burkitt lymphoma is type of lymphoma arising from undifferentiated B cells. It has been classified into three categories:

1. The endemic type is seen in young Africans in close association with Epstein-Barr virus and malaria
2. The sporadic type is seen in Europe and the United States
3. Lymphoma associated with human immunodeficiency virus.

Burkitt lymphoma of the breast affects pregnant or postpartum patients with massive enlargement of both breasts. Burkitt lymphoma of the breast is characterized by rapid spread and a poor prognosis. They are almost always bilateral. Mammography shows diffuse marked increase in parenchymal density. Massive bilateral involvement of the ovaries is common and tumors may develop in any of the abdominal organs, especially the liver, spleen and kidneys, and rarely in peripheral lymph nodes.

The majority of breast lesions encountered during pregnancy are benign. Physiological changes during pregnancy make evaluation of the breasts more difficult. Baseline and serial examinations are critical. Prompt and immediate biopsies of breast masses are important during pregnancy and benign-appearing or low-suspicion lesions should not be neglected.

REFERENCES

1. Cunningham F, Leveno K, Bloom S, et al. Maternal physiology. In: Cunningham F, Leveno K, Bloom S, Hauth J, Rouse D, Spong C, editors. Williams Obstetrics, 23rd edition. US: McGraw-Hill; 2010. pp.107.
2. Ayyappan AP, Kulkarni S, Crystal P, et al. Pregnancy-associated breast cancer: spectrum of imaging appearances. Br J Radiol. 2010;83(990):529-34.
3. Son EJ, Oh KK, Kim EK. Pregnancy-associated breast disease: radiological features and diagnostic dilemmas. Yousei Med J. 2006;47(1):34-42.
4. Magno S, Terribile D, Franceschini G, et al. Early onset lactating adenoma and the role of breast MRI: a case report. J Med Case Rep. 2009;3:43.
5. Sabate JM, Clotet M, Torrubia S, et al. Radiologic evaluation of breast disorders related to pregnancy and lactation. Radiographics. 2007;27(Suppl 1):S101-24.
6. O'Hara MF, Page DL. Adenomas of the breast and ectopic breast under lactational influences. Hum Pathol. 1985;16(17): 707-12.
7. Rosen PP. Fibroepithelial neoplasms. In: Rosen PP, editor. Rosen's breast pathology, 2nd edition. Philadelphia:lippincott-raven; 2001. pp.163-200.
8. Hoover HC Jr. Breast cancer during pregnancy and lactation. Surg Clin North Am. 1990;70(5):1151-63.
9. Clark RM, Chua T. Breast cancer and pregnancy: the ultimate challenge. Clin Oncol (R Coll Radiol). 1989;1(1):11-8.

Associated Gynecological Conditions

23

CHAPTER

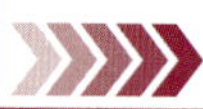

Rajat Ray, Yogita Dogra

INTRODUCTION

All gynecological conditions found in non-pregnant patients could be associated with pregnancy in first trimester. These conditions are described below.

VAGINITIS

Bacterial vaginosis (BV) is an extremely prevalent vaginal condition and the number one cause of vaginitis among both pregnant and nonpregnant women.[1] Current studies have found the prevalence of BV among pregnant women up to 50%.[2-5] The current predictors of BV have been limited to race, sexual activity, and socioeconomic status. Limited information exists concerning the factors or behaviors that increase a woman's risk for BV during pregnancy. BV has been related to many complications of pregnancy including amniotic fluid infection, preterm delivery, preterm labor, premature rupture of the membranes, and possibly spontaneous abortion (three- to fivefold increased risk).[6-11] One study examining several pregnancy outcomes related to BV diagnosed during the first trimester of pregnancy reported a 2.6-fold increased risk of preterm labor, a 6.9-fold increased risk of preterm delivery and a 7.3-fold increased risk of preterm premature rupture of the membranes.[10] Two diagnostic tests are commonly used for BV: (1) Amsel criteria and (2) Gram stain of vaginal fluid and use of Nugent criteria—this method has been shown to have a high sensitivity and specificity compared with Amsel criteria (89% and 83%, respectively).[12,13] The most common oral treatment in both pregnant and nonpregnant women is metronidazole.[14] It is a category B drug which means that no controlled studies have been done in pregnant women but no evidence of fetal risk appears to be present. Studies have shown no teratogenic effects.[15] The individual cure rate given a 7-day, twice-daily course of 500 mg ranges from 84% to 96%, and the cure rate given a 2 g single dose is 54–62%.[16] The other systemic treatment for BV is oral clindamycin 300 mg twice daily for 7 days with a cure rate of 94%.[16] The two topical treatments for BV include metronidazole 0.75% vaginal gel and clindamycin 2% vaginal cream.

CERVICAL INCOMPETENCE

It is difficult to diagnose cervical incompetence in first trimester. However, with a transvaginal scan in patients with recurrent miscarriages widening of internal os may be noted even before the cervical length is shortened. A significant proportion found to have a widened uterine isthmus at hysterosalpingography done before pregnancy show first trimester cervical effacement. A combination of medical progesterone and cervical cerclage begun during the first trimester results in successful term pregnancy.[17]

FIBROIDS

Only about 4% of pregnant women have sonographically evident uterine leiomyomas, about 12% of which are multiple.[18] They tend to become smaller during pregnancy, and fibroids initially less than 5 cm in diameter usually involute completely during pregnancy.[19] Complications occur in about 1 in 500 pregnancies.[20] Larger ones can undergo hemorrhagic infarction resulting in the painful myoma syndrome.[21] Symptoms may be minimal or may include severe abdominal pain, nausea, emesis, and pyrexia.[22] Ultrasonography and magnetic resonance imaging (MRI) are usually diagnostic.[23] Treatment consists of bed rest and nonsteroidal anti-inflammatory drugs (NSAIDs). Other complications are miscarriage, premature rupture of membranes, preterm delivery, placental abnormalities, uterine rupture (especially after prior myomectomy), dystocia, increased frequency of cesarean delivery, postpartum hemorrhage, and puerperal sepsis.[24] However, studies have reported successful myomectomy on symptomatic women in the first and second trimester of pregnancy, in whom pregnancies were completed without complications.[25]

PELVIC INFLAMMATORY DISEASE

Pelvic inflammatory disease (PID) rarely complicates pregnancy. It may lead to spontaneous abortion or intrauterine fetal demise. A diagnosis of suspected PID may be done by lower abdominal or adnexal tenderness or fullness and cervical motion tenderness as well as either a positive cervical specimen for *Neisseria gonorrhoeae* or *Chlamydia trachomatis*.[26] Successful pregnancy outcome can occur after treatment of PID in the first trimester.

TUBO-OVARIAN ABSCESS

Tubo-ovarian abscess is an emergency associated with maternal mortality and fetal wastage.[27] Abdominal pain, pyrexia, a palpable mass, and leukocytosis commonly occur. MRI, computed tomography (CT) scanning, or sonography, are helpful in the diagnosis, but laparoscopy is often required for confirmation. Treatment includes fluid, resuscitation, parenteral antibiotics, and expedient surgery unless the abscess is small, well contained, and amenable to radiologic drainage.[28]

PROLAPSE

Genital prolapse may be present prior to pregnancy or develop initially during pregnancy. However, in the majority of cases, pregnancy is superimposed on a pre-existing prolapse. The estimated incidence is one per 10,000–15,000 deliveries.[29] When some degree of prolapse is present before pregnancy, it usually will persist until the pregnancy progresses to the stage where spontaneous correction occurs which is due to the uterus becoming an abdominal organ in the second trimester, thereby pulling the cervix up into the vagina. The uterine descent, however, also may be aggravated by pregnancy as a result of physiologic increases in cortisol and progesterone, which leads to a concomitant softening and stretching of the pelvic tissues.

Pre-existing prolapse has been associated with infertility and spontaneous abortions. Spontaneous abortion may occur as a result of trauma and vascular congestion that accompany the prolapsed cervix. An impairment of blood flow and cervical edema with subsequent anoxia also may contribute to a higher incidence of abortion and preterm labor with prolapse. Literature review describes clinical features of pelvic pressure, lower back pain, urinary tract symptoms (e.g., acute retention and incontinence), cervical inflammation, and cervical mucosal ulcerations. Similarly, complications reported range from patient discomfort, cervical desiccation and ulceration, urinary tract infection, and acute urinary retention to miscarriage and even maternal death due to sepsis.[30]

Management depends on the degree of prolapse and gestational length. Pregnant women with prolapse may benefit from the use of a vaginal pessary to protect the cervix from local trauma associated with protrusion and for keeping the cervix in the vagina while ambulating. Pessary support, however, may be more beneficial in the woman with pre-existing prolapse rather than in those in whom the condition presents during mid to late pregnancy. An otherwise uncomplicated course and a vaginal delivery can be expected. However, it is essential to look out for the presence of cervical inflammation or edema which may complicate a vaginal delivery, where an elective caesarean section near term could be a valid and safe delivery option.

CERVICAL CARCINOMA *IN SITU* AND CARCINOMA

Five percent of pregnant women will develop abnormal cervical cytology. Cervical cancer is one of the most common malignancies in pregnancy, with an estimated incidence of 1–10 in 10,000 pregnancies.[31] Women with unexplained persistent bleeding in pregnancy, especially postcoital, should have a speculum examination, cytology, and colposcopy. When an abnormal Pap test is obtained on a woman who is pregnant, the evaluation is modified. In general, pregnancy has no effect on cervical carcinoma *in situ* (CIN) and the cervical lesion has no effect on the pregnancy. All that is really necessary is to exclude an invasive cancer because the treatment of invasive cancer takes precedence over pregnancy. However, in cases of high squamous intraepithelial lesion (HSIL) diagnosed before 16 weeks of pregnancy a colposcopic examination and laser vaporization/conization is recommended. In cases of low squamous intraepithelial lesion (LSIL), diagnosed after 16 weeks, colposcopic examination can be performed regularly but definitive treatment may be postponed to the postpartum period. The cervix is best not manipulated or biopsied during the first trimester because of the risk of spontaneous miscarriage. The atypical squamous cells of indetermined significance and LSIL lesions can easily wait until 6 weeks after the baby is born to evaluate and treat. Often this can be accomplished by a colposcopic examination, without the need for a biopsy. Colposcopy is, however, challenging in pregnancy as deciduosis can have an appearance suggestive of malignancy and the features of squamous metaplasia may be exaggerated, as are vascular changes. Sometimes biopsies and even cone biopsies must be done. The best time for these biopsies is the early second trimester because the risk for a spontaneous miscarriage has passed with the first trimester and cervical manipulation during the third trimester risks premature labor.

If an invasive cancer is diagnosed during pregnancy, the treatment is the same as for those not pregnant.

Women with The International Federation of Gynecology and Obstetrics (FIGO) stage IA1—disease can be treated by a shallow cone biopsy in the second trimester.[32] For more advanced disease, diagnosed in the first or second trimesters, staging is advised. Pelvic examination remains the basis, however, other techniques may be considered to evaluate the extent of the disease and assist decision-making. Since lymphatic spread is a major determinant of prognosis, it has recently been proposed that when pregnancy-sparing treatment is preferred, pelvic lymphadenectomy (either extra peritoneal or laparoscopic) should be considered in the second trimester to define lymph node status.[32,33] It is also suggested that sentinel node biopsy can be safely performed in pregnancy and this may play a role in the future.[33] For high-risk node positive disease it is advisable to terminate the pregnancy via hysterotomy and treat the women aggressively with standard chemoradiation.

For women with operable node negative cancers, FIGO less than or equals IB1: confined to the cervix and less than 4 cm is diameter there are several options. Trachelectomy has been performed in pregnancy, although associated with significant hemorrhage and pregnancy loss. Most frequently, a radical caesarean hysterectomy is considered once fetal maturity is reached.[33,34] The use of neoadjuvant chemotherapy (NACT) with paclitaxel and platinum chemotherapy during pregnancy has been reported in literature to shrink disease and theoretically minimize metastatic spread while awaiting fetal maturity.[35] Timing of delivery should be decided in conjunction with neonatal and obstetric advice. NACT may also be considered for more bulky higher stage disease (≥IB2) while awaiting fetal maturity, subsequent caesarean delivery and definitive treatment with chemoradiation. Vaginal delivery is seldom considered an option unless the cervix is free of tumor. Fatal recurrences in episiotomy scars have been reported. When continuation of pregnancy is desired, women should be informed of the "experimental nature" of the cancer treatment and associated risks for her and the pregnancy.

SEXUALLY TRANSMITTED DISEASES

Transmission of sexually transmitted diseases (STDs) from the pregnant women to her fetus or newborn infant can occur before, during, or after birth. Certain STDs, such as syphilis are able to cross the placenta and infect the fetus, potentially affecting fetal development. Other STDs including gonorrhea, chlamydia, hepatitis B, and genital herpes can be transmitted to the infant during vaginal delivery. Women who are human immunodeficiency virus (HIV) positive can transmit the virus to the fetus through the placenta during pregnancy. Infection can occur during the process of birth. Pregnant women infected with HIV who receive treatment during pregnancy can significantly reduce the risk of transmitting the virus to their infants. If a women infected by genital herpes has active genital herpes lesions at the time of delivery, a cesarean section is often recommended to protect the newborn against infection.

STDs in the prepregnancy period and pregnancy can cause:

- Miscarriage
- Ectopic pregnancy
- Preterm labor and delivery
- Low birth weight
- Birth defects, including blindness, deafness, bone deformities, and intellectual disability
- Stillbirth
- Illness in the newborn period (first month of life)
- Neonatal death.

Recommended screening tests:

- All pregnant women should be screened for HIV infection, syphilis and hepatitis B surface antigen (HBsAg) during an early prenatal visit. Women who are HBsAg positive should be provided with, or referred for, appropriate counseling and medical management
- All women at high risk for chlamydia, gonorrhea, and hepatitis C infection should be screened at the first prenatal visit
- Evidence does not support routine testing for BV, *Trichomonas vaginalis* and herpes simplex virus 2 (HSV-2).

OVARIAN CYSTS AND ADNEXAL MASSES

With the routine use of ultrasound in prenatal care, the finding of an "incidental" ovarian mass in pregnancy has become more common. In the first trimester, up to 8.8% of patients will have ovarian cysts or masses diagnosed by ultrasound, but it will persist in only 1–2% into the second trimester. Most first trimester masses are corpus luteal cysts that regress by the sixteenth week of pregnancy. Others are functional cysts, endometriosis, and benign ovarian neoplasms, cystic teratomas and cystadenomas are the most common.[36,37] Malignancies, including germ cell tumors, low-grade ovarian cancers, and invasive epithelial ovarian cancers, comprise 3% of ovarian masses during pregnancy, or an incidence of 1 in 5,000 pregnancies.[36,38] Most women with ovarian cancer present with stage I disease during pregnancy.[38] Cancers from the gastrointestinal tract or elsewhere rarely metastasize to the ovaries.[39] The pathology ranges from asymptomatic non-neoplastic ovarian cysts to the surgical emergencies of ovarian torsion, ruptured ovarian cyst, and tubo-ovarian abscess. About half of adnexal masses are less than 5 cm in diameter, about one quarter are between 5 cm and 10 cm in diameter, and about one quarter are more than 10 cm in diameter.[40] Ninety-five percent are unilateral.[41] Most adnexal masses are asymptomatic and are incidentally detected by sonography.[40,41,42] Even ovarian cancer is often asymptomatic.[36,43] Symptoms can include vague abdominal pain, abdominal distension, and urinary frequency.[36] Torsion, hemorrhage, or rupture produces severe abdominal pain. 10% to 15% of adnexal masses undergo torsion.[36] Ultrasound is the most important diagnostic tool used in the evaluation and management of adnexal masses in the pregnant patient. However, MRI has also been used to provide additional diagnostic information including the ability to develop three-dimensional images, delineate tissue planes, and characterize tissue composition, but is limited by cost and availability.

Management of adnexal masses in pregnancy can be expectant or surgical. A potential benefit for removal of the mass includes prevention of the complications and also preventing obstruction of labor at the time of delivery. Timing of surgery is important. Because most masses during early pregnancy are corpus luteum or other functional cysts that usually resolve, elective removal of an adnexal mass is generally recommended if it persists into the second trimester or is enlarging progressively. Delaying surgery may also decrease the rate of miscarriage from potential disruption of the corpus luteum and, prevents exposure of the fetus to anesthesia during organogenesis, which is typically complete by the end of the first trimester. Laparoscopic removal of adnexal masses in pregnancy is safe and is associated with decreased blood loss, shorter hospital stays, and reduced postoperative pain (*See* Chapter 28: Laparoscopic Surgery). No cervical or uterine instrumentation is performed. Excessive manipulation of the uterus during the procedure is also avoided to decrease uterine irritability.[44] When an ovarian malignancy is encountered, staging and debulking should be performed with minimum uterine manipulation, while preserving the uterus. Chemotherapy may be administered during the second and third trimesters of pregnancy in carefully selected patients.

Note: When performing laparoscopy during pregnancy, an open technique or left upper quadrant entry is used to decrease potential uterine injury.

ADNEXAL TORSION

Adnexal torsion occurs in about 1 of 1,800 pregnancies.[45] About one quarter of adnexal torsions occur during pregnancy,[46] because of the greater laxity of the tissue supporting the ovaries and oviducts during pregnancy.[47] It usually occurs between the sixth and fourteenth weeks of gestation. Both ovarian cysts and tumors, particularly the benign cystic teratoma, may undergo torsion, but many torsions are idiopathic or occur about extraovarian structures.[48] Right-sided torsion is more common than left sided torsion.[46,48] The clinical presentation is variable.[48,49] The lower abdominal pain is often sharp and sudden in onset and may last from several hours to days. Patients often have nausea and emesis. Signs include unilateral lower quadrant tenderness, a palpable adnexal mass, cervical tenderness, or rebound tenderness from peritonitis.[48] Leukocytosis is common. The diagnosis is often missed. Right-sided adnexal torsion may be difficult to differentiate from appendicitis. Other diagnostic considerations include a ruptured ovarian cyst or ectopic pregnancy. Adnexal torsion, diagnosed before tissue necrosis, is managed with adnexa-sparing laparoscopic detorsion. Salpingo-oophorectomy is necessary if necrosis or peritonitis has occurred, followed by progesterone therapy if the corpus luteum is removed.[50]

VESICOVAGINAL FISTULA

In a patient with vesicovaginal fistula (VVF) due to obstetric or gynecological causes, pregnancy rarely occurs. Congenital VVF may be misdiagnosed because of associated urinary tract abnormalities. Early diagnosis and identifying the location, size, and relationship with other tissues is important. Reasonable preoperative preparation, surgical, and postoperative surgical care are the key for treatment.

CONGENITAL ANOMALIES OF THE UTERUS

Uterine malformations with pregnancy are often revealed at the time of first sonographic examination in early pregnancy. An ideal method of imaging seems to be 3D ultrasonography. Patients with uterine malformations seem to have an impaired pregnancy outcome even as early as their first pregnancy. Overall term delivery rates in patients with untreated uterine malformations are only approximately 50% and obstetric complications are more frequent. Unicornuate and didelphys uterus have term delivery rates of approximately 45%, and the pregnancy outcome of patients with untreated bicornuate and septate uterus is also poor with term delivery rates of only approximately 40%. Arcuate uterus is associated with a slightly better but still impaired pregnancy outcome with term delivery rates of approximately 65%.[51] Pregnancy complications include early and late abortions, preterm delivery, intrauterine growth restriction and abnormal presentations.

When evaluating pregnancy during the first trimester, one should also look for associated gynecological pathologies and manage them accordingly as they may have a bearing on fetomaternal outcome.

REFERENCES

1. Rein MF, Holmes KK. Non-specific vaginitis, vulvovaginal candidiasis, and trichomoniasis clinical features, diagnosis and management. Curr Clin Top Infect Dis. 1983;4:281-315.
2. Fleury FS. Adult vaginitis. Clin Obstet Gynecol. 1981;24:407-38.
3. McGregor JA, French JI. Bacterial vaginosis in pregnancy. Obstet Gynecol Surv 2000;55(5 suppl 1):1-19.
4. Holzman C, Leventhal JM, Qiu H, et al. Factors linked to bacterial vaginosis in nonpregnant women. Am J Public Health. 2001;91:1664-70.
5. Cristiano L, Coffetti N, Dalvai G, et al. Bacterial vaginosis: prevalence in outpatients, association with some micro-organisms and laboratory indices. Genitourin Med. 1989; 65:382-7.
6. Eschenbach DA, Hillier S, Critchlow C, et al. Diagnosis and clinical manifestations of bacterial vaginosis. Am J Obstet Gynecol. 1988;158:819-28.
7. Abner KP, Hessol NA, Padian NS, et al. Risk factors for plasma cell endometritis among women with cervical Neisseria gonorrhoeae, cervica Chlamydia trachomatis, or bacterial vaginosis. Am J Obstet Gynecol. 1998;178:987-90.
8. Meis PJ, Goldenburg RL, Mercer B, et al. The preterm prediction study: significance of vaginal infections. Am J Obstet Gynecol. 1995;173:1231-5.
9. Hillier SL, Martius J, Krohn M, et al. A case-control study of chorioamniotic infection and histologic chorioamnionitis in prematurity. N Engl J Med. 1988;319:972-8.
10. Kurki T, Sivonen A, Renkonen OV, et al. Bacterial vaginosis in early pregnancy and pregnancy outcome. Obstet Gynecol. 1992;80:173-7.
11. Hay PE, Lamont RF, Taylor-Robinson D, et al. Abnormal bacterial colonization of the genital tract and subsequent preterm delivery and late miscarriage. BMJ. 1994;308:295-8.
12. Schwebke JR, Hillier SL, Sobel JD, et al. Validity of the vaginal Gram stain for the diagnosis of bacterial vaginosis. Obstet Gynecol. 1996;88:573-6.
13. Mastrobattista JM, Bishop KD, Newton ER. Wet smear compared with Gram stain diagnosis of bacterial vaginosis in asymptomatic pregnant women. Obstet Gynecol. 2000;96:504-6.
14. Joesoef MR, Schmid GP, Hillier SL. Bacterial vaginosis: review of treatment options and potential clinical indications for therapy. Clin Infect Dis. 1999;28(Suppl 1):S57-65.
15. Thapa PB, Whitlock JA, Brockman Worell KG, et al. Prenatal exposure to metronidazole and risk of childhood cancer: a retrospective cohort study of children younger than 5 years. Cancer. 1998;83:1461-8.

16. Greaves WL, Chungafung J, Morris B, et al. Clindamycin versus metronidazole in the treatment of bacterial vaginosis. Obstet Gynecol. 1988;72:799-802.
17. Fox NS, Chervenak FA. Cervical cerclage: a review of the evidence. Obstet Gynecol Surv. 2008;63(1):58-65.
18. Exacoustos C, Rosati P. Ultrasound diagnosis of uterine myomas and complications in pregnancy. Obstet Gynecol. 1993;82:97-101.
19. Strobelt N, Ghidini A, Cavallone M, et al. Natural history of uterine leiomyomas in pregnancy. J Ultrasound Med. 1994;13:399-401.
20. Katz VL, Dotters DJ, Droegemeuller W. Complications of uterine leiomyomas in pregnancy. Obstet Gynecol. 1989;73:593-6.
21. Rice JP, Kay HH, Mahony BS. The clinical significance of uterine leiomyomas in pregnancy. Am J Obstet Gynecol. 1989;160:1212-6.
22. Eichenberg BJ, Vanderlinden J, Miguel C, et al. Laparoscopic cholecystectomy in the third trimester of pregnancy. Am Surg. 1996;62:874-7.
23. Sherer DM, Maitland CY, Levine NF, et al. Prenatal magnetic resonance imaging assisting in differentiating between large degenerating intramural leiomyoma and complex adnexal mass during pregnancy. J Matern Fetal Med. 2000;9:186-9.
24. Coronado GD, Marshall LM, Schwartz SM. Complications in pregnancy, labor, and delivery with uterine leiomyomas: a population-based study. Obstet Gynecol. 2000;95:764-9.
25. Lolis DE, Kalantaridou SN, Makrydimas G, et al. Successful myomectomy during pregnancy. Hum Reprod. 2003;18(8): 1699-702.
26. Stitely ML, Gherman RB. Successful pregnancy outcome following first trimester pelvic inflammatory disease. ANZJOG. 2000;40:200-2.
27. Murthy JH, Hiremagalur SR. Differentiation of tubo-ovarian abscess from pelvic inflammatory disease, and recent trends in the management of tubo-ovarian abscess. J Ten Med Assoc. 1995;88(4):136-8.
28. Shulman A, Maymon R, Shapiro A, et al. Percutaneous catheter drainage of tubo-ovarian abscesses. Obstet Gynecol. 1992;80:555-7.
29. Guariglia L, Carducci B, Botta A, et al. Uterine prolapse in pregnancy. Gynecol Obstet Invest. 2005;60:192-4.
30. Daskalakis G, Lymberopoulos E, Anastasakis E, et al. Uterine Prolapse complicating pregnancy. Arch Gynecol Obstet. 2007;276(4):391-2.
31. Van Calsteren K, Vergote I, Amant F. Cervical neoplasia during pregnancy: diagnosis, management and prognosis. Best Pract Res Clin Obstet Gynaecol. 2005;19:611-30.
32. Yahata T, Numata M, Kashima K, et al. Conservative treatment of stage IA1 adenocarcinoma of the cervix during pregnancy. Gynecol Oncol. 2008;109(1):49-52.
33. Amant F, Van Calsteren K, Halaska MJ, et al. Gynaecological Cancers in Pregnancy: Guidelines of an International Consensus Meeting. Int J Gynaecol Cancer. 2009;19:S1-12.
34. Amant F, Brepoels L, Halaska MJ, et al. Gynaecologic Cancer complicating Pregnancy: An Overview. Best Pract Res Clin Obstet Gynaecol. 2010;24(1):61-79.
35. Li J, Wang LJ, Zhang BZ, et al. Neoadjuvant chemotherapy with paclitaxel plus platinum for invasive cervical cancer in pregnancy: two case report and literature review. Arch Gynecol Obstet. 2011;284(3):779-83.
36. Struyk AP, Treffers BE. Ovarian tumors in pregnancy. Acta Obstet Gynecol Scand. 1984;63:421-4.
37. Usui R, Minakami H, Kosuge S, et al. A retrospective survey of clinical, pathologic, and prognostic features of adnexal masses operated on during pregnancy. J Obstet Gynaecol Res. 2000;26:89-93.
38. Dgani R, Shoham Z, Atar E, et al. Ovarian carcinoma during pregnancy: a study of 23 cases in Israel between the years 1960 and 1984. Gynecol Oncol. 1989;33:326-31.
39. Cosme A, Ojeda E, Bujanda L, et al. Krukenberg tumor secondary to gastric carcinoma in a woman in her eighth month of pregnancy. Gastroenterol Hepatol. 2001;24:63-5.
40. Thornton JG, Wells M. Ovarian cysts in pregnancy: does ultrasound make traditional management inappropriate? Obstet Gynecol. 1987;69:717-21.
41. Hess LW, Peaceman A, O'Brien WF, et al. Adnexal mass occurring with intrauterine pregnancy: report of fifty-four patients requiring laparotomy for definitive management. Am J Obstet Gynecol. 1988;158:1029-34.
42. Derchi LE, Serafini G, Gandolfo N, et al. Ultrasound in gynecology. Eur Radiol. 2001;11:2137-55.
43. Hick JL, Rodgerson JD, Heegaard WG, et al. Vital signs fail to correlate with hemoperitoneum from ruptured ectopic pregnancy. Am J Emerg Med. 2001;19:488-91.
44. Giuntoli RL, Vang RS, Bristow RE. Evaluation and management of adnexal masses during pregnancy. Clin Obstet Gynecol. 2006:49(3):492-505.
45. Johnson Jr. TR, Woodruff JD. Surgical emergencies of the uterine adnexae during pregnancy. Int J Gynaecol Obstet. 1986;24:331-5.
46. McGowan L. Surgical diseases of the ovary in pregnancy. Clin Obstet Gynecol. 1983;26:843-52.
47. Mancuso A, Broccio G, Angio LG, et al. Adnexal torsion in pregnancy. Acta Obstet Gynecol Scand. 1997;76:83-4.
48. Houry D, Abbott JT. Ovarian torsion: a fifteen-year review. Ann Emerg Med. 2001;38:156-9.
49. Chen CP, Wang W, Wang TY. Adnexal torsion during late pregnancy. Am J Emerg Med. 1999;17:738-9.
50. Argenta PA, Yeagley TJ, Ott G, et al. Torsion of the uterine adnexa: pathologic correlations and current management trends. J Reprod Med. 2000;45:831-6.
51. Grimbizis G, Camus M, Tarlatzis B, et al. Clinical implications of uterine malformations and hysteroscopic treatment results. Hum Reprod. 2001;7:161-74.

Recurrent First Trimester Pregnancy Loss

24

CHAPTER

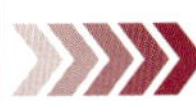

Mala Arora, Ritu Joshi

INTRODUCTION

Recurrent pregnancy loss (RPL) is a distressing problem that affects 1% of all women. Early pregnancy loss is unfortunately the most common complication of human gestation. Most of these losses are unrecognized and occur before or with the next expected menses. Miscarriage is defined as spontaneous loss of an intrauterine pregnancy prior to 24 weeks of gestation or before a fetal weight of 500 g is reached.[1] Recurrent miscarriage (RM) is defined by Stirrat as the spontaneous loss of three or more consecutive pregnancies.[2] The Royal College of Obstetricians and Gynecologists green top guidelines also endorses this definition.[3] However, the American College has recently redefined it as the loss of two consecutive pregnancies.[4] RM is a heterogeneous condition that has many possible causes; more than one contributory factor may be responsible in some while no cause may be identified in others.

ETIOLOGY

The causes of RMs are multiple and are listed in table 1. Consideration of timing of miscarriage is important, as different causes of miscarriage tend to manifest at different period of gestation. In first trimester miscarriages, important causes include chromosomal abnormalities (70% of cases), maternal diseases including poorly controlled diabetes mellitus, uncontrolled thyroid disease, severe systemic lupus erythematous, and antiphospholipid syndrome (APS); poor maternal lifestyle habits (including alcohol consumption, smoking and use of habit forming drugs); and exposure to nonsteroidal anti-inflammatory drugs at the time of conception.

Risk Factors

Age and success of previous pregnancies are two independent risk factors that affect the loss rate. It has been observed by many authors that there is an increasing risk of spontaneous abortion, with increasing maternal age, which may be due to association of maternal age with increased likelihood of chromosomal abnormalities in the embryo.

Genetic Factors

Most spontaneous miscarriages are caused by an abnormal karyotype (aneuploidy) of the embryo. At least 50% of all first-trimester spontaneous abortions are cytogenetically abnormal, the most common being monosomy X, trisomy 16, 13, 18, and 21.[5] Aneuploidies may cause sporadic miscarriage, however, a recent study has suggested that women with previous aneuploid

TABLE 1: Causes of recurrent pregnancy loss

Genetic	Parental translocations
	Embryo aneuploidies
	Skewed inactivation of X chromosomes
	Single gene disorders
Anatomical	Uterine mullerian anomalies
	Uterine polyps/adhesions
	Leiomyomas/adenomyosis
	Cervical incompetence
Endocrinological	Thyroid dysfunction
	Polycystic ovarian disease
	Poor ovarian reserve
	Uncontrolled diabetes mellitus
Infectious	Chlamydia
	Bacterial vaginosis
	Latent genital tuberculosis
	Nonspecific endometritis
Immunological—autoimmune	Antiphospholipid syndrome
	Systemic lupus erythematous
Immunological—alloimmune	
Lifestyle	Obesity
Environmental	Smoking
	Alcohol
	Radiation
	Anesthetic drugs
	Endocrine disrupters
Psychological	Stress
Unexplained	

fetus have an increased chance of recurrence.[6] The highest rate of cytogenetically abnormal conception occur earliest in gestation, with rates declining after the embryonic period (>30 mm crown-rump length).

Recurrent miscarriage may result due to the following reason.

Recurrent Aneuploidy

Numeric chromosomal abnormalities might be involved in both recurrent and sporadic losses. In order of frequency, the main chromosomal abnormalities are autosomal trisomies, polyploidy and monosomy X. Autosomal trisomy is involved in 50% of the cytogenetically abnormal abortuses in the first trimester. Most trisomies show maternal age effect, with chromosomes 16 being most commonly involved. Thirty percent of chromosomally abnormal spontaneous abortions are accounted by triploidy and tetraploidy which are not compatible with life. Tetraploidy rarely progress beyond 4 or 5 weeks gestation. Monosomy X (Turner's syndrome) is the single most common chromosomal abnormality among spontaneous abortions accounting for 20–25% of all abortions.

Structural Chromosomal Abnormality

It occurs in approximately 3% of cytogenetically abnormal abortuses. These abnormalities are thought to be most commonly inherited from the mother. Structural chromosomal problems found in males often leads to low sperm concentrations, male infertility, and therefore, a reduced likelihood of pregnancy and miscarriage. Chromosomal translocation is the most common structural rearrangement involved in RPL and has a prevalence of translocation in either parent of 3–5%, with the wife being affected twice as frequently as the husband.

Mendelian and Polygenic Factors

Single gene or polygenic factors involved in fundamental cellular and reproductive processes, are rarely detected, but could be causing recurrent euploid losses. Skewed X inactivation, defined as 90% inactivation of one specific parental allele, has also been found more frequently in women with recurrent abortion.

Management

Genetic counseling: The National Society of Genetic Counselors has published guidelines for counseling, based on recommendations of Inherited Pregnancy Loss Working Group.[7]

First trimester screening: Biochemical screening along with ultrasound is routinely offered for all pregnant women of advanced maternal age (older than 35 years). A woman's risk of having aneuploid fetus is 1 per 80, when she is older than 35 years and this is far greater than the risk of fetal loss after amniocentesis, which is 1 per 300–500.

Karyotype: Routine karyotype analysis after one miscarriage is not cost-effective or prognostic. However, after three spontaneous early miscarriages, it is useful.

Fluorescence in situ hybridization: Fluorescence *in situ* hybridization (FISH) is performed for five and maximum nine chromosomes. It has the advantage of quick reporting and is not dependent on successful culture. If an increased risk for future pregnancies is identified, all alternatives should be discussed, including foregoing any attempts at further conception, adopting, trying to conceive again with early prenatal testing, using donor gametes, or performing preimplantation genetic diagnosis.

Preimplantation genetic screening: The concept of preimplantation genetic screening, involves blastomere biopsy, analysis by FISH or comparative genomic hybridization, and replacing only normal gametes in women with advanced maternal age.[8]

Uterine Anomalies

There is no doubt that uterine defects can predispose women to first and second trimester pregnancy losses. Most commonly, the complications result from impaired vascularization at the implantation site. These anatomic abnormalities can be congenital, like septate uterus or acquired, such as intrauterine adhesions or leiomyoma. The incidence of uterine abnormalities is estimated to be 1 per 200–600, depending on the method used for diagnosis. Uterine abnormalities are present in approximately 10–15% of women with a history of pregnancy loss.[4]

Uterine mullerian anomalies: Women with certain Mullerian anomalies might be predisposed to RPL because of inadequate vascularity to the developing embryo and placenta, reduced intraluminal volume or cervical incompetence. The most common uterine defects include septate, unicornuate, and bicornuate uteri with unequal horns. Women with uterine septa have a 26% risk of reproductive loss, which improves after septum resection.[9]

Management: Accurate diagnosis is essential. Investigations include 2D and 3D transvaginal ultrasonography, hysteroscopy, hysterosalpingogram, and sonohysterograms. Findings may be confirmed by MRI. Prophylactic cervical cerclage may be considered although some authors support expectant management with serial assessment of cervical length by ultrasonographic examination. Data from retrospective and prospective trials have suggested that resection of uterine septum increases delivery rates (7085%).[10]

Immunological Causes

Immunological abnormalities could be classified as autoimmune or alloimmune.

Autoimmune Abnormalities

Recurrent pregnancy loss is associated with several autoimmune diseases. The most important is APS, also known as lupus anticoagulant (LAC) syndrome and Hughes syndrome. This disorder is characterized by the presence of antiphospholipid (APL) antibodies, which are frequently linked to pregnancy losses in the pre-embryonic (<6 weeks), embryonic (69 weeks) and fetal (≥10 weeks gestation) time periods. The APS is a broad heterogeneous entity encompassing patients with specific antibodies to both LAC and anticardiolipin (ACL), as well as nonspecific antinuclear antibodies. Three classes of clinically significant APL antibodies have been identified—ACL, LAC, and antibeta 2 glycoprotein 1 antibodies.[11]

Diagnosis is dependent on clinical and laboratory criterion (Box 1). Notably, the presence of the antibodies alone in the absence of other clinical symptoms does not define the syndrome.

Box 1: Diagnostic criterion for antiphospholipid syndrome (APS)

Diagnosis of APS requires the presence of at least one clinical criteria and one laboratory criteria

Clinical criteria

- Vascular thrombosis
- Pregnancy morbidity
  - Three or more unexplained consecutive miscarriages with anatomic, genetic, and hormonal causes excluded
  - One or more unexplained death(s) of a morphologically normal fetus at or after 10 weeks gestation
  - One or more premature birth(s) of a morphologically normal neonate at or before 34 weeks gestation, associated with severe pre-eclampsia or severe placental insufficiency

Laboratory criteria

- ACL: immunoglobulin G (IgG) and/or immunoglobulin M (IgM) isotype is present in medium or high titer on two or more occasions, 6 or more weeks apart
- Demonstration of a prolonged phospholipid-dependent coagulation or screening test (e.g., activated partial thromboplastin time, dilute Russell's viper venom time and texatarin time)
  - Failure to correct the prolonged screening test result by mixing with normal platelet-poor plasma
  - Shortening or correction of the prolonged screening test result with the addition of excess phospholipids
  - Exclusion of other coagulopathies as clinically indicated (e.g., factor VIII inhibitor) and heparin

Box 2: Treatment options for autoimmune disorders

- Low molecular weight or unfractionated heparin
- Low dose aspirin
- Immunoglobulins in cases with very high titers of antibodies
- Combination of above therapies

Systemic lupus erythematosis: Systemic lupus erythematosis (SLE) is the most common disease associated with APS and may lead to RPL. Patients with SLE have 12% prevalence for ACL antibodies, and 15% for LAC antibodies.

Management: Treatment options are shown in box 2.

Alloimmune Abnormalities

It has been speculated that a defect in the maternal immune response to the semi allogeneic fetal graft could be involved in the mechanism of recurrent abortion. Because the fetus is a semi allograft, some protective immunologic mechanisms should be involved to prevent maternal rejection. HLA-G and HLA-E are expressed on invasive trophoblast cells. This expression pattern is unique among HLA genes and suggests that HLA-G might be involved in interactions that are critical in establishing or maintaining pregnancy.

Implantation of the embryo is associated with reduction in the level of proinflammatory cytokines like interleukin 1 and TNF alpha (Th1 response) and activation of anti-inflammatory cytokines like interleukin 4, 6, 10, 11, and 13 (Th2 response) in the endometrium. Failure to achieve this change in cytokine pattern will result in unexplained RM. Activation of the maternal rejection response is associated with activation of natural killer cells in the endometrium which are embryotoxic.[12]

Currently, there are no clinical tests to confirm alloimmune rejection and these patients are treated as unexplained RM. Treatment with paternal leucocyte transfusion, third party donor leucocytes, trophoblast membranes, and intravenous immunoglobulins has shown no benefit in this subgroup.[13] However, the search is on for new immune potentiators that may prove useful.

Infectious Causes

Numerous organisms have been implicated in sporadic causes of miscarriages, but common microbial causes of RPL have not been confirmed. The presence of bacterial vaginosis in the first trimester of pregnancy has been reported as a risk factor for second-trimester miscarriage and preterm delivery but the evidence for an association with first-trimester miscarriage is inconsistent. Latent genital tuberculosis can cause RPL. Diagnosis is by identification of *Mycobacterium tuberclosis* by DNA/RNA polymerase chain reaction (PCR) on endometrial biopsy. Chlamydia endometritis is also shown to be associated with RMs.

Note: Toxoplasmosis, rubella, cytomegalovirus, herpes, and listeria infections are only implicated in sporadic miscarriage and are not responsible for RM. Routine TORCH screening is not recommended in these cases.

Endocrine and Metabolic Disorders

Ovulation, implantation, and the early stages of pregnancy depend on an intact maternal endocrine regulatory system. Diabetes mellitus, hypothyroidism, polycystic ovarian syndrome (PCOS), luteal phase defect, and obesity are classically associated with an increased risk of miscarriage.

Diabetes Mellitus

Women with poorly controlled diabetes, as evidenced by high glycosylated haemoglobin (HbA1c) levels in the first trimester are at a significantly increased risk of both miscarriage (23 times more than general population) and fetal malformation.

Thyroid Dysfunction

Antithyroid antibodies and subclinical hypothyroidism may be markers for an increased risk for miscarriage.

Low Progesterone Levels and Luteal Phase Defects

Progesterone is the principal hormone responsible not only for rendering the endometrium receptive to embryo implantation, but also for positive immunomodulation in early pregnancy. Low progesterone levels have been associated with miscarriage but whether they are the cause nhyhb or result of a failing pregnancy is still uncertain. Supplementation of progesterone in patients with RM is currently empirical and results of the progesterone in recurrent miscarriages (PROMISE) trial are eagerly awaited.[14]

Polycystic Ovarian Syndrome and Obesity

Both insulin resistance and hyperandrogenemia are responsible for increased incidence of abortion in patients with PCOS.[15] Obese women independently have a high-risk of RM.[16] Weight reduction and metformin seems to improve pregnancy outcome.

Inherited Thrombophilia

Recurrent miscarriages are often characterized by defective placentation and microthrombi in the placental vasculature. In addition, certain inherited disorders that predispose women to venous and/or arterial thrombus formation are associated with pregnancy loss. Abnormal gestations have abnormal fibrin distribution in chorionic villi that make allogeneic contact with maternal tissue making the area more prone to clot formation.

Activated protein C resistance (*Factor V Leiden*): Patients with a single point mutation in the gene coding for Factor V produce a mutated

Factor V (called Factor V Leiden) that is resistant to inactivation by *Activated protein C*, resulting in increased thrombin production and a hypercoagulable state. This mutated gene is inherited as an autosomal dominant trait and is the most common cause of thrombosis and familial thrombophilia, with a prevalence of 3–5% in the general population and could be responsible for RPL.[17]

Coagulation inhibitors: Little data exists evaluating deficiencies of antithrombin III, protein S or protein C and pregnancy loss.

Specific coagulation factor deficiencies: The deficiency of Factor XII (Hageman) is associated with both systemic and placental thrombosis, leading to RM in as many as 22% of patients.

Abnormal homocysteine metabolism: Hyper-homocysteinemia, which may be congenital or acquired, is also associated with thrombosis, premature vascular disease, and pregnancy loss. The most common acquired form is due to folate deficiency.[18] In those patients, folic acid replacement helps achieve normal homocysteine levels within a few days.

Therapy:

- Aspirin: Low dose aspirin 60–150 mg/day irreversibly inhibits the enzyme cyclooxygenase in platelets and macrophages, resulting in inhibition of thromboxane synthesis without affecting prostacyclin production. This can be started in the prepregnancy period in order to facilitate implantation. It is ideally stopped 1 week prior to delivery.
- Heparin: Inhibits blood coagulation and does not cross the placenta; therefore, presents no risk to the fetus. Low molecular weight heparin has a convenient once a day dosage and has been found to be as effective as heparin which needs to be administered twice daily. Therapy is started with a positive pregnancy test and continued till 36 weeks of pregnancy.

Lifestyle and Environmental Factors

Couples experiencing RM are often concerned that toxins in the environment could contribute to their reproductive difficulty. Heavy metals (such as lead and mercury), organic solvents, alcohol, and ionizing radiations are confirmed environmental teratogens and exposure to them may contribute to pregnancy loss. Cessation of smoking is associated with reduction in miscarriage rates. High doses of caffeine and hyperthermia are suspected teratogens, and the teratogenic impact of pesticides remains unknown.

Psychological Cause

It has been seen that stress plays an important role and simple psychological support has led to successful pregnancy outcomes.[19]

The spectrum of etiologies for RM is diverse. Multiple causes may contribute to RM in some patients while no cause may be identified in 40% of patients. Treatment in this subgroup is largely empirical and sometimes frustrating. Role of *in vitro* fertilization is emerging in these patients.[20] It helps to identify aneuploidies in the embryo. Some of these patients will benefit by ovum donation and embryo donation. Others with incorrectable defects in the endometrium may require surrogacy. Assisted reproductive technologies has opened up new vistas in the treatment of patients with RM that were do not respond to other treatment modalities.

REFERENCES

1. WHO recommended definitions, terminology and format for statistical tables related to the perinatal period and use of a new certificate for cause of perinatal deaths. Modifications recommended by FIGO as amended October 14, 1976. Acta Obstet Gynecol Scand. 1977;56(3):247-53.
2. Stirrat GM. Recurrent miscarriage I: definition and epidemiology. Lancet. 1990;336(8716):673-5.
3. RCOG. Green Top Guideline No17. The investigation and treatment of couples with recurrent miscarriage.[online] Revised May 2011 Available from: http://www.rcog.org.

uk/resources/Public/pdf/Recurrent_Miscarriage_No17.pdf [Accessed November, 2013].

4. Practice Committee for the American Society for Reproductive Medicine. Definitions of infertility and recurrent pregnancy loss. Fertil and steril. 2008;89(6):1603.
5. Carp J, Toder V, Aviram A, et al. Karyotype of the abortus in recurrent miscarriage. Fertil Steril. 2001;75:675-82.
6. Warburton D, Dallaire L, Thangavelu M, et al. Trisomy recurrence: a reconsideration based on North American data. Am J Hum Genet. 2004;75(3):376-85.
7. Laurino MY, Bennet RL, Saraiya DS, et al. Genetic evaluation and counselling of couples with recurrent miscarriage:recommendations of the National Society of genetic Counselors. J Genet Couns. 2005;14(3):165-81.
8. Almousawa S, Lavery SA. Preimplantation Genetic Screening-Time to re-evaluate. In: Arora M, editor. World Clinics Obstetrics & Gynecology. 2011.
9. Salim R, Regan L, Woelfer b, et al. A comparative study of morphology of congenital uterine anomalies in women with or without a history of recurrent first trimester miscarriage. Hum Reprod. 2003;18(1):162-6.
10. Shokier T, Abdelshaheed M, El Shafie M, et al. Determinants of fertility and reproductive success after hysteroscopic septoplasty for women with unexplained primary infertility: a prospective analysis of 88 cases. Eur J Obstet gynecol Reprod Biol. 2011;155(1):54-7.
11. Empson M, Lassere M, Craig JC, et al. Recurrent pregnancy loss with antiphospholipid antibody: a systematic review of therapeutic trials. Obstet Gynecol. 2002;99:135-44.
12. Moffett A, Reagan L, Braude P. Natural Killer cells, miscarriage, and infertility. BMJ. 2004;329(7477):1283-85.
13. Porter TF, La Coursiere Y, Scott JR. Immunotherapy for recurrent miscarriage. Cochrane Database Syst Rev. 2006;(2): CD000112.
14. Progesterone in Recurrent miscarriage study (PROMISE trial) ISRCTN 92644181.
15. Rai R, Backos M, Rushworth F, et al. Polycystic ovaries and recurrent miscarriage—a reappraisal. Hum Reprod. 2000;15(3):612-5.
16. Pandey S, Bhattacharys S. Obesity & miscarriage. In: Arora M, editor. World Clinics in Obstetrics & Gynecology. 2011.
17. ACOG. Practice bulletin no 113: inherited thrombophilias in pregnancy. Obstet Gynecol. 2010;116(1):212-22.
18. Arora M, jain R, Gover S. Incidence of hyperhomocysteinemia in Recurrent miscarriage. In: Arora M, editor. World clinics in Obstetrics & Gynecology. 2011.
19. Arck PC, Knackstedt MK. Role of stress in recurrent pregnancy loss. In: Arora M (Ed). Recurrent Pregnancy loss. pp. 206.
20. Go KJ, Patel JC, Cunningham DL. The role of assisted reproductive technology in the management of recurrent pregnancy loss. Curr Opin Endocrinol Diabetes Obes. 2009;16:459-63.

In Vitro Fertilization Conception

25

CHAPTER

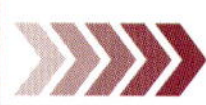

Bharati Dhorepatil, Arati Rapol

INTRODUCTION

Since the birth of the first *in vitro* fertilization (IVF) child in 1978, have occured in fertility techniques. Availability and easy accessibility of treatment, is resulting in many couples conceiving by assisted reproductive technologies. With IVF, the pregnancy rate is approximately 40%, with a live birth rate of 23%. Thus, with routine first trimester screening, one will undoubtedly encounter patients who have undergone some form of assisted conception techniques.

The data required for those patients who have undergone fertility treatment varies considerably from those conceiving naturally and as a result can markedly affect screening results. In the pregnancies conceived by assisted reproductive technology, compared to spontaneous conceptions, there is a higher risk of stillbirth, preeclampsia, gestational hypertension, gestational diabetes mellitus, delivery of small for gestational age neonates, and cesarean section. However, multiple regression analysis showed that after taking into account maternal characteristics, the only significant contributions of IVF were for preeclampsia and elective cesarean section and the contributions of ovulation induction (OI) were for miscarriage, spontaneous early preterm delivery, and small for gestational age. So the conception by IVF and OI is associated with increased risk for adverse pregnancy outcome and screening plays a very crucial role in predictions of those.

Dating

A recent, well-referenced editorial by Gardosi discusses the inaccuracy of last menstrual period dating and advocates routine ultrasound confirmation of dates.[1] Crown-rump measurements at 6–10 weeks are accurate in assigning gestational age. In patients who have undergone any assisted reproductive technology (ART) procedure the pregnancy should be dated by crown rump length (CRL) between 11 weeks and 14 weeks according to National Institute for Health and Clinical Excellence (NICE) guidelines.

A simple rule at early gestation is that a 7 mm embryo is about 7 menstrual weeks and grows about 1 mm/day for the next 3 weeks. CRLs at gestational ages greater than 10 weeks are less accurate.[2]

Ultrasound: Normal Landmarks

Warren and associates described the orderly appearance of gestational sac, yolk sac, and embryo with heartbeat at a given number of days from the onset of the last menstrual period[3] (Table 1).

TABLE 1: The appearance of early gestational structures

Days from LMP gestational sac	*28–35 100%*	*35–42*	*42–49*	*49–56*
Yolk sac	0%	91%	100%	
Embryo with + FHTs	0%	0%	86%	100%

LMP, last menstrual period; FHTs, fetal heart tones.

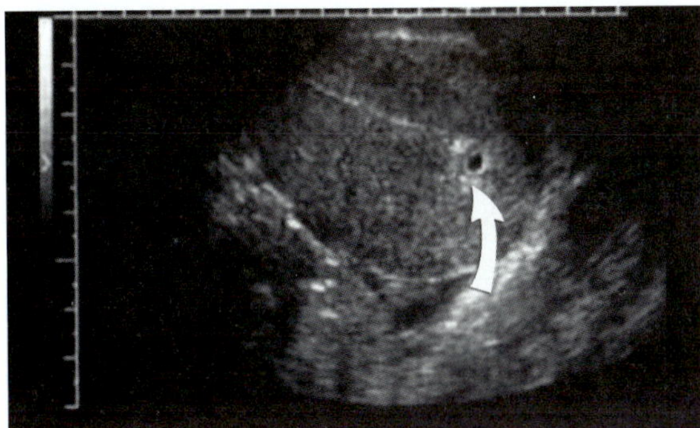

FIGURE 1 A very early (3 mm mean diameter) intrauterine gestational sac at 5 weeks post-menstruation (arrow).

With a transvaginal probe, a 3–4 mm gestational sac can usually be seen by 5 weeks from the last menstrual period (Fig. 1). A yolk sac or small fetal pole is usually seen by 6 menstrual weeks, when the mean diameter of the sac

TABLE 2: Correlation between beta-human chorionic gonadotropin levels and appearance of early gestational structures4

Structure	*Days from LMP*	*hCG (mIU/mL)*	*Second IS β-hCG (mIU/mL) IRP*
Sac	35	1,400	914
Fetal pole	40	5,100	3,800
Heart motion	47	17,200	13,200

LMP, last menstrual period; IRP, International Reference Preparation; IS, International Standard; hCG, human chorionic gonadotropin.

has reached 10 mm. As shown by Fossum and colleagues, the appearance of these structures can be correlated with beta-human chorionic gonadotropin (β-hCG) levels[4] (Table 2).

Considerable caution must be exercised not to confuse collections of fluid within a decidualized endometrium with early gestational sacs. These “pseudogestational sacs” can lead to a missed diagnosis of ectopic pregnancy. Normal early gestational sacs are seen eccentrically-placed, adjacent to the echogenic central stripe (Fig. 2).

Approximately 15-20% of women have a spontaneous, clinically recognized pregnancy loss in the first trimester. A subchorionic bleed (identified on ultrasound) is associated with an

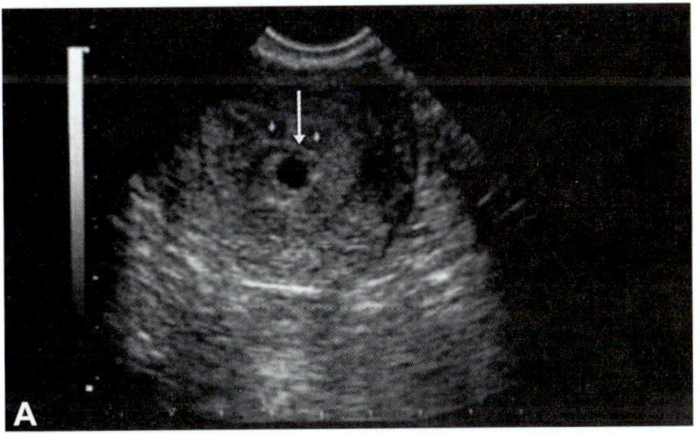

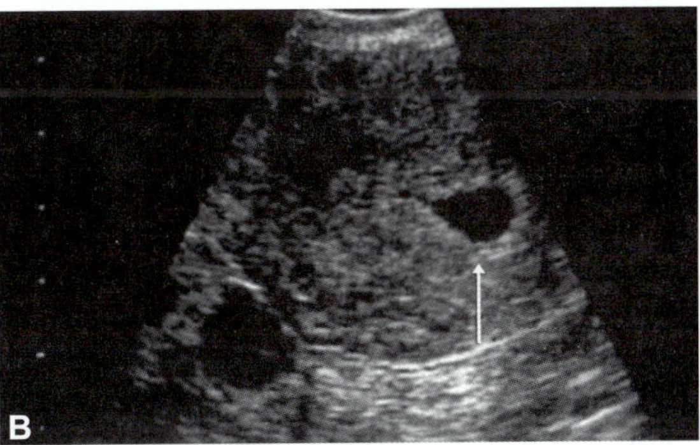

FIGURE 2 A, An eccentrically-placed intrauterine gestational sac 6 weeks post-menstruation (arrow). **B,** A pseudosac (arrow) in a patient with ectopic pregnancy representing a collection of blood or fluid collected within the endometrial cavity.

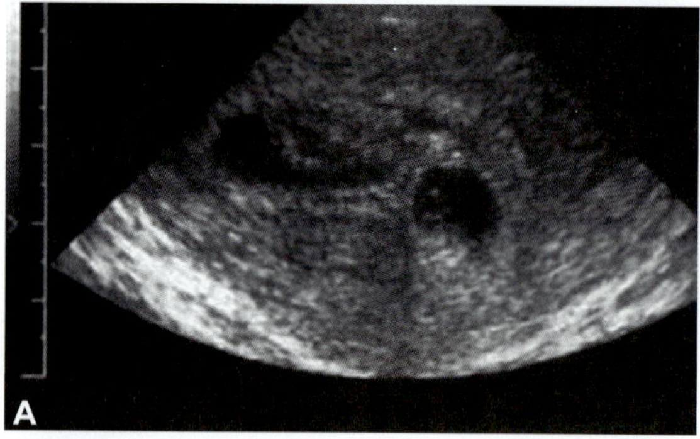

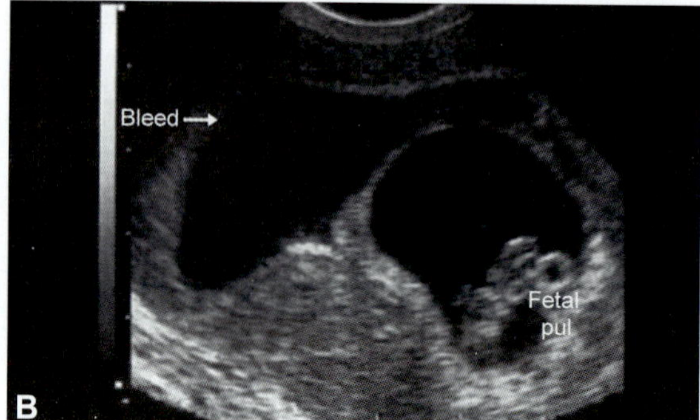

FIGURE 3 **A,** A 7-week intrauterine gestational sac with a large subchorionic bleed and clot. **B,** Ten days later, the clot has resolved but a residual subchorionic bleed is noted.

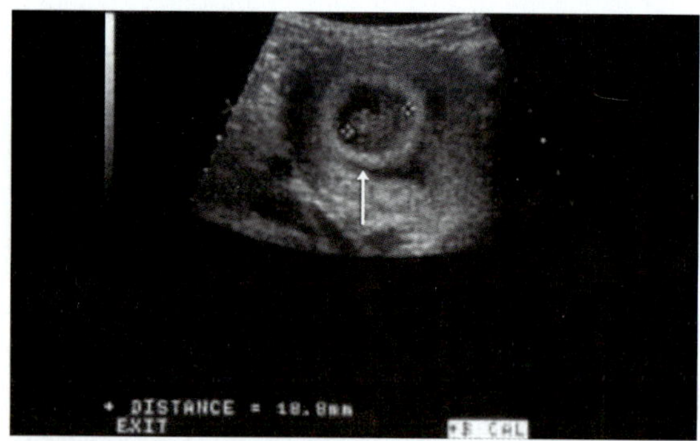

FIGURE 4 An 8-week fetal pole crowded into the gestational sac with a subchorionic bleed (arrow).

increased risk of miscarriage, stillbirth, abruptio placentae, and preterm labor (Fig. 3). The risk of spontaneous abortion increased in proportion to an increase in the size of the subchorionic bleeds. Bradycardic fetal heart rates, small sac size, abnormal yolk sacs (Fig. 4), and large subchorionic bleeds have all been associated with an increased risk of first-trimester pregnancy loss.

Missed Abortion

Pennell and associates, using transvaginal scanning (TVS), found that a 12 mm mean sac diameter (MSD) is seen at approximately 6+ menstrual weeks.[5] Failure to see a yolk sac or small fetal pole when the sac size reaches this diameter should heighten concern of a loss. If a TVS repeated 7–10 days later fails to reveal embryonic structures, the diagnosis of missed abortion can be made unequivocally.

By TVS, fetal heart motion should be seen 100% of the time when the fetal pole reaches 5 mm.[5] Absence of fetal heart motion at this stage is a strong indication of missed abortion. By transabdominal scan (TAS), fetal heart motion should be seen when the fetal pole reaches 12 mm. The reliability of TAS can be compromised by maternal obesity, obscuring leiomyomas, and retroversion. Goldstein and colleagues, using TVS, found that fetal heart motion should be seen when the mean sac diameter reaches 20 mm.[6] Absence of fetal heart motion at this stage is consistent with a missed abortion. By TAS, fetal heart motion is usually seen at a diameter of 25 mm.

For patients who appear not to believe the diagnosis of pregnancy loss, a repeat scan at an appropriate interval may be indicated.

Ectopic Pregnancy

The sensitivity of TVS in detecting actual ectopic adnexal masses is probably dependent on both β-hCG levels and the skill of the sonographers. Stovall and co-workers, visualized 94% of the ectopic adnexal masses in patients with a mean pretreatment β-hCG level of 4,558 mIU/mL.[7] They noted a fetal heartbeat in 20% of the ectopic pregnancies (Fig. 5).[7] A large percentage of the time, identification of an ectopic adnexal mass is based on the findings of a tubal ring or complex adnexal mass (Fig. 6) (*See* Chapter 16: Ectopic Pregnancy).

The fallopian tube is outlined by fluid collection, which was found to represent hemoperitoneum at laparoscopy.

Trisomy Screening

In chromosomally normal pregnancies conceived after IVF and intracytoplasmic sperm injection (ICSI), the pregnancy-associated plasma protein median value was significantly decreased when compared with that of pregnancies conceived spontaneously (0.78 and 0.79 vs. 0.98), while there was no difference in the group treated by frozen embryo replacement. There was no difference in the level of free β-hCG between groups. The median nuchal translucency thickness was smaller in the overall ART group compared with controls. The false-positive rate of first-trimester combined screening in the overall ART group, adjusted for maternal age, was significantly higher. It seems advisable to use a population of IVF/ICSI pregnancies to establish median curves for the first-trimester serum screening parameters and perhaps also for nuchal translucency thickness. However, care must be taken, as different ART treatment methods and aspects of medical history seem to alter the screening parameters in different ways.

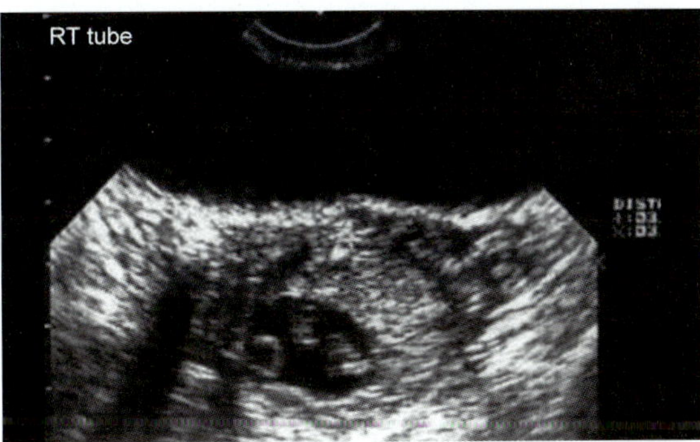

FIGURE 5 A tubal pregnancy with fetus and yolk sac.

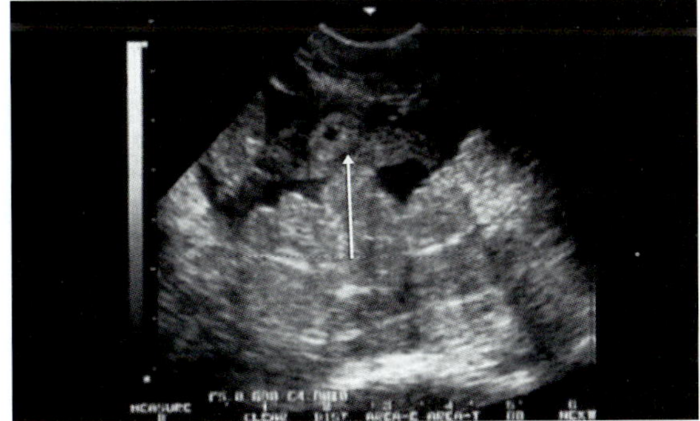

FIGURE 6 An ectopic pregnancy identified by a small tubal ring (arrow).

Multiple Gestation

The single greatest risk associated with fertility treatment is multiple births.

The determination of chorionicity of multiple gestations is of obvious interest to the obstetrician because of the greatly increased morbidity and mortality in monochorionic pregnancies and in particular monoamniotic-monochorionic twin pregnancies. Chorionicity and zygosity should be ascertained in the first trimester screening (*See* Chapter 2: Dating and Chorionicity).

Progesterone Support

Recently there is a lot of debate over the need of continuation of progesterone support in patients who conceive after IVF. No difference in the ongoing pregnancy rate has been seen by continuing progesterone beyond 12 weeks. Recommendations after IVF procedure are vaginal progesterone 200 mg twice daily or vaginal progesterone gel 8% once daily and/or injection hCG 2,000 IU intramuscularly weekly

Finally, couples having come on a very long journey to reach first trimester screening, their perception of high and low risk may differ markedly from the general pregnant population. It is the role of the clinician to allow them to make an informed choice having received a clear explanation of the facts (NICE guidelines 2008).

REFERENCES

1. Gardosi J. Dating of pregnancy: time to forget the last menstrual period. Ultrasound Obstet Gynecol. 1997;9(6):367-8.
2. MacGregor SN, Tamura SK, Sabbagha RE, et al. Underestimation of gestational age by conventional crown-rump length dating curves. Obstet Gynecol. 1987;70(3 Pt 1):344-8.
3. Warren WB, Timor-Trisch I, Peisner DB, et al. Dating the early pregnancy by sequential appearance of embryonic structures. Am J Obstet Gynecol. 1989;161(3):747-53.
4. Fossum GT, Davajan V, Kletzky OA. Early detection of pregnancy with transvaginal ultrasound. Fertil Steril. 1988;49(5):788-91.
5. Pennell RG, Needleman L, Pajak T, et al. Prospective comparison of vaginal and abdominal ultrasound in normal early pregnancy. J Ultrasound Med. 1991;10(2):63-7.
6. Goldstein I, Zimmer EA, Tamir A, et al. Evaluation of normal gestational sac growth: Appearance of embryonic heartbeat and embryo movements using transvaginal technique. Obstet Gynecol. 1991;77(6):885-8.
7. Stovall TG, Ling FW, Gray LA, Carson SA, Buster JE. Methotrexate treatment of unruptured ectopic pregnancy: a report of 100 cases. Obstet Gynecol. 1991;77(5):749-53.

Twin Pregnancy

26

CHAPTER

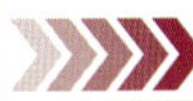 *Krishna Kavita Ramavath*

INTRODUCTION

Twin gestation has been a long interested topic in obstetrics. It has stimulated more interest in recent years as the rate of twinning has profoundly changed by iatrogenic methods. Given that medical treatments of Infertility and Assisted Reproductive Techniques (ART) have had a long-term success to date, there is an epidemic of multiple gestations globally.

According to a study published in the *Lancet*, preterm birth rates increased from 1990 to 2010 in 48 of 65 countries and decreased in only three. In addition, increased preterm birth rates were experienced in high-income as well as lower-income countries. So, one of the causes could be multiple gestations.

Undoubtedly, these pregnancies have high risk of perinatal morbidity and mortality. Maternal and fetal complications are unusually high. Mothers with multiple gestations are at increased risk of anemia and preterm labor, and also present with an increased incidence of malpresentations and medical complications.

The important fetal risks are prematurity, congenital anomalies, and unique complications, such as monoamnionicity, discordant growth, twin to twin transfusion syndrome (TTTS), acardiac twin, and vanishing twin.[1]

This chapter focuses exclusively on the first trimester in twin pregnancies like determination of zygosity and chorionicity, diagnostic role of ultrasound, vanishing twin syndrome, management of twin pregnancies, the unique complications and special nutritional care.

INCIDENCE AND EPIDEMIOLOGY

About 1.1% of all pregnancies are twins. Dizygotic twins are more common about two thirds, and monozygotic twins are about a third.

Natural occurrence of twins by Hellin's law is at a rate of 1:86. According to encyclopedia of multiple birth records throughout the world, there are more than 125 million twins.

There is significant variation among different countries and different races. Yoruba (African tribe in Nigeria) has 45 twins per 1,000 live births which is highest rate of twinning in the world. The twin birth rate in USA was 32.2 per 1,000 in 2007.

The incidence of monozygotic twins is uniform throughout the world, 3.5 per 1,000 live births. The incidence of dizygotic twins is affected by many factors and varies between 4 per 1,000 and 50 per 1,000 live births. This ranges from about 6 per 1,000 births in Japan to 15 per 1,000 in India and up to 24 in USA. This wide variation is attributed to variables like *in vitro* fertilization (IVF), maternal age, and ethnic differences.

ZYGOSITY AND CHORIONICITY

Classification of Twins by Zygosity

There are two types of twins:
1. Monozygotic, identical, uniovular, or single-egg twins.
2. Dizygotic, fraternal, biovular, nonidentical, or two-egg twins.

Monozygotic Twins

- They have identical genotypes and, therefore are of same sex
- Because of the early division of the ovum after fertilization by a single sperm, they contain identical genetic information.

Dizygotic Twins

- They are the result of the fertilization of two ova by two different sperms resulting in separate maternal and paternal genetic contribution to each infant
- Spontaneous dizygotic twins can be familial, and increased levels of follicle stimulating hormone may have a role
- Dizygotic twins have two placentas. They are always dichorionic-diamniotic (di-di).

The chorionicity and amnionicity of monozygotic twins is certainly complex and is considered by the time of zygote cleavage:[2]
- *Dichorionic-diamniotic twins*: Result with the cleavage by day 3. The sites of implantation are two with two separate blastocysts
- *Monochorionic-diamniotic twins* (*mono-di*): Result with the cleavage after day 3. Here, one placenta is shared by two fetuses as blastocyst is already formed. Each twin will have a separate amnion and a chorion, when cleavage is between days 4 and day 8
- *Monochorionic-monoamniotic pregnancy* (*mono-mono twins*): Result of cleavage between days 8 and day 13. These twins will have one chorion and one amnion. This is generally considered to be rare and seen only in 2% of monozygotic twins. Umbilical cord entanglement is the well-known risk and poses high mortality for both the twins in this situation
- *Conjoined twins*: Result from incomplete division of the fertilized egg after day 13. Considered to be very rare and seen one per 200 monozygotic pregnancies and one per each 50,000 live births.

Zygosity

Although DNA fingerprinting is beneficial in determination of zygosity, this prenatal testing is an invasive procedure to sample amniotic fluid (amniocentesis), placental tissue [chorionic villous sampling (CVS)], or fetal blood (cordocentesis). It has a potential to pose risk to fetuses.[3]

Classification of Twins by Chorionicity and Amnionicity

It is particularly important to the healthcare professionals to determine the chorionicity and amnionicity in multiple gestations due to the unique complications. This helps in classifying multiple gestations by the number of placentas (chorionicity) and the number of amniotic sacs (amnionicity).
- Determination of chorionicity by an ultrasound relies on the factors like visualization of fetal gender, placental number, amniotic sacs, and the membrane in between
- Dichorionic twins have different sex and are dizygotic
- The best modality to determine chorionicity in early pregnancy at 6–9 weeks is by an ultrasound

- In dichorionic twins, the intertwin membrane is clearly visualized
- Monochorionic twins have no chorionic layer
- After 9 weeks, this septum is seen as a triangular tissue projection at the base and is called a lambda sign.[4] At 11–14 weeks, due to suboptimal visualization, the presence pregnancies or absence of the lambda sign provides a reliable interpretation between dichorionic pregnancies and monochorionic pregnancies.

So the most relevant signs in early twin gestation are evaluation of the total number of gestational sacs at 7–10 weeks and the presence of a lambda sign between 11 weeks and 14 weeks.

BEST NONINVASIVE DIAGNOSTIC MODALITY—THE ULTRASOUND

From the conception until delivery, the use of ultrasound in the management of twins is very much recommended by all obstetricians and gynecologists. Use of ultrasound virtually helps not only in the accurate diagnosis but also helps to know the fetal progress. It is safe and reliable method and may be done repeatedly throughout pregnancy.

The most appropriate uses of ultrasound in the first trimester are accurate confirmation of gestational age, determination of chorionicity, measurement of cervical length, visualization of both fetal hearts and intertwin membrane, and assessment of amniotic fluid in both gestational sacs.

The most important diagnostic points of twins on an ultrasound are as follows:[5]

- Ultrasound diagnosis of dichorionic twins
  - Visualization of two separate placentas
  - Detection of two separate genders
  - Two amniotic sacs with a sandwiched thick intertwin membrane
  - "Lambda" or "triangle" signs
- Ultrasound diagnosis of monochorionic twins
  - Documentation of a single placenta
  - Thin intertwin membrane
  - Identical genders
  - Insertion of the intertwin membrane directly into the placenta which is called a "T-sign"
  - No "lambda" sign
- Ultrasound diagnosis of monoamniotic twins
  - An intertwin membrane will not be visualized
  - The most definitive finding is umbilical cord entanglement
  - Color Doppler has a specific and valuable role
  - Considered to be rare (0.4–1.4% of all twins).

TWIN REVERSED ARTERIAL PERFUSION SYNDROME AND ACARDIAC TWIN

Twin reversed arterial perfusion (TRAP sequence) is indeed a rare syndrome that occurs only in the monochorionic twin pregnancies. It has an incidence of 1 in 35,000 births. In this condition, the acardiac twin and "pump twin" coexist. With the use of advanced ultrasound equipment, it is now possible to diagnose cases of TRAP syndrome at 8 weeks of gestation using transvaginal three-dimensional color Doppler. Reversed arterial perfusion on Doppler is the most important diagnostic finding.

Early diagnosis and confirmation of acardiac twins with TRAP syndrome in the first trimester allows for early treatment and better outcome of pregnancy which would otherwise cause high output cardiac failure in pump fetus.[6,7]

VANISHING TWIN SYNDROME

Vanishing twin syndrome is first described by Stoeckel in 1945.[8] This finding is unique to multifetal gestations. Disappearance of one or more fetuses after their identification may be the result of miscarriage of one twin or multiple fetuses.

Use of ultrasonography in early pregnancy allows accurate diagnosis. Its frequency is observed in 20–30% of multiple pregnancies.

Review of literature relating to vanishing twin shows that 10–15% of singleton births were initially twin gestations. The fetus may be completely reabsorbed with the formation of a fetus papyraceus (i.e., a flattened or parchment like compressed fetus), or there may be an abnormality on the placenta suggesting a cyst, subchorionic fibrin, or amorphous material. Significant genetic or chromosomal abnormalities are frequently revealed in the analysis of fetal tissue.

Maternal morbidity in first trimester is less adverse. Mild vaginal bleeding and cramping are noted.

Major complications noted in second and third trimesters are premature labor, infection, postpartum hemorrhage, disseminated intravascular coagulation (DIC), and obstruction of labor by a low-lying fetus papyraceus causing dystocia. Such complications may lead to a cesarean delivery.

Fetal Morbidity and Mortality

It is reported that the surviving fetus has good prognosis if the vanishing twin syndrome occurred in first trimester. An increased risk of neurological impairment which presents as cerebral palsy is noted in the second half of pregnancy.

- Transfusion of thromboplastic proteins to the surviving twin may lead to DIC
- Aplasia cutis or areas of skin necrosis is also frequently noted.

Work-up

- Increased levels of specific biochemical parameters like pregnancy associated plasma protein-A and free beta human chorionic gonadotropin (β-hCG) are documented
- Alpha-fetoprotein levels are elevated
- The rate of rise of β-hCG is significantly reduced than in a normal twin pregnancy.

Antenatal Care in Vanishing Twin

- Close follow-up of pregnancy with serial ultrasonographic evaluations of the live fetus
- The surviving fetus is recognized to be at risk for low birth weight and small for gestational age
- No special medical care is needed for uncomplicated vanishing twin syndrome.

SURVIVAL OF THE EARLY TWIN PREGNANCY AND COMPLICATIONS

- Growth abnormalities or congenital anomalies are high in twins which in turn increase the risk of fetal death rates
- Monochorionic twins show a higher neurological morbidity, discordancy, and death. Ten to fifteen percent of mono-di twins develop twin to twin transfusion syndrome (TTTS)
- Monoamniotic twin pregnancies have number of complications like cord entanglements, abdominal wall and renal malformations which result in fetal demise. The death of one fetus, results in more than 20% risk for adverse neurologic outcome in a co-twin survivor
- The principal risk for the surviving twin is preterm delivery[9]
- A practical approach to evaluate cerebral lesions in the survivors is by ultrasound and fetal cerebral magnetic resonance imaging.[9]

PRENATAL DIAGNOSIS

Aneuploidy Screening

Recommended first trimester screening test for aneuploidies in twin pregnancies is nuchal translucency combined with maternal age. It is important for the clinicians to be aware that aneuploidies increase with maternal age. To reduce the false positive rates, first trimester serum screening should be combined with nuchal translucency.

The nuchal fold thickness of each fetus must be documented in monochorionic pregnancies as increased thickness is an indicator of TTTS and chromosomal abnormalities.[9]

Fetal Sampling Technique: Chronic Villous Sampling or Amniocentesis?

- Studies have shown that the outcomes of fetal loss with sampling in twins is slightly higher
- CVS is considered to be the procedure of choice and favored over amniocentesis[10]
- The preferred route is transabdominal as compared to transcervical
- Its performance after 70 days of gestation carries minimal or no risks and between 11 weeks and 14 weeks provides a safe and early result
- It helps in decision making of selective pregnancy reduction with minimal risk.

MANAGEMENT OF MULTIPLE PREGNANCIES

- *Pregnancy symptoms*: Typical signs and symptoms of pregnancy can be more intense
- *Morning sickness*: Tends to be exaggerated in some women
- *Measuring large for gestational age*: Increased uterine size is a significant indicator
- *Heart beats*: An ultrasound best detects two or more heartbeats as early as 10–12 weeks
- *Edema*: Extreme fatigue and water retention in the form of pedal edema is common
- *More frequent antenatal visits*: Monthly in the first trimester, twice in a month during the second trimester, and every week during the third trimester are recommended
- *Nutrients*: Iron, folic acid, calcium, protein, and other essential nutrients intake is increased due to the increased demand
- *Weight gain*: Expected weight gain of 10 pounds in the first trimester can be due to increased blood volume, tissue, and uterine growth. Women in singleton pregnancies typically gain around 30 pounds for entire 9 months. For twins, the recommendation is often 35–45 pounds (16–20 kg).[11]

Dichorionic-diamniotic Twin Gestations

- Management includes a monthly follow-up. Recommended weight gain is around 10 pounds in the first trimester
- Periodic ultrasound every month for estimation of fetal weight is advised
- First trimester early Doppler umbilical artery study is also recommended keeping in view of unique complications
- It is recommended to plan delivery of uncomplicated di-di twin pregnancies from 38 weeks and before 40 weeks.

Monochorionic-diamniotic Twin Gestations

- Because of the increased risks obstetric ultrasound is performed twice monthly
- The recommended time of delivery of an uncomplicated pregnancy is from 36 weeks to 38 weeks.

Monochorionic-monoamniotic Twin Pregnancies

- A standard protocol has to be followed regarding first trimester prenatal diagnosis and should be managed carefully with intensified surveillance for cord entanglement
- The recommended time of delivery is after 32 weeks and before 36 weeks by a caesarean section.

FOCUS ON NUTRITION IN FIRST TRIMESTER OF TWIN PREGNANCY

Special attention to nutrition and nutritional counseling should be part of first trimester care of twin pregnancy. Neonatal outcomes are highly improved with appropriate maternal weight gain in early pregnancy.

Nausea and vomiting are intensified in first trimester and they should be managed aggressively with intravenous fluids, thiamine vitamin B_1 (vit B_1) and vitamin B_6. Electrolyte imbalances should be promptly recognized and corrected.

It is important for the practicing clinician to recognize poor intake which further leads to poor weight gain. Hence, a well-balanced diet with micro- and macro-nutrient supplementation is suggested by the Michigan multiple clinical experience study.

Reasonable approach early in pregnancy would be to give a prenatal vitamin, calcium, zinc, magnesium with iron, and folate. Omega 3-fatty acids and vitamin D are also advised if well tolerated to have favorable outcomes.

With available data on twin pregnancies and increased risks of low birth weight and prematurity, pregnant women should be counseled to focus on body mass index specific weight gain rather than high calorie intake.[11]

Serum ferritin levels are the best guide to iron deficiency during the early visits and early iron supplementation helps to cope up the demands.

Mothers with twins are recommended to consume 3,000–4,000 kcal per day.

Finally, maternal education regarding a healthy balanced diet, lifestyle modifications, and taking appropriate supplements result in a favorable outcome.

KEY POINTS FOR CLINICAL PRACTICE

- First trimester ultrasound is the best diagnostic modality for all women with twin pregnancies and measurement of crown-rump length is the best parameter
- Amnionicity and chorionicity have to be documented in women with twin pregnancy
- Accurate pregnancy dating is important by first trimester ultrasound. In twin pregnancies as a result of IVF, this is calculated from the date of embryo transfer. It helps in evaluation of fetal growth and intrauterine growth restriction
- Nuchal translucency thickness measurement should be an integral part of the first trimester scanning in both mono- and dichorionic twins
- Monochorionic gestations should have serial ultrasound surveillance from 16 weeks and are to be evaluated every 2 weeks for evidence of TTTS and other complications
- Early diagnosis of acardiac twin and TRAP syndrome is done by Doppler evaluation which shows characteristic reversed arterial perfusion
- Serial ultrasounds are also necessary in cases of vanishing twins, to watch carefully for signs of infection in the survivor like cerebral calcifications, echogenic bowel, or abnormalities in amniotic fluid
- In case of diagnostic sampling a trans-abdominal, CVS is recommended over amniocentesis
- Specific nutritional interventions for mothers of twin gestation should be emphasized early in first trimester. Adequate weight gain in early pregnancy effectively improves the outcomes of twins.

The unique experience of having twins is carried forward and beyond by the collective team-work of healthcare professionals. A special focus not only in first trimester but at every trimester is important to have an excellent outcome.

REFERENCES

1. Hayes EJ. Review of Multiple Pregnancy: Epidemiology, Gestation & Perinatal Outcome. 2nd ed. J Exp Clin Assist Reprod. 2005;2:12.
2. Carroll SG, Tyfield L, Reeve L, et al. Is zygosity or chorionicity the main determinant of fetal outcome in twin pregnancies? Am J Obstet Gynecol. 2005;193(3 Pt 1):757-61.
3. Fox, Traci B. (2006). "Multiple Pregnancies: Determining Chorionicity and Amnionicity" Department of Radiologic Sciences Faculty Papers. Paper 1.[online] Available from http://jdc.jefferson.edu/rsfp/1 [Accessed November, 2013].
4. Wood SL, St Onge R, Connors G, et al. Evaluation of the twin peak or lambda sign in determining chorionicity in multiple pregnancy. Obstet Gynecol. 1996;88(1):6-9.

5. Morin L, Lim L. Ultrasound in twin pregnancies. J Obstet Gynaecol Can. 2011;33(6):643-56.
6. Podobnik M, Podobnik P, Brlecic I. First-trimester diagnosis of acardiac twins by three-dimensional ultrasound: case report-Ultrasound in Obstet Gynecol. 2006;28(4):557.
7. Rohilla M, Chopra S, Suri V, et al. Acardiac-acephalus twins: a report of 2 cases and review of literature. Medscape J Med. 2008;10(8):200.
8. Landy HJ, Keith LG. The vanishing twin:a review. Hum Reprod Update. 1998;4:177-83.
9. Vayssière C, Benoist G, Blondel B, et al. Twin pregnancies: guidelines for clinical practice from the French College of Gynecologists and Obstetricians (CNGOF). Eur J Obstet Gynecol Reprod Biol. 2011;156(1):12-7.
10. Simonazzi G, Curti A, Farina A, et al. Amniocentesis and chorionic villus sampling in twin gestations: which is the best sampling technique? Am J Obstet Gynecol. 2010;202(4):365.
11. Goodnight W, Newman R, Society of Maternal-Fetal Medicine. Optimal nutrition for improved twin pregnancy outcome. Obstet Gynecol. 2009;114(5):1121-34.

Surgery and Anesthesia

27

CHAPTER

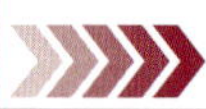

Suchitra N Pandit, Deepali P Kale

INTRODUCTION

Surgery in pregnancy involves the care of two patients, i.e., mother and fetus. Approximately 1 in 500 to 1 in 635 women require nonobstetrical abdominal surgery during their pregnancy.[1]

Close liason between the surgeon and obstetrician is necessary. The problems in the management of acute abdomen during pregnancy are:

- Expanding uterus displacing the intra-abdominal organs thus rendering the physical examination difficult
- Higher prevalence of nausea and vomiting, abdominal pain in normal obstetric population, masking the features of acute abdomen
- General reluctance to operate on a gravid patient

Elective surgery in first trimester should be avoided due to the risk of teratogenicity and miscarriage. Nonobstetric surgeries performed in the first trimester are only emergency surgeries. Semi-emergency procedures should be deferred till the second trimester. The risk of surgery and anesthesia to mother and fetus should be weighed against the disadvantages of conservative treatment modalities.

The most common nonobstetrical surgical emergencies complicating pregnancy are acute appendicitis, cholecystitis, and intestinal obstruction.[1] Other conditions necessitating surgery during pregnancy include ovarian cysts, masses or torsion, symptomatic cholelithiasis, adrenal tumors, splenic disorders, symptomatic hernias, complications of inflammatory bowel diseases, and acute abdominal pain of unknown etiology.

SURGERIES PERFORMED DURING THE FIRST TRIMESTER

Gynecological Surgeries

- Adnexal torsion
- Ovarian cyst rupture
- Torsion of pedunculated subserous myoma
- Heterotopic pregnancy.

For these surgeries *See* Chapter 28: Laparoscopy.

Nongynecological Surgeries

- Acute appendicitis
- Acute cholecystitis
- Bowel obstruction
- Bowel perforation
- Meckel's diverticulitis
- Acute pancreatitis
- Blunt trauma
- Penetrating trauma
- Surgery for breast cancer.

ANATOMICAL AND PHYSIOLOGICAL CHANGES IN PREGNANCY

Before arriving at the clinical diagnosis of acute abdomen in pregnancy, the obstetrician must be aware of the anatomical and physiological alterations in the intra-abdominal organs. Physical examination findings may be less prominent compared to nongravid patients.

The uterine size gradually increases thereby making the palpation of abdominal masses difficult. Anatomical changes may modify clinical signs, like tenderness at Mcburneys point due to displacement of the appendix. The changes in relationship of ureters have to be kept in mind. The uterus can also obstruct and inhibit the movement of omentum to an area of inflammation, distorting the clinical picture. To distinguish the extra-uterine tenderness from uterine tenderness, palpation has to be done in right or left lateral decubitus position, thus displacing the gravid uterus to one side.

Physiological changes in the maternal respiratory system like alterations in the vital capacity and tidal volume are important from anesthesia point of view. It is imperative to prevent maternal hypoxia during surgery. The maternal circulatory system changes like increase in blood volume may necessitate higher drug dosages.

Peritoneal signs are often absent in pregnancy because of lifting and stretching of abdominal wall. The underlying inflammation has no direct contact with the parietal peritoneum, which precludes muscular response like guarding and rigidity that would be otherwise expected.

MATERNAL SAFETY DURING NON-OBSTETRIC SURGERY IN PREGNANCY

Alteration in Laboratory Values

Due to physiologic consequences of pregnancy, laboratory parameters are altered, so interpretation of results must be done with reference to normal range for pregnancy. For example, normal white blood cell count in pregnancy ranges from 6,000–16,000/mm^3 in second and third trimester and from 20,000–30,000/mm^3 during labour.

Use of Imaging Technique

Managing abdominal pain in the gravid patient presents a dilemma in which the clinician must consider the risks and benefits of diagnostic modalities and therapies to both the mother and the fetus. An underlying principle to the workup of abdominal pain was stated by Sir Zachary Cope in 1921, "Earlier diagnosis means better prognosis." In pregnant women with abdominal pain, fetal outcome depends on the outcome of the mother. Optimal maternal outcome may require radiologic imaging, sometimes with ionizing radiation. A risk-benefit discussion with the patient should occur prior to any diagnostic study.

Medications During Pregnancy

Some medications are contraindicated in pregnancy. Benefits should be carefully weighed against the risks. Due to hemodynamic and physiological changes in pregnancy, drug doses may need to be altered.

IMAGING TECHNIQUES

Ultrasound

Ultrasonographic (USG) imaging during pregnancy is safe and useful in identifying the etiology of acute abdominal pain which may be gynecological or nongynecological in etiology. No adverse effects to mother or fetus from ultrasound have been reported. It is the initial radiographic test of choice for most gynecologic causes of abdominal pain including adnexal mass, torsion, and cyst rupture. Ultrasound is also a useful study for many non-gynecologic causes of abdominal pain, including symptomatic gallstones and appendicitis.[2-4]

Risk of Ionizing Radiation

Expeditious and accurate diagnosis should take precedence over concerns for ionizing radiation. Cumulative radiation dosage should be limited to 5–10 rads during pregnancy.

Significant radiation exposure may lead to chromosomal mutations, neurologic abnormalities, mental retardation, and increased risk of childhood leukemia. Although cumulative radiation dosage is the primary risk factor for adverse fetal effects, fetal age at exposure is also important.[5-7] Fetal mortality is greatest when exposure occurs within the first week of conception. It has been recommended that the cumulative radiation dose to the conceptus during pregnancy be less than 5–10 rads.[8] As an example, the radiation dose to the conceptus for a plain abdominal radiograph averages 0.1–0.3 rads, while a computed tomography (CT) of the pelvis yields up to 5 rads of fetal exposure.[9]

The most sensitive time period for central nervous system teratogenesis is between 10 and 17 weeks gestation, and routine radiographs should be avoided during this time. In later pregnancy, the concern shifts from teratogenesis to increasing the risk of childhood hematologic malignancy. The background incidence of childhood cancer and leukemia is approximately 0.2–0.3%. Radiation may increase that incidence by 0.06% per 1 rad delivered to the fetus.[8]

Exposure of the conceptus to 0.5 rad increases the risk of spontaneous abortion, major malformations, mental retardation, and childhood malignancy to one additional case in 6,000 above baseline risk.[9] It has been suggested that the risk of aberrant teratogenesis is negligible at 5 rads or less and that the risk of malformation is significantly increased at doses above 15 rads. No single diagnostic study should exceed 5 rads.[6-12]

Computed Tomography

Contemporary multidetector CT protocols deliver a low radiation dose and may be used judiciously during pregnancy. Radiation exposure to the fetus may be as low as 2 rads for pelvic CT scans but can reach 5 rads when a full scan of the abdomen and pelvis is performed. This radiation dose is considered safe but may cause teratogenesis and increase the risk of developing childhood hematologic malignancies.[9] CT protocols and radiation doses vary by institution, and the individual practitioner should be aware of the radiation exposure at his or her institution and attempt to minimize fetal radiation exposure as far as possible.

Magnetic Resonance Imaging

Magnetic resonance imaging without the use of intravenous gadolinium can be performed at any stage of pregnancy. MRI provides excellent soft tissue imaging without ionizing radiation and is safe to use in pregnant patients.[13] Some authors express concern about the detrimental effects of the acoustic noise to the fetus, but no specific adverse effects of MRI on fetal development have been reported. Intravenous gadolinium agents cross the placenta and may be detrimental; therefore, their use during pregnancy should be confined to select cases where it is considered imperative.[14]

Nuclear Medicine

Administration of radionucleotides for diagnostic studies is generally safe for mother and fetus.[15] Radiopharmaceuticals, including technetium-99m, can generally be administered at doses that provide whole fetal exposure of less than 0.5 rad well within the safe range of fetal exposure.[16] Consultation with a nuclear medicine radiologist or technologist should be considered prior to performing the study.

Cholangiography

Intraoperative and endoscopic cholangiography exposes the mother and fetus to minimal radiation and may be used selectively during pregnancy. The lower abdomen should be shielded when performing cholangiography during pregnancy to decrease the radiation exposure to the fetus.[17]

Radiation exposure during cholangiography is estimated to be 0.2–0.5 rads.[17] Fluoroscopy generally delivers a radiation dose of up to 20 rads/minute, but varies depending on the X-ray equipment used, patient positioning, and patient size. Efforts should be made to shield the fetus from radiation exposure without compromising the field of view necessary for proper imaging. No adverse effects to pregnant patients or their fetuses have been reported specifically from cholangiography.

The radiation exposure during endoscopic retrograde cholangiopancreatography (ERCP) averages 2–12 rads, but can be substantially higher for long procedures.[18] ERCP also carries risks beyond radiation exposure of bleeding and pancreatitis. In non-pregnant patients, the risk of bleeding is 1.3% and risk of pancreatitis is 3.5–11%.[19] These additional risks warrant the same careful risk-benefit analysis and discussion with the patient as other operative and procedural interventions. Alternatives to fluoroscopy include intra-operative ultrasound and choledochoscopy. These are both acceptable methods provided the surgeon has the appropriate equipment and skills to accurately perform the examinations.

Magnetic resonance cholangiopancreatography is an alternative approach that is gaining widespread acceptance. It is a useful diagnostic tool but offers no therapeutic capability. It has not been studied specifically in pregnant women.

The use of radiography is worrisome due to potential fetal adverse effects. However, risk benefits should be weighed to avoid misdiagnosis. USG is the most preferred imaging modality in a pregnant woman because of its noninvasiveness, speed, and accuracy. MRI is used if diagnosis is not confirmed by USG. Both USG and MRI are not associated with known fetal adverse effects. Proper shielding of maternal abdomen is indicated if X-ray exposure is necessary. Consultation with an expert in dosimetry calculation may be helpful in a calculating estimated fetal dose when multiple diagnostic radiographs are required.

PRINCIPLES OF GENERAL SURGERY IN FIRST TRIMESTER OF PREGNANCY

- As per hospital infection control policy, use broad spectrum antibiotics, e.g., cefuroxime, ampicillin, and metronidazole preoperatively
- Preoxygenation, intubation, and ventilation to prevent fetal hypoxia and resuscitation in case of hypovolemia
- Copious irrigation and use of intraperitaoneal drain.

LAPAROSCOPIC SURGERY DURING PREGNANCY

During its infancy, some argued that laparoscopy was contraindicated during pregnancy due to concerns for uterine injury and fetal perfusion. As surgeons have gained more experience with laparoscopy, it has become the preferred treatment for many surgical diseases in the gravid patient.

DIAGNOSTIC LAPAROSCOPY

Diagnostic laparoscopy is safe and effective when used selectively in the workup and treatment of acute abdominal processes in pregnancy. Diagnostic laparoscopy provides direct visualization of intra-abdominal organs. While not enough data are available to recommend this as a primary diagnostic approach in the pregnant patient, it is a reasonable alternative to radiologic imaging. The benefits of operative exploration are avoidance of ionizing radiation, diagnostic accuracy, and the capability to treat a surgical problem at the same time. Furthermore, it has been shown that laparoscopy can be performed safely during any trimester of pregnancy with minimal morbidity to the fetus and mother.[20-24]

LAPAROSCOPY VERSUS LAPAROTOMY

Laparoscopic treatment of acute abdominal disease has the same indications in pregnant as in nonpregnant patients.

Once the decision to operate has been made, the surgical approach (laparotomy vs. laparoscopy) should be determined based on the skills of the surgeon and the availability of the appropriate staff and equipment. An appropriate discussion with the patient regarding the risks and benefits of surgical intervention should be undertaken. Benefits of laparoscopy during pregnancy appear similar as in nonpregnant patients including less postoperative pain, less postoperative ileus, decreased length of hospital stay, and faster return to work.[20-27] For details on laparoscopic surgery *See* Chapter 28: Laparoscopy.

NONGYNECOLOGICAL SURGERIES

Acute Cholecystitis

Cholecystectomy is required in 1 in 1,600–10,000 pregnancies. The symptomatology of acute cholecystitis is identical in pregnant and nonpregnant women. Murphy's sign is less common in pregnant women with cholecystitis.

Laparoscopic cholecystectomy is the treatment of choice in the pregnant patient with gallbladder disease, regardless of trimester.

In the past, nonoperative management of symptomatic cholelithiasis in pregnancy has been recommended.[28-30] At present, early surgical management is the treatment of choice. This is supported by data showing recurrence of symptoms in 92% of patients managed nonoperatively, when they presented in the first trimester, 64% when presenting in the second trimester, and 44% when presenting in the third trimester.[31-32] The delay in surgical management results in increased rates of hospitalizations, spontaneous abortions, preterm labor, and preterm delivery compared to those undergoing cholecystectomy.[19,21,26]

Nonoperative management of symptomatic gallstones in gravid patients result in recurrent symptoms in more than 50% of patients, and 23% of such patients develop acute cholecystitis or gallstone pancreatitis. Gallstone pancreatitis results in fetal loss in 10% to 60% of pregnant patients.[33-35]

The significant morbidity and mortality associated with untreated gallbladder disease in the gravid patient favors surgical intervention preferably by the laparoscopic route.[36-40]

Choledocholithiasis during pregnancy may be managed with preoperative ERCP with sphincterotomy followed by laparoscopic cholecystectomy, laparoscopic common bile duct exploration, or postoperative ERCP.[33-35]

Complications associated with choledocholithiasis are relatively uncommon during pregnancy.[41,42] However, these complications can result in significant morbidity and mortality making appropriate management of these patients important. There have been no trials comparing common bile duct exploration at the time of laparoscopic cholecystectomy to ERCP followed by cholecystectomy in pregnant patients. Good outcomes have been described with intraoperative common bile duct exploration, but very few cases have been reported. Multiple studies have demonstrated safe and effective management of common bile duct stones with preoperative ERCP with fetal shielding, followed by laparoscopic cholecystectomy.[43]

Acute Appendicitis

The pregnant patient with appendicitis presents unique challenges to both the surgeon and gynaecologist.

- Firstly early pregnancy needs confirmation at the time of presentation
- Secondly, the anemia and physiological changes that normally occur during pregnancy alter the physical findings and laboratory values that are often used for diagnosis of appendicitis

- Thirdly, cases of appendicitis that occur during pregnancy can produce significant morbidity and mortality if not promptly identified and treated
- Fourthly, the treating surgeon has limitations in the use of certain diagnostic procedures because of possible teratogenicity like X-ray abdomen
- Finally, the surgeon is treating two patients simultaneously, the mother and the fetus and must be aware of the potential effects of treatment on both patients at all times.[44]

Recent studies have shown that approximately 30% of cases occur during the first trimester, 45% during the second trimester, and 25% during the third trimester, labor, or puerperium.[44] The incidence of appendicitis during pregnancy is equal to nonpregnant women of the same age. During the first six months of pregnancy, symptoms of appendicitis are same as in nonpregnant woman. But in pregnancy, these can be confused with morning sickness, ectopic pregnancy, and twisted ovarian cyst in the first trimester. During the third trimester, patient complains of pain, higher and more lateral in the abdomen or right flank as enlarged uterus leads to displacement and lateral rotation of cecum and appendix.

The appendix remains in the right iliac fossa during the first trimester, moves to the pelvic brim during second trimester and reaches the lower right upper quadrant in the third trimester. Incidence of perforated diffuse peritonitis is high as infection cannot be localized due to Braxton Hicks uterine contractions and the inability of the omentum to reach the inflamed appendix. Guarding and rigidity are difficult to elicit in the third trimester due to stretched abdominal muscles.[4] Laboratory examination of blood and urine may be of little diagnostic aid. Premature labour is seen in about half the women. Fetal mortality is high due to septicaemia and prematurity. Appendectomy should be performed on suspicion of appendicitis just as if pregnancy was not present. If surgery is performed before the appendix ruptures, pregnancy outcomes are better. Hence, if acute appendicitis is suspected in a pregnant patient, we recommend a close working relationship between the surgeon, obstetrician, and anesthesiologist to minimize maternal and fetal morbidity and mortality. Due to difficulty in the diagnosis of acute appendicitis in a pregnant patient, a higher negative laparotomy rate in these patients (20–35%) is acceptable as compared to nonpregnant patients (15%). An aggressive surgical approach seems justified since the incidence of perforation increases to 66% if there is delay in removing the appendix after diagnosis has been made.[45]

Selecting the type and location of incision depends on the:

- Uterine size
- Gestational age
- Location of abdominal pain
- Presence of peritonitis.

There is often a tendency amongst obstetricians to relate cases of pain abdomen during pregnancy with the genital organs leading to late referrals and diagnosis. Maternal mortality from appendicitis is now almost zero, and is nearly always associated with perforation and peritonitis. Overall, fetal mortality reported is 2–8.5% but it increases to 35% in perforation and peritonitis.[44,46]

To conclude, appendicitis in pregnancy has always been a difficult problem compared to nonpregnant patients. Early appendectomy is the treatment of choice recommended at all stages of pregnancy. However, if appendix ruptures or abscess forms, emergency exploration by a midline or right paramedian abdominal incision is recommended.

There is a definite role of diagnostic laparoscopy in patients with right lower quadrant abdominal pain with positive pregnancy test in patients with past history of pelvic inflammatory disease.

Laparoscopic Appendectomy

Laparoscopic appendectomy is the preferred approach in pregnant patients with appendicitis. This retrospective series of 45 patients has shown very low rates of preterm delivery and no reports of fetal demise.[47]

In some circumstances, clinical findings may be sufficient for diagnosis. When the diagnosis remains uncertain, prompt ultrasound, CT, or MRI are useful adjuncts to more accurate diagnosis. However, the false negative rates of CT and MRI studies have yet to be fully evaluated in the gravid patient, and some hospitals may not have immediate access to these radiologic modalities. A diagnostic laparoscopy may be both diagnostic as well as therapeutic in these caeses even in the third trimester of pregnancy.[48]

A recent meta-analysis comparing laparoscopy versus open appendectomy in pregnancy concluded that fetal loss may be slightly greater with laparoscopic procedures.[49]

However, laparoscopy can be the gold standard diagnostic tool that will reduce rate of negative laparotomy as well as rule out ectopic pregnancy and salpingitis. CT of the appendix should be performed judiciously during pregnancy because of radiation exposure to the fetus.[50,51] If laparoscopic appendectomy is performed early in pregnancy, it is associated with negligible maternal and fetal complications.

Intestinal Obstruction

Bowel obstruction occurs with frequency of 1 in 1,500-16,000 pregnancies. Intra-abdominal adhesions (due to previous abdominal/pelvic surgery or pelvic inflammatory disease) and volvulus are common causes. Cecal volvulus is somewhat less common in first trimester, but may occur in the third trimester of pregnancy.

Patient will present with crampy abdominal pain, constipation, and vomiting. Plain abdominal X-ray with presence of air fluid level or progressive bowel dilatation in serial films at 4-6 hours interval are diagnostic. Initial conservative treatment consists of fluid and electrolyte replacement, nasogastric suction for bowel decompression, montoring maternal oxygen saturation and fetal heart rate. If conservative management fails, surgical exploration is warranted. A midline vertical incision is recommended with resection of gangrenous segment and primary anstomosis. Fetal mortality rate after maternal intestinal obstruction is 20–26%. Maternal mortality can range from 6 to 20%.[52]

Breast Cancer Surgery in Pregnancy

Surgery is usually the first treatment option for pregnant women with breast cancer. A lumpectomy or mastectomy and lymph node removal, may be done to remove the tumor.

GYNECOLOGICAL SURGERIES IN PREGNANCY

Adnexal Masses

Laparoscopy is safe and effective treatment in gravid patients with symptomatic ovarian cystic masses. Observation is acceptable for all other cystic lesions provided ultrasound does not show solid components and vascular flow and tumor markers are normal. Initial observation is warranted for most cystic lesions <6 cm in size.

The incidence of adnexal masses during pregnancy is 2%.[53] Most of the adnexal masses discovered during the first trimester are functional cysts that resolve spontaneously by the second trimester. Eighty to ninety-five percent of adnexal masses ≤6 cm in diameter in pregnant patients spontaneously resolve; therefore nonoperative management is warranted in such cases.[53]

Persistent masses are most commonly functional cysts or mature cystic teratomas with the incidence of malignancy reported at 2 to 6%. Historically, the concern over malignant potential and risks associated with emergency surgery have led to elective removal of masses that persist after

16 weeks and are >6 cm in diameter.[54-57] Recent literature supports the safety of close observation in these patients when ultrasound findings are not suggestive for malignancy, tumor markers (CA125/LDH) are normal, and the patient is asymptomatic. In the event that surgery is indicated, various case reports[58-60] support the use of laparoscopy in the management of adnexal masses in every trimester.

Adnexal Torsion

Adnexal torsion involves the ovary, fallopian tube, and broad ligament. Laparoscopy is recommended for both diagnosis and treatment unless clinical severity warrants laparotomy.

Ten to fifteen percent of adnexal masses undergo torsion.[52] Laparoscopy is the preferred method of both diagnosis and treatment in the gravid patient with adnexal torsion. Multiple case reports have confirmed safety and efficacy of laparoscopy for adnexal torsion in pregnant patients.[61] If diagnosed before tissue necrosis, adnexal torsion may be managed by simple laparoscopic detorsion. However, with late diagnosis of torsion adnexal infarction may ensue, which can result in peritonitis leading to spontaneous abortion. The gangrenous adnexa should be completely resected and progesterone therapy initiated after removal of the corpus luteum, if less than 12 weeks gestation. Laparotomy may sometimes be necessary as dictated by the patient's clinical condition and operative findings.

Ovarian Torsion During Pregnancy

Ovarian torsion is an uncommon cause of acute abdominal pain in nonpregnant women but is more common during pregnancy, especially in the first trimester as compared to the second and is rare in the third trimester. Ovarian torsion occurs in the enlarged ovary, secondary to cysts or neoplasms. The most common cause in pregnancy is a corpus luteum cyst, which usually regresses spontaneously by the second trimester. The incidence of ovarian torsion rises fivefold during pregnancy to approximately 5 per 10,000 pregnancies. When present, it manifests as acute onset, severe, and colicky unilateral pelvic pain. Pain is usually unremitting but can wax and wane in cases of incomplete or intermittent torsion. It may be accompanied with fall in blood pressure and heart rate.[61,62]

Earlier, the treatment of choice for ovarian torsion was salpingooophorectomy, with care to avoid untwisting the ovarian pedicle to prevent emboli and toxic substances related to hypoxia from entering the peripheral circulation. Current recommendations are to untwist the ovarian pedicle, to re-establish ovarian circulation, and to conserve viable ovarian tissue on the affected side, with no systemic complications reported to date. This also helps to preserve fertility, even in adnexa that initially appear nonviable, purple, or black in color.[63]

Ovarian torsion can usually be managed laparoscopically.[64] In case of an ovarian cyst, a simple cystectomy can be performed. If a dermoid, endometrioma, functional cyst (corpus luteum cyst), or a malignant cyst is accidentally ruptured, every effort should be made to avoid spilling the very irritating sebaceous contents, or malignant cells into the peritoneal cavity. If this occurs, prolonged peritoneal irrigation with warm saline will prevent peritonitis. Complete internal examination of cyst for excrescences, microscopic examination of frozen section, and intraoperative staging wherever required should be resorted to.

Red Degeneration of Fibroid

Occurs commonly in pregnancy more so in second trimester but it is managed conservatively.

POST OPERATIVE CARE

- Adequate maternal hydration should be maintained with balance between the input and output

- Post-operative documentation of fetal cardiac activity on ultrasonographyor fetal heart sounds on Doppler is mandatory. Vigilant follow-up through the antenatal period is recommended due to the risk of preterm labour.
- Close monitoring of vital signs, recurrence of pain, and vaginal bleeding
- Regional anesthesia should be used whenever possible to decrease postoperative pain and subsequent release of catecholamines, which can stimulate uterine contractility. Continued epidural infusion of narcotics for up to 72 hours is an excellent way to minimize postoperative pain.

ANESTHETIC CONSIDERATIONS

In order to provide safe anesthesia to mother and fetus, it is essential to remember the physiological and pharmacological changes in pregnancy.[65-72]

The anesthetist has the following goals:

- Optimize and maintain normal maternal physiological function
- Optimize and maintain uteroplacental blood flow and oxygen delivery
- Avoid unwanted drug effects on the fetus
- Avoid stimulating the myometrium (oxytocic effects)
- Avoid awareness during anaesthesia
- Use regional anaesthesia, wherever possible.

Ideal anesthetic technique should not interfere with early embryonic development, should result in minimal nausea, sedation, postoperative pain, and psychomotor impairment.

Between the 15th and 56th days of gestation, the human embryo is said to be most vulnerable to the teratogenic effects of drugs.[66] Also, secondary effects of drugs on the fetus should be considered (e.g., vasoactive drugs affecting placental blood flow).

Maternal Safety

Cardiovascular Changes

Maternal cardiac output increases in pregnancy by 50% and peaks by the end of the second trimester.[70] This is due to a combination of an increased heart rate (25%) and stroke volume (30%). The increase in heart rate is a reflex response to a lowered systemic vascular resistance caused by circulating estrogen and progesterone. Left ventricular hypertrophy and dilatation facilitate the increase in stroke volume but myocardial contractility remains unchanged.

Electrocardigram changes that occur in pregnancy and are entirely normal include left axis deviation and minor ST/T wave changes. Heart murmurs are also common due to turbulence associated with increased blood flow.

Aortocaval Compression

As the enlarging uterus moves out of the pelvis, it can compress the inferior vena cava and the descending aorta in the supine position.[72] The compression of the inferior vena cava causes decreased venous return and hence preload, which reduces cardiac output by up to 20%. This is known as *supine hypotension syndrome*. Pregnant patients compensate for hypotension by an increase in sympathetic tone causing vasoconstriction and tachycardia. This may divert blood away from organs such as the uterus, with subsequent fetal distress. The compression of the aorta can cause a further reduction in uterine blood flow. Aortocaval compression becomes clinically relevant from approximately 20 weeks gestation. It is also important in the first trimester if the uterus is unduly enlarged with myomas, molar pregnancy, or multifetal pregnancy. It can be relieved by a left lateral tilt of 15°, which is therefore essential in all pregnant patients in the supine position after 20 weeks. This is especially important to remember when a patient is under regional anesthesia/analgesia since hypotension is potentiated by sympathetic block.

There is an increase in blood volume in pregnancy of between 35–50% at term. There is both an increase in plasma volume and red cell volume, but a greater increase in plasma volume, which leads to a dilutional anaemia. The reduced blood viscosity aids flow through the uteroplacental circulation and the increase in volume serves as a protective measure against haemorrhage at delivery. It must be remembered that because of the increase in blood volume, along with a resting tachycardia, there may be delay in the onset of the classical symptoms and signs of hypovolaemia.

Pregnancy is a hypercoaguable state with an increase in most clotting factors. The platelet count may fall but there is actually an increase in production and consumption. Pregnancy is a significant risk factor for thromboembolism and, therefore, thromboprophylaxis is essential in the postoperative period when the risk is further increased by immobility and dehydration.

Respiratory Changes

The respiratory changes of pregnancy are perhaps the most important for anesthetists to note. There is an increased oxygen demand of up to 60% at term. This is met by an increased cardiac output and an increase in minute ventilation (MV). MV increases early due to an increase in respiratory rate and tidal volume and is up by 45% at term. This increase in MV is mediated by progesterone, which acts as a respiratory stimulant. The increased MV causes a mild respiratory alkalosis ($PaCO_2$ decreases by 1 kPa). The increase in pH is limited by increased renal bicarbonate excretion. Relative hypocapnia should be maintained when artificially ventilating pregnant patients. An increase in maternal $PaCO_2$ limits the gradient for CO_2 diffusion from fetal to maternal blood leading to fetal acidosis. The functional residual capacity (FRC), which is the main oxygen reserve in the apnoeic patient, is decreased in pregnancy due to the enlarging uterus displacing the diaphragm upwards. This is further exacerbated in the supine position and increases as the pregnancy progresses. Airway management may be challenging during pregnancy. Bag-mask ventilation may be more difficult due to increased soft tissue in the neck. Laryngoscopy can be hindered by weight gain. Increased edema of the vocal cords due to increased capillary permeability can hinder intubation and increase the risk of bleeding. This may make further attempts at intubation more difficult and increase the incidence of failed intubation. Increased maternal oxygen consumption and reduced FRC results in rapid oxygen desaturation during attempts at intubation. Smaller sized endotracheal tubes may be needed and all anesthetists should be familiar with a failed intubation drill. Nasal intubation should be avoided due to increased vascularity of mucous membranes. Given the combination of these changes, careful pre-oxygenation is essential prior to induction of anaesthesia. This should be confirmed if possible by monitoring the end tidal oxygen fraction which should always be >0.9. Pre-oxygenation can be less efficient in the term parturient in the supine position because the closing volume of the alveoli may be greater than the FRC. Pre-oxygenation in a slightly head up position may help this.

Gastrointestinal Changes

Circulating progesterone reduces the lower esophageal sphincter (LOS) tone, increasing the incidence of esophageal reflux. This is further exacerbated by anatomical changes. The gravid uterus is displaced upwards and to the left pushing the intra-abdominal part of the oesophagus into the thorax in most pregnant women. This often makes the LOS incompetent and lowers the barrier pressure. These factors, along with a lowered stomach pH, increase the risk and severity of aspiration pneumonitis under general anaesthesia.

It is recommended that from 16 weeks gestation patients undergoing general anes-thesia should be given prophylaxis against aspiration pneumonitis. This usually includes a nonparticulate antacid, such as sodium citrate 0.3 M 30 mL and an H2 receptor antagonist, e.g., ranitidine 150 mg orally or 50 mg intravenously. Some anesthetists may also choose to give a prokinetic such as metoclopramide. Induction of anesthesia should be by a rapid sequence technique with cricoid pressure and a fast acting muscle relaxant, such as suxamethonium. A cuffed endotracheal tube should be used. At the end of the procedure patients, should be extubated fully awake in the lateral position.

Remember:
- Left lateral tilt to prevent aortocaval compression
- Meticulous pre-oxygenation to prevent hypoxia
- Antacid prophylaxis and rapid sequence induction to reduce risk of aspiration.

Altered Pharmacokinetics/Pharmacodynamics of Drugs

Pharmacokinetic and pharmacodynamic profiles are altered in pregnancy and drugs should be titrated accordingly. The minimum alveolar concentration (MAC) of volatile agents is reduced by 30% under the influence of progesterone and endogenous endorphins. There is a decrease in plasma cholinesterase levels by 25% from early pregnancy, but prolonged neuromuscular blockade with suxamethonium is uncommon due to increased blood volume causing an increased volume of distribution. Non-depolarising muscle relaxants have a prolonged duration of action. Neuromuscularmonitoringwithanervestimulator is recommended. The increased blood volume causes a physiological hypoalbuminaemia. This alters the plasma protein binding and increases the free or unbound fraction of drugs. An example of this is local anesthetics. There is also increased neural tissue sensitivity. These factors decrease the therapeutic doses and also the toxic plasma levels of local anaesthetic agents.

The volume of the epidural and subarachnoid spaces is reduced due to the gravid uterus compressing the inferior vena cava causing distension of the epidural venous plexus. This leads to a more extensive spread of local anaesthetic agents administered during central neuraxial blockade and also increases the risk of inadvertent intravascular injection. Careful aspiration prior to injection should always be performed.

Fetal Safety

Prevention of Fetal Asphyxia

One of the most serious risks to the fetus during maternal surgery is intrauterine asphyxia. This must be avoided by maintaining maternal oxygenation and hemodynamic stability. It is extremely important to avoid hypoxia, extreme hyper- and hypocarbia, hypotension, and uterine hypertonus. Maternal hypoxemia causes uteroplacental vasoconstriction and decreased perfusion, causing fetal hypoxia, acidosis, and ultimately death. There is a linear relationship between maternal and fetal $PaCO_2$. Maternal hypercarbia limits the gradient for CO_2 diffusion from fetal to maternal blood and leads to fetal acidosis. Therefore, endtidal carbon dioxide monitoringshouldbeusedtoguideventilationand arterial blood gas analysis should be considered during prolonged or laparoscopic surgery. Hypocarbia is also problematic, potentially causing uteroplacental vasoconstriction and fetal acidosis, although the mild hypocapnia that occurs with the physiological changes of pregnancy should be maintained ($PaCO_2$ around 4 kPa). Uteroplacental circulation is not autoregulated and hence perfusion is entirely dependant on the maintenance of an adequate maternal blood pressure and cardiac output. Hypotension can be caused by anesthetic drugs, central neuraxial blockade, hypovolemia, or aortocaval compression. Maternal hypotension needs to be treated aggressively by ensuring left lateral tilt and boluses of intravenous fluids. Additional vasopressors may be required and currently it is felt alpha agonists, such as phenylephrine and metaraminol produce a better fetal acid balance than indirect sympathomimetic agents, such as ephedrine. Ephedrine also has a relatively slow onset and long duration of action and tachyphylaxis can occur making titration difficult.

Drugs and Teratogenicity

Teratogenicity is defined as the observation of any significant change in the function or form of a child secondary to prenatal treatment. The teratogenicity of a drug depends upon the dose administered, the route of administration and the timing of fetal exposure.

The period from the 3rd to the 8th week of gestation represents the most important time for organogenesis during which drugs can exert their most serious teratogenic effects. After this, drug exposure should not cause organ abnormalities, but fetal growth retardation may occur. Although most anesthetic agents are safe in humans, their doses should be kept minimum. The fetus is at more risk from asphyxia than the teratogenic effect of anesthetic drugs. Studies looking at the outcomes of women who underwent surgery during pregnancy suggest no increase in congenital anomalies in their offspring but an increase in fetal loss, growth restriction, and low birth weight attributed to the requirement for surgery. There is some concern from animal and epidemiological studies that exposure to general anesthetic agents may cause neurodevelopmental delay in infants. It is difficult to extrapolate animal findings to humans and in epidemiological studies it is difficult to distinguish the potential confounding effects of anesthesia, reason for surgery and underlying medical conditions. Nitrous oxide inhibits methionine synthetase, and therefore, there is concern it could affect DNA synthesis in the developing fetus. It has also been shown to be teratogenic during peak organogenesis in rodents, but there is no evidence in humans. Anesthesia can be safely delivered without nitrous oxide and, therefore, many would avoid its use during nonobstetric surgery in the pregnant woman. Another drug of concern is ketamine. This causes increased uterine tone and fetal asphyxia and should not be used in the first two trimesters. The effect is not seen in the third trimester. Benzodiazepines have been associated with a cleft lip and palate in animal studies. The association in humans is controversial. A single dose has not been associated with teratogenicity and may be useful to provide anxiolysis preoperatively.

Prevention of Preterm Labour/Fetal Monitoring

Surgery during pregnancy increases the risk of spontaneous abortion, preterm labour, and preterm delivery. This risk is increased with intra-abdominal procedures. Uterine manipulation should be kept to a minimum and drugs that increase uterine tone (e.g., ketamine) should be avoided. Prophylactic tocolytic therapy is controversial as there are associated maternal side effects and its efficacy during nonobstetric surgery has not been proven. Perioperative fetal monitoring is also an area of controversy. From 18 to 22 weeks fetal heart rate (FHR) monitoring is feasible and from 25 weeks, heart rate variability can be observed. Continuous monitoring may be technically difficult during abdominal operations or in cases of maternal obesity. Anesthetic agents reduce both baseline FHR and FHR variability and, therefore, interpretation is difficult and may lead to unnecessary interventions. Anesthetic agents do not cause decelerations or persistent fetal bradycardia and these changes may indicate fetal distress. Monitoring may enable swift action to be taken such as the optimisation of maternal haemodynamics, oxygenation, and ventilation.

Laparoscopic Surgery

There were previous concerns regarding fetal safety during laparoscopic surgery. These included fears of direct uterine and fetal trauma, fetal acidosis due to absorbed carbon dioxide, and decreased maternal cardiac output secondary to the increased intra-abdominal pressure and positioning with a subsequent decrease in utero-placental perfusion. There are advantages to laparoscopic surgery for both the mother and the fetus, such as decreased post-operative pain (and, therefore, less need for analgesics), shorter recovery times, and a lower risk of thromboembolic events. A Swedish study[75] compared laparotomy and laparoscopy performed in pregnancy in over 2 million deliveries. Premature delivery, growth restriction and low birth weight were more common in both groups compared to the general population but there were no differences between the laparotomy and laparoscopy groups. Pregnancy should, therefore, not be seen as a contraindication to laparoscopic surgery if surgery is required. Certain precautions should be taken. Pneumatic stockings should be used to promote venous return and the lowest pressure pneumoperitoneum (<12 mmHg) should be used where possible.

Aortocaval compression should be avoided and changes in position should be undertaken slowly. $PaCO_2$ should be closely monitored by the routine use of end tidal carbon dioxide monitoring and consideration of arterial blood gas analysis in selected cases. FHR monitoring may be advisable to detect fetal compromise early allowing optimization of maternal hemodynamics. FHR changes may indicate the need for temporary deflation of the pneumoperitoneum.

Deep Venous Thrombosis Prophylaxis

As previously stated, pregnancy induces a hyper-coaguable state and the risk of thromboembolic disease is further increased by postoperative venous stasis. Attention to thromboprophylaxis is, therefore, essential. This should include early mobilisation, maintaining adequate hydration, thromboembolus deterrent stockings, and other calf compression devices and consideration of pharmacological prophylaxis (e.g., subcutaneous low molecular weight heparin).

Analgesia

Adequate analgesia is important as pain will cause increased circulating catecholamines which will impair uteroplacental perfusion. Analgesia may mask the signs of early preterm labour and, therefore, tocometry is useful to

TABLE 1: Food and Drug Administration classification of fetal risk from drugs

Category A	Adequate and well controlled studies have failed to demonstrate a risk to the fetus in the first trimester of pregnancy (and there is no evidence of risk in later pregnancies)
Category B	Animal reproduction studies have failed to demonstrate a fetal risk but there are no controlled studies in pregnant women, OR animal reproduction studies have shown an adverse effect, but adequate well controlled studies in pregnant women have failed to demonstrate a risk to the fetus in any trimester
Category C	Animal reproduction studies have shown an adverse effect on the fetus and there are no adequate well controlled studies in humans, or studies in animals and humans are not available. Potential benefits of drugs may warrant its use in pregnant women despite potential risks
Category D	There is positive evidence of human fetal risk, but the benefits from use in pregnant women may be acceptable despite the risk (e.g., life threatening situation or serious disease for which safer drugs are not available)
Category X	Studies in animals or humans have demonstrated fetal abnormalities, or evidence based on human experience, and the risk of use of the drug in pregnant women clearly outweighs any possible benefit. The drug is contraindicated in women who are or may become pregnant

detect contractions. This will enable tocolysis to be administered without delay. If a pregnancy continues beyond the first postoperative week, the incidence of premature labour is no higher than the nonsurgical pregnant patient. The US FDA introduced a classification system in 1979 of drug risk to the fetus. This runs from category A (safest) to category X (known danger) as shown in table 1.

There are other classification systems from other countries. However, the FDA requires a relatively large amount of high quality data for a drug to be classified as category A. As a result many drugs which are classified as category A in other countries are classified as category C by the FDA.

CONCLUSION

Nonobstetric surgery during pregnancy is not uncommon and anesthetists should be aware of the implications for management. The physiological changes of pregnancy need to be considered, especially the avoidance of aortocaval compression, antacid prophylaxis, and adequate preoxygenation. The airway needs careful evaluation preoperatively.

The main risk to the fetus is asphyxia. This can be avoided by ensuring adequate maternal oxygenation and ventilation, avoiding hypotension, and drugs that increase uterine tone. This should ensure adequate uteroplacental perfusion. Perioperative fetal heart rate monitoring may be useful. Regional anesthesia is likely to have benefits over general anesthesia. Attention should be paid to thromboprophylaxis, analgesia, and signs of preterm labour in the postoperative period. When caring for pregnant ladies undergoing nonobstetric, surgery a multidisciplinary team is essential. This should include surgeons, anesthetists, obstetricians, midwives, and nurses. Elective surgery should be postponed until 6 weeks postpartum when possible. Nonelective surgery should be delayed until the second trimester when organogenesis has occurred and the risk of teratogenicity decreases but this may not always be possible.

REFERENCES

1. Kammerer WS. Nonobstetric surgery during pregnancy. Med Clin North Am. 1979;63:1157-64.
2. Lim HK, Bae SH, Seo GS. Diagnosis of acute appendicitis in pregnant women: value of sonography. Am J Roentogenol. 1992;159:539-42.
3. Manmoodian S. Appendicitis complicating pregnancy. South Med J. 1992;85:19-24.
4. Masters K, Levine BA, Gaskill HV, Sirinek KR. Diagnosing appendicitis during pregnancy. Am J Surg. 1984;148:768-71.
5. Chen MM CF, Kaimal A, Laros Jr RK. Guidelines for computed tomography and magnetic resonance imaging use during pregnancy and lactation. Obstet Gynecol. 2008;112:(2 Pt 1): 333-40.
6. National Council on Radiation Protection and Measurements. Medical radiation exposure of pregnant and potentially pregnant women. NCPR No. 54. Bethesda, MD. 1977.
7. Menias CO, Elsayes KM, Peterson CM, Huete A, Gratz BI, Bhalla S. CT of pregnancy-related complications. Emerg Radiol. 2007;13(6):299-306.
8. Hurwitz LM, Yoshizumi T, Reiman RE, Goodman PC, Paulson EK, Frush DP, et al. Radiation dose to the fetus from body MDCT during early gestation. AJR Am J Roentgenol. 2006;186:871-6.
9. Forsted DH, Kalbhen CL. CT of pregnant women for urinary tract calculi, pulmonary thromboembolism, and acute appendicitis. AJR Am J Roentgenol. 2002;178(5):1285.
10. Patel SJ, Reede DL, Katz DS, Subramaniam R, Amorosa JK. Imaging the pregnant patient for nonobstetric conditions: algorithms and radiation dose considerations. Radiographics. 2007;27:1705-22.
11. De Wilde JP, Rivers AW, Price DL. A review of the current use of magnetic resonance imaging in pregnancy and safety implications for the fetus. Prog Biophys Mol Biol. 2005;87 (2-3):335-53.
12. Garcia-Bournissen F, Shrim A, Koren G. Safety of gadolinium during pregnancy. Can Fam Physician. 2006;52:309-10.
13. McKenna DA, Meehan CP, Alhajeri AN, Regan MC, O'Keeffe DP. The use of MRI to demonstrate small bowel obstruction during pregnancy. Br J Radiol. 2007;80:e11-4.
14. Birchard KR, Brown MA, Hyslop WB, Firat Z, Semelka RC. MRI of acute abdominal and pelvic pain in pregnant patients. AJR Am J Roentgenol. 2005;184:452-8.
15. Adelstein SJ. Administered radionuclides in pregnancy. Teratology. 1999;59:236-9.

16. Schaefer C, Meister R, Wentzeck R, Weber-Schoendorfer C. Fetal outcome after technetium scintigraphy in early pregnancy. Reprod Toxicol. 2009;28:161-6.
17. Karthikesalingam A, Marker SR, Weerakkody R, Walsh SR, Carroll N, Praseedom RK. Radiation exposure during laparoscopic cholecystectomy with routine intraoperatinve cholangiography. Surg Endosc. 2009;23:1845-8.
18. Jorgensen JE, Rubenstein JH, Goodsitt MM, Elta GH. Raidation doses to ERCP patients are significantly lower with experienced endoscopists. Gastrointest Endosc. 2010;72:58-65.
19. Andriulli A, Loperfido S, Napolitano G, Niro G, Valvano MR, Spirito F, et al. Incidence rates of post-ERCP complications: a systematic survey of prospective studies. Am J Gastroenterol. 2007;102(8):1781-8.
20. Al-Fozan H, Tulandi T. Safety and risks of laparoscopy in pregnancy. Curr Opin Obstet Gynecol. 2002;14:375-9.
21. Conron RW Jr, Abbruzzi K, Cochrane SO, Sarno AJ, Cochrane PJ. Laparoscopic procedures in pregnancy. Am Surg. 1999;65:259-63.
22. Amos JD, Schorr SJ, Norman PF, Poole GV, Thomae KR, Mancino AT, et al. Laparoscopic surgery during pregnancy. Am J Surg. 1996;171:435-7.
23. Rizzo AG. Laparoscopic surgery in pregnancy: long-term follow-up. J Laparoendosc Adv Surg Tech A. 2003;13(1):11-5.
24. Shay DC, Bhavani-Shankar K, Datta S. Laparoscopic surgery during pregnancy. Anesthesiol Clin North America. 2001;19: 57-67.
25. Barone JE, Bears S, Chen S, Tsai J, Russell JC. Outcome study of cholecystectomy during pregnancy. Am J Surg. 1999;177:232-6.
26. Rollins MD, Chan KJ, Price RR. Laparoscopy for appendicitis and cholelithiasis during pregnancy: a new standard of care. Surg Endosc. 2004;18(2):237-41.
27. Muench J, Albrink M, Serafini F, Rosemurgy A, Carey L, Murr MM. Delay in treatment of biliary disease during pregnancy increases morbidity and can be avoided with safe laparoscopic cholecystectomy. Am Surg. 2001;67:539-42; discussion 542-33.
28. Visser BC, Glasgow RE, Mulvihill KK, Mulvihill SJ. Safety and timing of nonobstetric abdominal surgery in pregnancy. Dig Surg. 2001;18:409-17.
29. Geisler JP, Rose SL, Mernitz CS, Warner JL, Hiett AK. Non-gynecologic laparoscopy in second and third trimester pregnancy: obstetric implications. JSLS. 1998;2:235-8.
30. Graham G, Baxi L, Tharakan T. Laparoscopic cholecystectomy during pregnancy: a case series and review of the literature. Obstet Gynecol Surg. 1998;53:566-74.
31. Tuech JJ, Binelli C, Aube C, Pessaux P, Fauvet R, Descamps P, et al. Management of choledocholithiasis during pregnancy by magnetic resonance cholangiography and laparoscopic common bile duct stone extraction. Surg Laparosc Endosc Percutan Tech. 2000;10:323-5.
32. Baillie J, Cairns SR, Putman WS, Cotton PB. Endoscopic management of choledocholithiasis during pregnancy. Surg Gynecol Obstet. 1990;171:1-4.
33. Sungler P, Heinerman PM, Steiner H, Waclawiczek HW, Holzinger J, Mayer F, et al. Laparoscopic cholecystectomy and interventional endoscopy for gallstone complications during pregnancy. Surg Endosc. 2000;14:267-71.
34. Cosenza CA, Saffari B, Jabbour N, Stain SC, Garry D, Parekh D, et al. Surgical management of biliary gallstone disease during pregnancy. Am J Surg. 1999;178:545-8.
35. Scapa E. To do or not to do an endoscopic retrograde cholangiopancreatography in acute biliary pancreatitis? Surg Laparosc Endosc. 1995;5:453-4.
36. Stepp K, Falcone T. Laparoscopy in the second trimester of pregnancy. Obstet Gynecol Clin North Am. 2004;31:485-96, vii.
37. Pucci RO, Seed RW. Case report of laparoscopic cholecystectomy in the third trimester of pregnancy. Am J Obstet Gynecol. 1991;165:401-2.
38. Weber AM, Bloom GP, Allan TR, Curry SL. Laparoscopic cholecystectomy during pregnancy. Obstet Gynecol. 1991;78: 958-9.
39. Williams JK, Rosemurgy AS, Albrink MH, Parsons MT, Stock S. Laparoscopic cholecystectomy in pregnancy. A case report. J Reprod Med. 1995;40:243-5.
40. Costantino GN, Vincent GJ, Mukalian GG, Kliefoth WL Jr. Laparoscopic cholecystectomy in pregnancy. J Laparoendosc Surg. 1994;4:161-4.
41. Andreoli M, Sayegh SK, Hoefer R, Matthews G, Mann WJ. Laparoscopic cholecystectomy for recurrent gallstone pancreatitis during pregnancy. South Med J. 1996;89:1114-5.
42. Schwartzberg BS, Conyers JA, Moore JA. First trimester of pregnancy laparoscopic procedures. Surg Endosc. 1997;11: 1216-7.
43. Thomas SJ, Brisson P. Laparoscopic appendectomy and cholecystectomy during pregnancy: six case reports. JSLS. 1998;2:41-6.
44. Weingold AB. Appendicitis in pregnancy. Clin Obstet Gynecol. 1983;26:801-10.
45. Chawla S, Vardhan S, Jog S. Appendicitis during pregnancy. MJAFI. 2003;59:212-5.
46. Doberneck RC. Appendectomy during pregnancy. Am Surg. 1985;51:265-73.
47. Lemieux P, Rheaume P, Levesque I, Bujold E, Brochu G. Laparoscopic appendectomy in pregnant patients: a review of 45 cases. Surg Endosc. 2009;23:1701-5.
48. Donkervoort SC, Boerma D, Suspicion of acute appendicitis in the third trimester of pregnancy: pros and cons of a laparoscopic procedure. JSLS. 2011;15(3):379-83.
49. Wilasrsmee C, Sukrat B, McEvoy M, Attia J, Thakkinstian A. Systematic review and metaanalysis of safety of laparoscopic versus open appendicectomy for suspected appendicitis in pregnancy. Br J Surg. 2012;99(11):1470-78.

50. Rao PM, Rhea JT, Novelline RA, Mostfavi AA, McCabe CJ. Effect of computed tomography of the appendix on treatment of patients and use of hospital resources. N Engl J Med. 1998;338:141-7.
51. Castro MA, Shipp TD, Castro EE, Ouzounian J, Rao P. The use of Helical computed tomography in pregnancy for the diagnosis of acute appendicitis. Am J Obstet Gynaecol. 2001;184:954-60.
52. Tarraza HM, Moore RD. Gynecologic causes of the acute abdomen and the acute abdomen in pregnancy. Surg Clin North Am. 1997;77:1371-94.
53. American College of Obstetricians and Gynecologists. ACOG Practice Bulletin. Management of adnexal masses. Obstet Gynecol. 2007;110:201-14.
54. Nezhat F, Nezhat C, Silfen SL, Fehnel SH. Laparoscopic ovarian cystectomy during pregnancy. J Laparoendosc Surg. 1991;1:161-4.
55. Parker WH, Levine RL, Howard FM, Sansone B, Berek JS. A multicenter study of laparoscopic management of selected cystic adnexal masses in postmenopausal women. J Am Coll Surg. 1994;179:733-7.
56. Tazuke SI, Nezhat FR, Nezhat CH, Seidman DS, Phillips DR, Nezhat CR. Laparoscopic management of pelvic pathology during pregnancy. J Am Assoc Gynecol Laparosc. 1997;4:605-8.
57. Chung MK, Chung RP. Laparoscopic extracorporeal oophorectomy and ovarian cystectomy in second trimester pregnant obese patients. JSLS. 2001;5:273-7.
58. Yuen PM, Chang AM. Laparoscopic management of adnexal mass during pregnancy. Acta Obstet Gynecol Scand. 1997;76:173-6.
59. Loh FH, Chua SP, Khalil R, Ng SC. Case report of ruptured endometriotic cyst in pregnancy treated by laparoscopic ovarian cystectomy. Singapore Med J. 1998;39:368-9.
60. Stepp KJ, Tulikangas PK, Goldberg JM, Attaran M, Falcone T. Laparoscopy for adnexal masses in the second trimester of pregnancy. J Am Assoc Gynecol Laparosc. 2003;10:55-9.
61. Chapron C, Capella-Allouc S, Dubuisson JB. Treatment of adnexal torsion using operative laparoscopy. Hum Reprod. 1996;11:998-1003.
62. Chapron C, Capella-Allouc S, Dubuisson JB. Treatment of adnexal torsion using operative laparoscopy. Hum Reprod. 1996;11:998-1003.
63. Zweizig S, Perron J, Grubb D, et al. Conservative management of adnexal torsion. Am J Obstet Gynecol. 1993;168:1791-5.
64. Pan HS, Huang LW, Lee CY, et al. Ovarian pregnancy torsion. 2004;270:119-21.
65. Goodman S. Anaesthesia for non obstetric surgery in the pregnant patient. Semin Perinatol. 2002;26:136-45.
66. Koren G, Pastuszak A, Ito S. Drugs in pregnancy. N Engl J Med. 1998;338:1128-37.
67. Mhuireachtaigh RN, O'Gorman DA. Anesthesia in pregnant patients for nonobstetric surgery.Review Article. J Clin Anesth. 2006;18:60-6.
68. Walton NKD, Melachuri VK. Anaesthesia for non-obstetric surgery during pregnancy. Continuing Education in Anaesthesia, Critical Care and Pain. 2006;6:83-85.
69. Rosen MA. Management of Anesthesia for the Pregnant Surgical Patient. Anesthesiology. 1999;91:1159-63.
70. Heidemann BH, McClure JH. Changes in maternal physiology during pregnancy. Continuing Education in Anaesthesia, Critical Care. 2003;3:65-8.
71. Van de Velde M, De Buck F. Anesthesia for non-obstetric surgery in the pregnant patient. Minerva Anestesiologica. 2007;73:235-40.
72. Hool A. Anaesthesia in pregnancy for non-obstetric surgery. Anaesthesia Tutorial of the Week 185. 2010:6-9.

Laparoscopic Surgery

28

CHAPTER

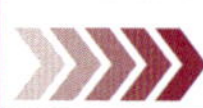

Punita Bhardawaj

INTRODUCTION

Laparoscopic surgery during pregnancy becomes a challenge due to pregnancy associated changes in physiology and anatomy. The gestational age and viability should be determined and surgical risks should be explained to the patient and the partner prior to the operative procedure.

Laparoscopic procedures commonly performed during pregnancy are as follows:

- Laparoscopic cholecystectomy
- Resection of ectopic/heterotopic pregnancy
  - Abdominal pregnancy
  - Corpus luteum hemorrhage
- Adnexal torsion
- Appendectomy
- Termination of cesarean scar ovarian rudimentary horn pregnancy

Increased fetal risk in laparoscopic surgery can be due to:

- *Effects of pneumoperitoneum in pregnancy during laparoscopic procedure:* Pneumoperitoneum rise in intra-abdominal pressure which decreases vena cava return and hence the cardiac output. Trendelenburg position further decreases the cardiac output. This decreases the cardiac index. This combined with maternal hypoxia may cause fetal death.[1]

  Rise in intra-abdominal pressure decreases uterine blood flow which may cause fetal hypoxia and fetal death.[2] Pneumoperitoneum decreases movement of the diaphragm due to splinting which increases peak airway pressure, decrease in functional reserve capacity, increases ventilation perfusion mismatch, and decreases thoracic cavity compliance.[3]

  Pneumoperitoneum with carbon dioxide (CO_2) leads to hypercarbia and further hypoxemia. Peritoneal absorption of CO_2 leads to respiratory acidosis in the pregnant woman and her fetus. Fetal tachycardia and hypotension may be due to fetal hypercarbia. This can be corrected by hyperventilation which maintains mild maternal alkalosis
- *Effect of increased intra-abdominal pressure*: Keep the intra-abdominal pressure to below 15 mmHg with adequate visualization to prevent ventilatory and circulatory complications, and gas embolism[4]
- *Pneumoperitoneum increases venous stasis*: Pneumatic compression devices reduce the risk of thromboembolism along with early mobilization in laparoscopic surgery
- *Decreased uterine blood flow*: Decreased uterine blood flow from pneumoperitoneum may be hypothetical. However, if venous return is compromised, decreased uterine blood flow will ensue

- *Effect of anesthesia and anesthetic drugs*: Certain anesthetic drugs may be teratogenic and should be avoided in pregnancy. Hypercarbia should be avoided and oxygenation should be strictly maintained
- *Maternal organ injury*: Uterine injuries are uncommon in first trimester pregnancy surgery. However, an enlarged uterus may be easily punctured by the veress needle or trocar. Stomach and small bowel needle injuries heal and go unrecognized. Significant undetected bowel injury can present as late sepsis and peritonitis leading to fetal/maternal mortality and morbidity[4]
- *Fetal effects of laparoscopy*: Visser in his study states that there is no teratogenicity, fetal loss, preterm labor in nonobstetric abdominal surgery in the first and second trimester. Third trimester surgery may be associated with preterm labor but not fetal loss.[5] Surgical interventions may result in low birth weight/intrauterine growth restriction in babies. There are few studies on long-term follow-up of babies, one such study found no long-term effects in babies.[6] Nevertheless, surgery during pregnancy for nonobstetric, nonemergency abdominal disorders should ideally be postponed after delivery.

ADVANTAGES OF LAPAROSCOPY IN PREGNANCY

- Decreased fetal respiratory depression in third trimester surgeries, due to decreased postoperative narcotic requirement
- Decreased risk of wound complications
- Diminished postoperative maternal hypoventilation
- Decreased risk of thromboembolic events
- Decreased postoperative ileus
- Improved visualization decreasing the requirement of uterine manipulation.
- Decreased uterine irritability results in lower rates of spontaneous abortion and preterm delivery
- Short hospital stay
- Early mobilization and return to work.

PRECAUTIONS TO BE OBSERVED FOR LAPAROSCOPIC SURGERY IN PREGNANCY

Use of Diagnostic Modalities

- Ultrasonographic imaging is safe and useful in identifying the etiology of acute abdominal pain, and hemoperitoneum in the pregnant patient. It is the initial radiographic test of choice
- Expeditious and accurate diagnosis should take precedence over concerns for ionizing radiation if an X-ray is warranted. Cumulative radiation dosage should be limited to 5–10 rads during pregnancy. Fetal mortality is greatest when exposure occurs within the first week of conception. The most sensitive time period for central nervous system (CNS) teratogenesis is 10–17 weeks of gestation. No single diagnostic study should exceed 5 rads
- Contemporary multidetector computed tomography (CT) protocols deliver a low radiation dose and may be used judiciously during pregnancy[7]
- Magnetic resonance imaging (MRI) without the use of intravenous gadolinium can be performed at any stage of pregnancy. MRI provides excellent soft tissue imaging
- Administration of radionucleotides for diagnostic studies is generally safe for mother and fetus provided whole fetal exposure is less than 0.5 rads[8]
- Intraoperative and endoscopic cholangiography exposes the mother and fetus to minimal radiation and may be used selectively during pregnancy. The lower abdomen should be shielded when performing cholangiography during pregnancy to decrease the radiation exposure to the fetus. Radiation exposure during cholangiography is (0.2–0.5 rads)[9]

- Fluoroscopy delivers a radiation dose of up to 20 rads/min depending on the X-ray equipment, patient positioning, and patient size. Radiation dose during endoscopic retrograde cholangiopancreatography (ERCP) is 2–12 rads, but can be higher for long procedures. Hence both fluroscupy and ERCP should not be routinely performed during pregnancy.

Diagnostic Laproscopy

Diagnostic laparoscopy is safe and effective when used selectively in the work-up and treatment of acute abdominal processes in pregnancy. The surgical approach avoids ionizing radiation, diagnoses the problem, and can treat at the same sitting. Laparoscopy can be performed in any trimester of pregnancy with minimal morbidity to mother and fetus.[9]

Patient Selection

Laparoscopic treatment of acute abdominal disease has the same indication in pregnant and nonpregnant patients. Benefits of laparoscopy during pregnancy are similar to those in nonpregnant patient including less postoperative pain, less postoperative ileus, decreased length of hospital stay, and faster returns to work.[10,11] The same patients selection criteria are used as for non pregnancy patients.

Laparoscopy and Trimester of Pregnancy

Laparoscopy can be safely performed during any trimester of pregnancy. However, the second trimester is safest with regard to risk of teratogenicity and preterm labor.

Patient Positioning

Gravid patients should be placed in the left lateral decubitus position to minimize compression of the vena cava. This improves the venous return and cardiac output. This precaution may not observed in first trimester surgery.

Initial Port Placement

Initial abdominal access can be safely accomplished with an open (Hassan) technique, veress needle, or optical trocar. The port location is adjusted according to fundal height and previous incisions.

Insufflation Pressure

Carbon dioxide insufflation of 10–15 mmHg can be safely used for laparoscopy in the pregnant patient. There are no data showing detrimental effects to human fetuses from CO_2 pneumoperitoneum.[12]

Intraoperative CO_2 Monitoring

Intraoperative CO_2 monitoring by capnography is recommended during laparoscopy in the pregnant patient. Ventilation can be adjusted according to end tidal (ET) CO_2 levels to prevent fetal hypercarbia.

Venous Thromboembolic Prophylaxis

Intraoperative and postoperative pneumatic compression devices, and early postoperative ambulation are recommended as prophylaxis for deep venous thrombosis (DVT) in the gravid patient. Pregnancy is a hypercoagulable state with 0.1–0.2% incidence of DVT.[13] CO_2 pneumoperitoneum may increase the risk of DVT by predisposing to venous stasis. Insufflation pressure of 12 mmHg causes a significant decrease in blood flow that cannot be completely reversed by intermittent pneumatic compression device.[14] Hence, intermittent release of pneumoperitoneum is recommended if the surgery is prolonged.

There are no data regarding use of heparin in patients undergoing laparoscopy, though its use has been suggested in patients undergoing extended major operations.[15] In patients who require anticoagulation during pregnancy, heparin has proven safe and is the agent of choice.[16]

Safety of Laparoscopic Surgery

Laparoscopic *cholecystectomy* is the treatment of choice in the pregnant patient with gall bladder diseases regardless of trimester. Early surgical management is the treatment of choice in symptomatic gall stones. Recurrent symptoms occur in 92% of patients managed nonoperatively in the first trimester, 6.4% in the second trimester, and 44% in the third trimester.[17]

The delay in surgical management results in increased rates of hospitalization, spontaneous abortions, preterm labor, and preterm delivery compared to those undergoing cholecystectomy.[18]

Nonoperative management of symptomatic gallstones in gravid patients results in recurrent symptoms in more than 50% of patients and 23% of such patients develop acute cholecystitis or gallstone pancreatitis.[19] Gallstone pancreatitis results in fetal loss in 10–60% of pregnant patients.[20] Decreased rates of spontaneous abortion and preterm labor have been reported in laparoscopic cholecystectomy when compared to laparotomy.[21]

Laparoscopic *appendectomy* may be performed safely in pregnant patients with appendicitis. Timely diagnosis in pregnant patients may decrease the risk of fetal loss and improve outcomes. When diagnosis is uncertain, ultrasound and/or MRI help in establishing diagnosis and decrease rate of negative laparoscopy.

Laparoscopy is safe and effective treatment in gravid patients with symptomatic *ovarian cystic masses* in every trimester. Initial observation is warranted for most cystic lesions less than 6 cm in size. Observation is acceptable in all cystic lesions where tumor markers are normal and ultrasound does not suggest malignancy. Most adnexal masses diagnosed in the first trimester are functional cysts that resolve by second trimester.[22] Persistent masses are most commonly functional cysts or mature cystic teratomas with incidence of malignancy in 2–6% cases.[23]

Laparoscopy is recommended for both diagnosis and treatment of *adnexal torsion* unless clinical severity warrants laparotomy. Ten to fifteen percent adnexal masses undergo torsion. If diagnosed before tissue necrosis, adnexal orsion can be managed by simple untwisting laparoscopically.[24]

With late diagnosis, adnexal infarction may occur resulting in peritonitis, spontaneous abortion, preterm delivery, and death.[25] The gangrenous adnexa should be completely resected[26] and progesterone therapy initiated after removal of corpus luteum, if less than 12 weeks gestation.[24]

Perioperative Care

Fetal heart monitoring should occur pre- and postoperatively in the setting of urgent abdominal surgery during pregnancy. Obstetric opinion can be taken pre and postoperatively based on severity of disease and gestational disease. Delaying the treatment of an acute abdominal process to obtain such a consultation should be avoided as treatment delay may increase the risk of morbidity and mortality to the mother and the fetus.[27]

Tocolytics should not be used prophylactically in pregnant women undergoing surgery but should be considered perioperatively when signs of preterm labor are present. The agent and dosage of tocolytics should be individualized.[28]

LAPAROSCOPIC MANAGEMENT OF SURGICAL DISEASE DURING PREGNANCY

One in 500–635 women will require nonobstetrical abdominal surgery during their pregnancy.[29,30]

Nonobstetrical surgical emergencies commonly complicating pregnancy are appendicitis, cholecystitis and intestinal obstruction,[29] others being ovarian masses, adrenal tumor, splenic problems, and hernia which are symptomatic, gallbladder stones which are symptomatic, inflammatory bowel diseases, and idiopathic abdominal pain. The surgical approach is decided by surgeon skills and availability of equipment. Pregnant patient may undergo laparoscopic surgery safely during any trimester without any appreciated increase in risk to the mother or fetus.[10,11,19, 31-35]

Gallbladder Disease

Conservative management of acute cholecystitis is advocated in pregnancy unless there is pancreatitis, ascending cholangitis, or common bile duct obstruction. If conservative management fails, recurrent biliary colics and gallstone pancreatitis or cholangitis that is not corrected by ERCP occurs, surgical option should be chosen. Laparoscopic cholecystectomy during pregnancy is the most common laparoscopic procedure, best done in second trimester. Muench et al. report cases performed in the first trimester.[36] Delay in surgical treatment may result in increased hospitalizations, spontaneous abortions, preterm labor, and preterm delivery.[13,35-39]

Choledocholithiasis

Multiple studies have demonstrated safe and effective management of common bile duct stones in pregnancy with ERCP and sphincterotomy with subsequent laparoscopic cholecystectomy.[40,41]

Appendectomy

Appendicitis in pregnant patient can be difficult to diagnose as symptoms cannot be differentiated by gastrointestinal (GI) tract symptoms, location of pain, or physical examination. Leukocytosis is commonly seen in pregnancy. A negative exploration rate of 35–50% is seen in pregnancy. Pregnant patient with suspicion of appendicitis should undergo immediate laparoscopy/exploration in any trimester of pregnancy. Early diagnosis and intervention reduces the rates of perforation. Pregnant patient with appendicitis will have perforation in 25% cases.[42,43] Perforation rates increase to 66% cases if treatment is delayed more than 24 hours.[44]

Perforation occurs twice as often in the third trimester (69%) compared to first and second trimester.[45]

Adrenal, Kidney, and Spleen Removal

Laparoscopic adrenalectomy during pregnancy has been effective in management of primary hyperaldosteronism,[46] Cushing's syndrome, and pheochromocytoma.[47-50]

Laparoscopic splenectomy[51,52] has been performed in hereditary spherocytosis and auto-immune thrombocytopenic purpura.[53,54]

Laparoscopic nephrectomy has been reported in first and second trimester without associated complications.[55,56]

Surgery during pregnancy should minimize maternal risk without compromising the safety of the fetus. Gasless laparoscopic surgery has been advocated by some for lengthy surgeries.[57]

Adnexal Mass

Diagnosis of adnexal mass increases with routine use of ultrasound in first trimester. Reported incidence is 1 in 600 (1 in 81–1 in 2,500 live births). Corpus luteum accounts for 33% of adnexal masses, benign cystic teratoma (dermoid) 33%, and malignancy in 2–5% of these patients.[58] Conservative management of simple cyst is recommended till the second trimester. Masses which persist are removed to prevent torsion/rupture during pregnancy, to prevent obstruction at delivery if cyst is large and to rule out malignancy. Elective removal of persistent adnexal mass during pregnancy is better than removal of symptomatic mass in an emergency.

It is advisable to remove persistent mass of more than 6 cm in the second trimester irrespective of ultrasound picture, though surgery for benign adnexal mass in pregnancy is associated with a higher rate of preterm labor than that with expectant management.[59] Laparoscopic surgery in the first and second trimester of pregnancy for any gynecologic condition is reasonably safe.

Ovarian cystectomy/oophorectomy (if malignancy is suspected) is performed laparoscopically as in nonpregnant patients. No uterine handling is done vaginally. A 10 mm umbilical port and two 5 mm ports are placed ipsilaterally or contralaterally. Cytology is taken. Cyst wall is removed through the umbilical port. Ovarian base hemostasis is ensured. Cautery to the uterus is avoided.

Torsion

Ovarian torsion in pregnancy can be confused with other abdominal emergencies. The differential diagnosis includes ectopic pregnancy, ruptured hemorrhagic cyst, appendicitis, endometrioma, and degenerating fibroid. Ultrasound and Doppler help in diagnosis. Presence of Doppler flow does not exclude torsion.[60] Torsion is often a complication of ovarian hyperstimulation syndrome. 75% of patients complicated by torsion were pregnant.

Detorsion is the procedure of choice. This can be easily carried out laparoscopically and the ovaries are then placed anatomically. Aspiration of cysts can be carried out simultaneously. Single site laparoscopic surgery has also been described.[61,62] Laparoscopy is well suited for diagnosis and treatment of adnexal torsion occurring during the first trimester of pregnancy[63] (Figs. 1 and 2).

Ectopic Pregnancy

Ectopic pregnancy is a gynecologic emergency, the leading cause of death in the first trimester accounting for up to 13% of all pregnancy, related

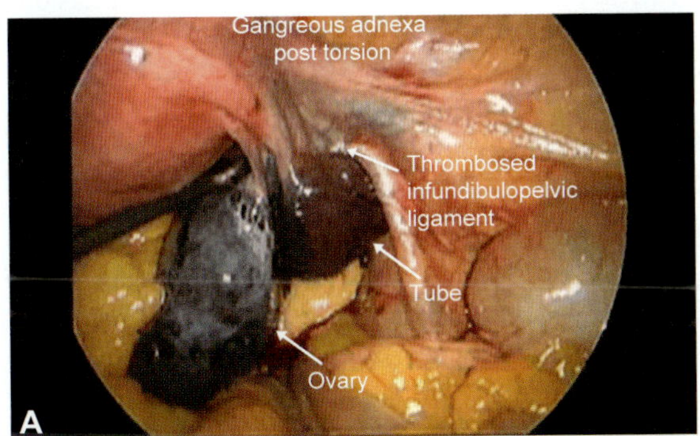

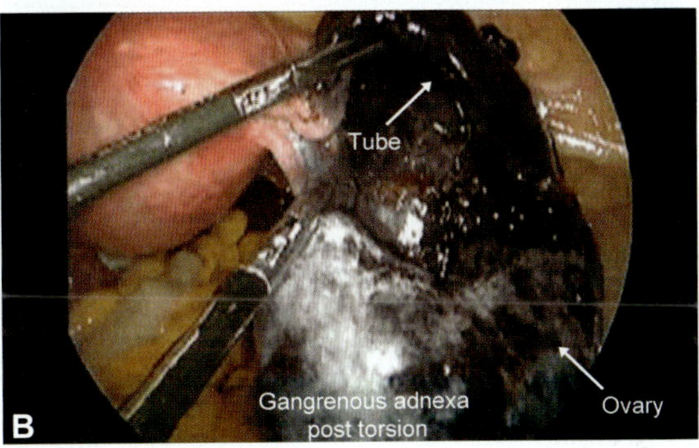

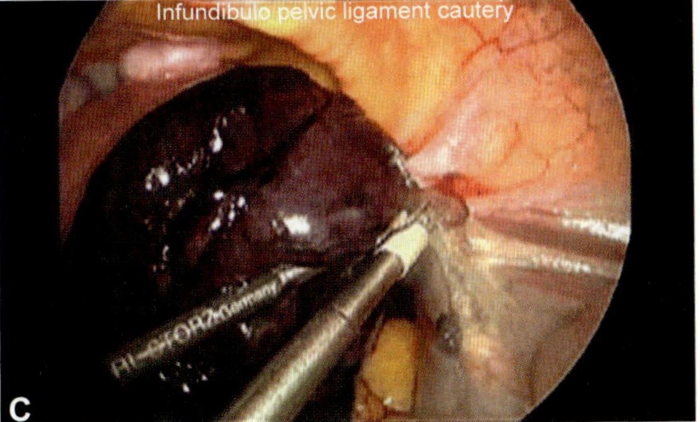

FIGURE 1 Dissection of gangrenous adnexa after torsion. **A, B,** Thrombosed infundibulopelvic ligament is seen; **C,** Cautery of infundibulopelvic ligament.

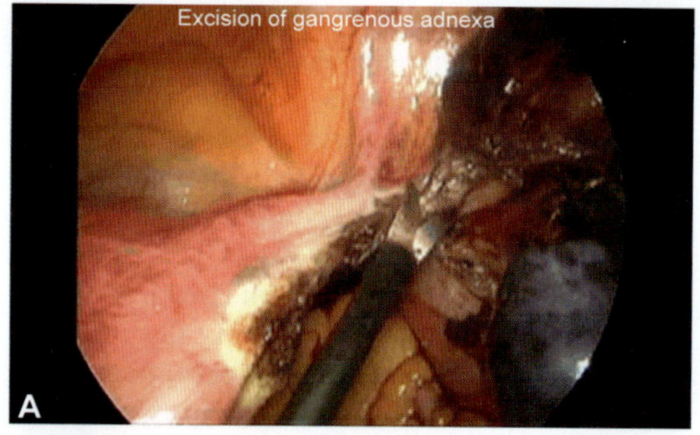

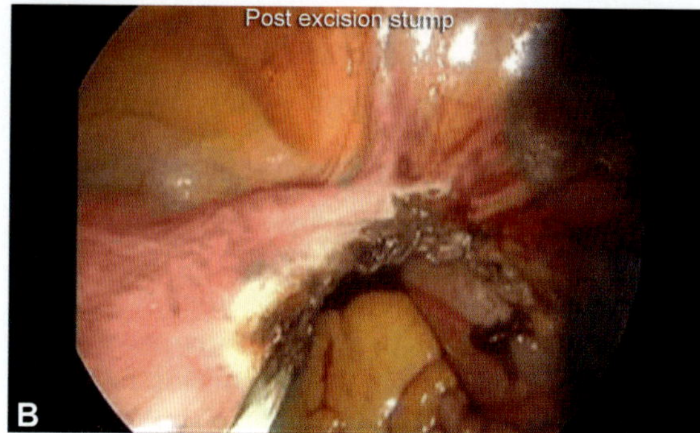

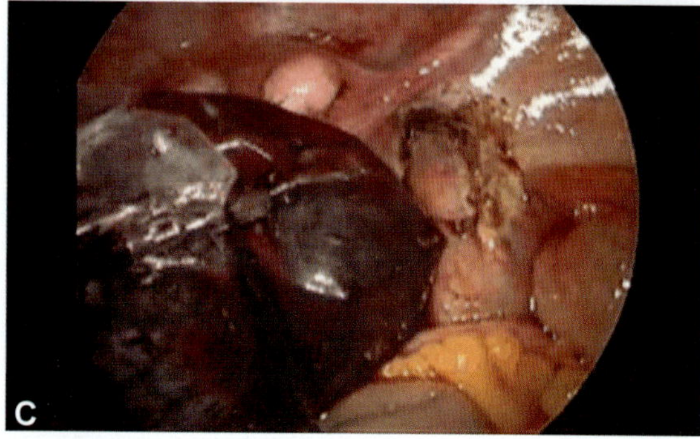

FIGURE 2 Removal of gangrenous adnexa post torsion.

deaths.[64] Implantation of the zygote outside the uterus occurs in 1:200 pregnancies. The incidence of ectopic pregnancies has been increasing in the past two decades correlating with increased accuracy of diagnosis, late age of first pregnancy, increased incidence of sexually transmitted diseases, and an increased number of *in vitro* fertilization (IVF) cycles.

Women with ectopic pregnancies are at risks of subsequent infertility and recurrence.[65] The risk of recurrence of ectopic pregnancy is approximately 10% in women with one previous ectopic pregnancy and at least 25% in women with more than two previous ectopic pregnancies.[66] The associated mortality markedly decreased to 0.5 deaths per 1,000 pregnancies because of early diagnosis and treatment before rupture.[67] Ruptured ectopics continue to occur because patients and sometimes doctors do not recognize the early signs and symptoms of the condition.[68] Early diagnosis has led to the development of minimally invasive surgical and nonsurgical options. The choice of treatment including expectant, medical, and surgical management depends on the location of the ectopic pregnancy, symptoms, gestational age, and desire to preserve fertility.[65] Surgical intervention is still the mainstay of treatment especially when a women is not a good candidate for medical therapy.[69,70] The advantages of surgical treatment include less time for resolution of an ectopic pregnancy and avoidance of the need for prolonged monitoring.[70] Surgical treatment of an ectopic pregnancy may also affect the prognosis for subsequent fertility.[65] The surgical approach to ectopic pregnancy has traditionally been salpingectomy by laparotomy till Shapiro and Adler performed the first laparoscopic salpingectomy in 1973.[71] Since then laparoscopy has been the procedure of choice due to its numerous benefits for the patient: faster recovery, less pain, decreased blood loss, and better quality of life after surgery.[72]

Laparoscopic treatment of ectopic pregnancy has been associated with decreased morbidity rates, lower cost, and shorter hospital stay. However, laparoscopic approach is associated with higher persistent trophoblast rate.[73]

Early diagnosis of ectopic pregnancy can be made with the combination of transvaginal ultrasound and measurement of beta human chorionic gonadotropin (β-hCG). The sensitivity of β-hCG allows the diagnosis to be made only 10–15 days after ovulation. A delayed increase in β-hCG should raise the suspicion of extra uterine pregnancy. Ultrasound allows visualization and localization of the gestational sac before the 6th week in 98% of cases. Early diagnosis allows treatment of ectopic pregnancy with methotrexate. In certain centers, 50% ectopic pregnancies can be managed medically. Changing trends of laparoscopic management of ectopic pregnancy has been seen in the past decade.[74] Laparoscopy has become the standard approach for surgically managing ectopic pregnancies if adequate expertise and equipment are available.

The patient is positioned on the table in the lithotomy position with legs on stirrups and back brought to the edge of the table. Bladder is catheterized. Intrauterine manipulator is used. Primary trocar 10 mm is placed at the umbilicus. Two accessory 5 mm trocars are placed on the same side or one each on contralateral side. Surgical expertise and good anesthesia back-up allows even patent with large hemoperitoneum to be managed laparoscopically.

Salpingectomy is the method of choice in women who have completed child bearing and in cases of tubal rupture. Other indications for salpingectomy are:

- Extrauterine pregnancy following sterilization
- Blocked tubes
- Previous tubal surgery
- Desiring sterilization
- Persistent bleeding following salpingotomy
- β-hCG more than 100,000 mIU/mL
- Recurrent tubal pregnancy
- Tubal pregnancy more than 5 cm size.

After introducing the laproscope hemoperitoneum is cleared from the pelvis to allow rapid visualization of the bleeding area. Bipolar forceps and scissors are introduced to coagulate and dissect the tube and mesosalpinx. The tube containing the gestational sac is removed through the 10 mm umbilical port. If the tube is dilated and very friable one can remove it in an endobag. Thorough lavage is then carried out to remove collected blood in the abdominal cavity. Tubal stump is inspected to ensure hemostasis. One must make sure that the proximal tubal stump is coagulated to prevent occurrence of future stump ectopics (Fig. 3).

Salpingotomy: Preservation of the tube should be tried in all patients who have not completed child bearing, have no evidence of tubal rupture, and have stable hemodynamic status. The size of ectopic pregnancy should be less than 5 cm. Hemostasis can be achieved by infiltrating the mesosalpinx with vasopressin 10 units in 100 cc normal saline using 22 gauge needle or using the outer sheath of veress needle. One has to be careful about avoiding intravascular injection. Vasopressin injection apart from providing hemostasis also reduces the risk of persistent ectopic by 15% due to its anoxic effect on the trophoblast. Vasopressin is contraindicated in patients with coronary artery disease. Incision over the maximum area of distension is made at the antimesenteric tubal wall. One can also use a monopolar knife electrode using a cutting or blended current (20 or 70 w). Ectopic pregnancy is then identified and removed with grasping/biopsy forceps or with the aid of pressurized irrigation. The saline wash from salpingotomy site should come out of the fimbrial end. Dye test will demonstrate tubal patency. Ectopic pregnancy in the extraluminal space will exhibit tubal dilatation without intraluminal involvement. It is easier to evacuate intraluminal ectopics compared to extraluminal which are small in size, poorly visible

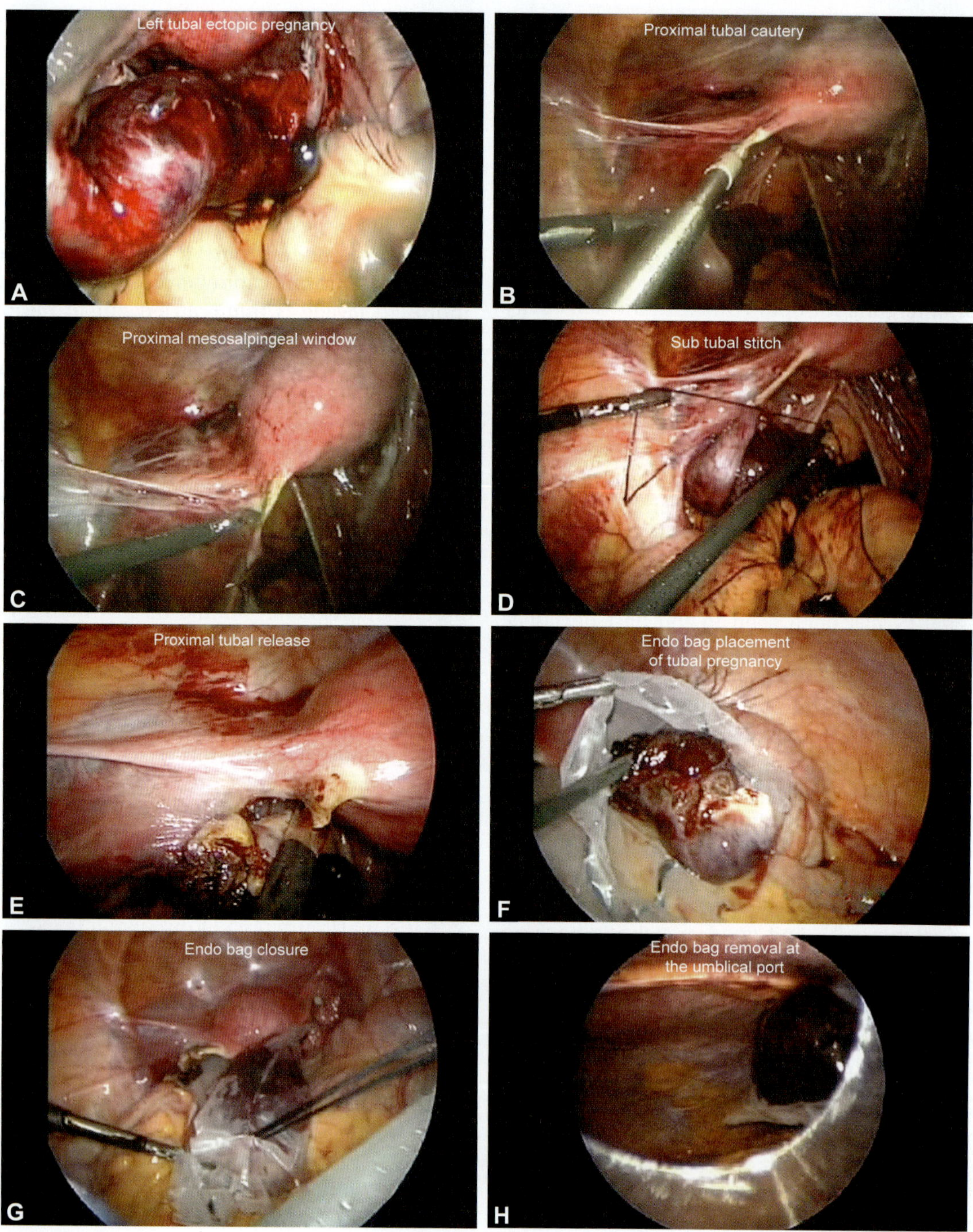

FIGURE 3 Left tubal ectopic pregnancy-salpingectomy. **A,** Left tubal ectopic pregnancy; **B,** Proximal tubal cautery; **C,** Proximal mesosalpingeal window; **D,** Sub-tubal stitch, **E,** Proximal tubal release; **F,** Endo bag placement of tubal pregnancy; **G,** Endo bag closure; **H,** Endo bag removal at the umbilical port.

in the thickness of the tubal wall. As soon as the serosa is incised, the products slip out without needing to enlarge the opening. Irrigation will not allow the saline to flow through the distal part of the tube.

The salpingotomy incision does not require suturing unless there is mucosal eversion. Bleeding from the base and tubal margins can be managed with hemostatic tamponade by grasping forceps. Precise coagulation can be done if pressure does not work. Arterial bleeding can be controlled by targeted use of bipolar current. Diffuse venous bleeding specially from the base of implantation in the muscle layers in case of extraluminal location can be controlled with bipolar forceps. The superficial scar in the extraluminal space does not come in the way of tubal healing. Too much coagulation is avoided. If bleeding persists, mesosalpingeal vessels may be tied selectively (Fig. 4).

The patient should be followed with serial β-hCG measurements. Methotrexate can be used as adjuvant treatment.

Milking of tubal pregnancy can be done through the fimbrial end. Since many ectopic pregnancies have not implanted in the intraluminal tubal portion, this procedure is associated with incomplete removal of the trophoblast and damage to tubal wall. Hence, it is not recommended. The technique may be applied in selected cases where removal of products of conception (POC's) located at the fimbrial end or in the distal tubal segment.

Interstitial or Cornual Ectopic Pregnancy

These account for 3% of ectopic gestations. The mortality rate for a woman diagnosed with such a pregnancy is 2–2.5%.[75,76] This is because of increased incidence of hemorrhage. Medical management is a useful option for treating cornual pregnancies, but is not without its drawbacks. With methotrexate treatment, neither gestational sac size nor serum β-hCG levels can be used to predict success for cornual gestations.[77] Overall failure rate for methotrexate treatment is as high as 35%[78,79] (Fig. 5).

Because of the potential for catastrophic outcomes associated with failure of medical management, surgery remains the mainstay of treatment. Resection of the cornual region of the uterus along with the ipsilateral fallopian tube has been the option of choice in women interested in future fertility. As both technology and surgical skills have improved, this resection has been performed laparoscopically with good outcomes.[79-,83] Even with cornual rupture, expert laparoscopists have used laparoscopic sutures os stapling device to perform a cornual wedge resection.[84,85] Cornual resection uses full thickness uterine incision. Future cesarean deliveries are recommended to decrease the risk of uterine rupture.

Recent years have seen the use of conservative surgical alternatives to cornual resection, to increase future fertility and decrease risk of uterine rupture. Such methods include the use of cornuostomy rather than cornuectomy.[84,86,87]

Combination surgical approach consists of performing laparoscopy and hysteroscopy followed by dilatation and evacuation, and a final hysteroscopy.[88-90]

In stable patients with small cornual ectopic pregnancy (CEP) of size 1–2 cm and low hCG concentration (<5,000 IU), systemic methotrexate in a single dose of 50 mg/m^2 can be an option. In stable patients with large CEP or high hCG concentration, elective surgical treatment (Wedge resection) is preferred. Medical treatment may require multiple doses, may be prolonged, and run the risk of rupture and severe bleeding. In unstable patients, surgery should be performed after quick resuscitation. A laparoscopic approach is preferable to open approach, however, laparotomy should not be delayed when expedient laparoscopic services are not available. Cornuostomy is carried out for small, less than 3 cm, CEP's and wedge resection for larger or

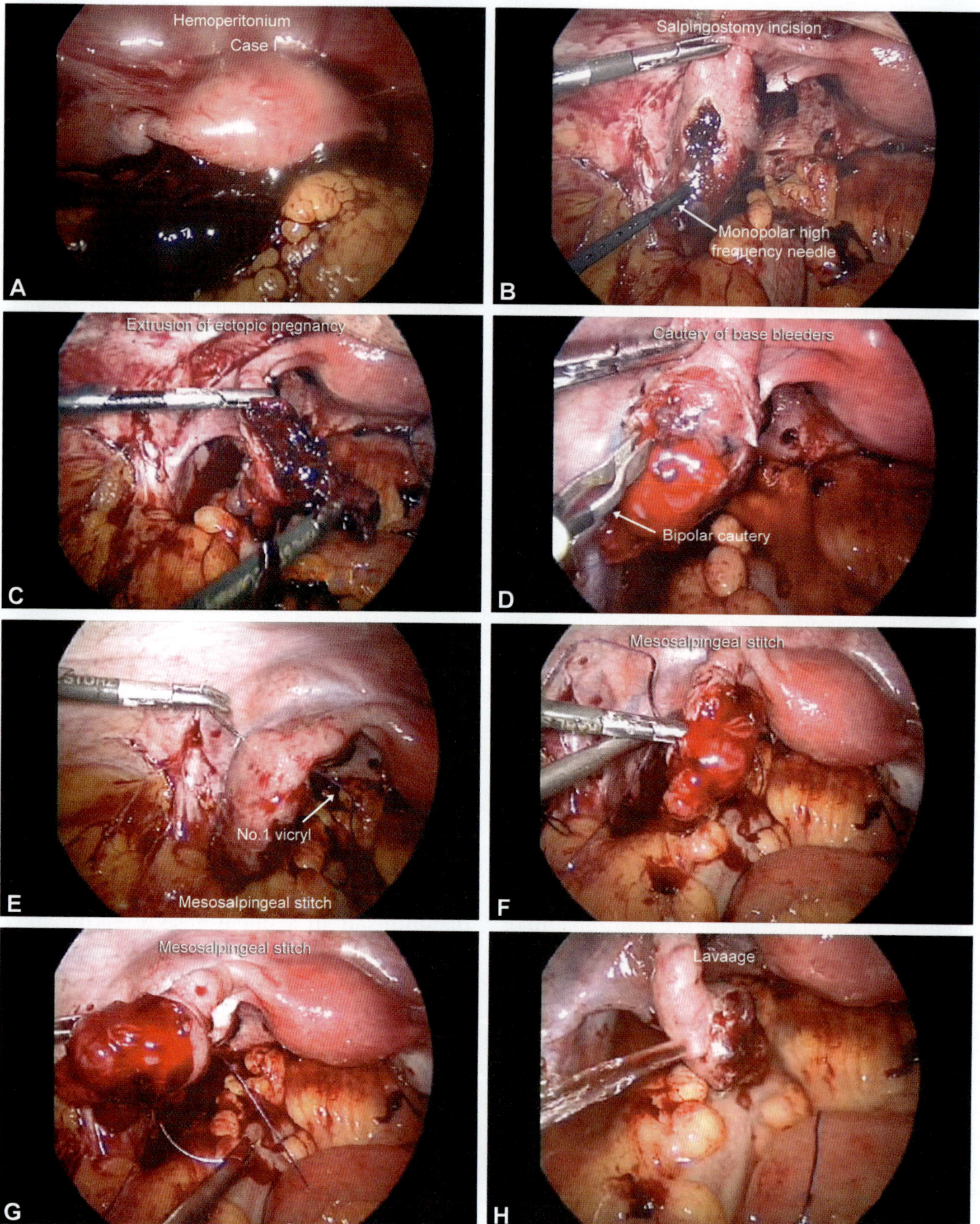

FIGURE 4 Right tubal ectopic pregnancy-salpingostomy. **A,** Hemoperitoneum; **B,** Salpingostomy incision; **C,** Extrusion of ectopic pregnancy; **D,** Cautery of base bleeders; **E, F, G,** Mesosalpingeal stitch; **H,** Lavage.

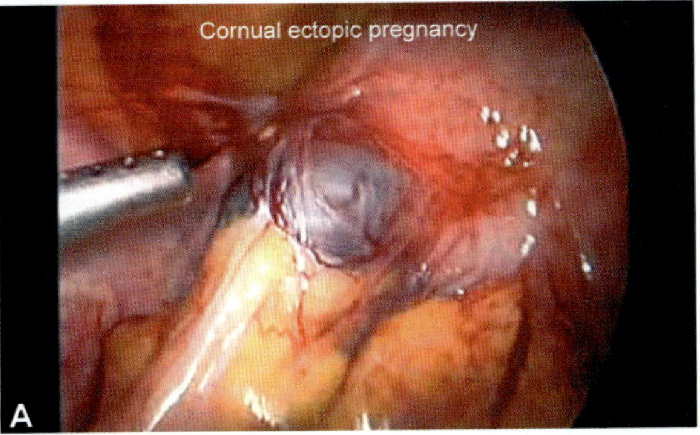

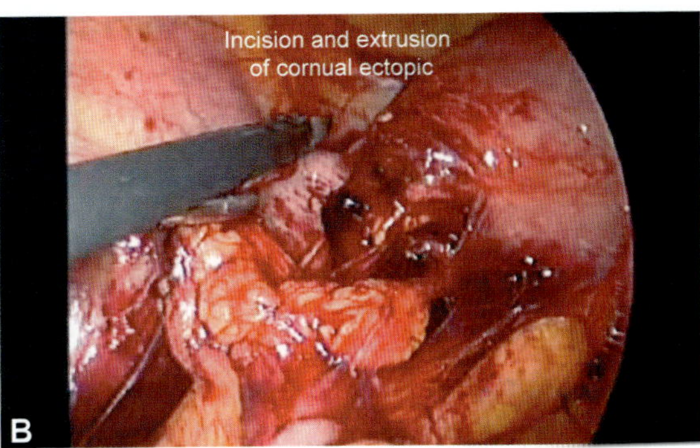

FIGURE 5 Cornual ectopic pregnancy excision. **A,** Cornual ectopic pregnancy; **B,** Incision and extrusion of cornual ectopic pregnancy.

recurrent CEP's. Vasopressin can be used to reduce bleeding and minimal electrosurgery is used to reduce thermal tissue damage. Vasopressin 20 U in 80 cc saline is injected into the myometrium at the base of cornual pregnancy. This can be done transabdominally using a long 21 gauge spinal needle connected to a syringe under laparoscopic vision. Anterior and posterior aspects of CEP are injected. Number of injection sites are limited to reduce puncture site bleeding. Vasopressin is injected till blanching occurs. Monopolar diathermy with 30 W cutting current can be used for cornuostomy or wedge resection. Cornuostomy is carried out in cases of CEP's smaller than 3 cm. A small incision is made over the most prominent point till the conceptus protrudes. The CEP is lifted off or expelled via hydrodissection. The implantation site is inspected for remnants and bleeds. Cornual wedge resection is carried out in large CEP's (>3 cm) and in recurrent CEP's. A circumferential incision is given around the CEP midway between the base and the top. One or two mattress sutures are adequate for cornuostomy and 2–4 for cases of wedge resection. Braided polyglactin 910 or vicryl sutures are used to achieve hemostasis keeping diathermy to the minimum. Postoperative follow-up is by serial hCG measurements. Methotrexate is given postoperatively if hCG concentrations do not decrease by 15% within 48 hours.[91]

Abdominal Ectopic Pregnancy

This is a rare event and accounts for 1.1% of all ectopic pregnancies. It is a condition with high maternal and fetal morbidity and mortality. Early diagnosis using ultrasound, MRI, and laparoscopy is essential. This can be treated readily by laparoscopy if done in early weeks of pregnancy. In case of advanced abdominal pregnancy with live fetus laparotomy would be required.

Cesarean Scar Ectopic Pregnancy

Pregnancy implantation within the scar of a previous cesarean delivery is one of the rarest locations of an ectopic pregnancy. The time interval between the last cesarean section and the cesarean scar ectopic pregnancy (CSP) is usually 6 months to 1 year.[92,93] The gestational age at diagnosis ranges from 5 weeks to 12^{+4} weeks. It has also been reported after IVF and embryo transfer.[94] A delay in diagnosis can lead to uterine rupture and significant maternal morbidity. Vial et al. proposed two different types of CSP's.

1. The first is an implantation in the prior cesarean scar with progression toward the cervicoisthmic space or the uterine cavity. This may progress to a viable birth with the risk of life threatening bleed.

2. The second is a deep implantation into a caesarean section defect toward the bladder and abdominal cavity a type that is more prone to rupture.[95]

The therapeutic approach of CSP is still a dilemma. Earlier the diagnosis the more minimal is the therapeutic approach. The risk of bleeding in viable pregnancy increases with gestational age. Bleeding mainly results from the placental invasion into the myometrium, which prevents complete separation and removal of placenta. Moreover, a deficient scarred myometrium does not have the ability to contract which further aggravates blood loss. Medical treatment is considered the management of choice. Apart from anesthetic risks surgical treatment involves operative risk, especially massive bleeding. Measures to reduce bleeding include:

- Local injection of vasopressin and tamponade of intra-abdominal pressure of laparoscopy decreases bleeding during the procedure[96]
- Use of uterotonics along with surgical hemostatic measures is more effective[97]
- Bilateral uterine artery embolization to minimize bleeding has been proposed[98]
- Insertion of a Shirodhkar cervical suture during the evacuation of CSP is an effective method of hemostasis[99]
- Bilateral uterine artery ligation also reduces perioperative bleeding.[100,101]

Surgical treatment involves removal of gestation mass and repair of defect. But no treatment modality can guarantee uterine integrity.[102] Surgical repair of scar can be offered as a primary treatment or as secondary operation after initial treatment. Many would still consider laparotomy and hysterotomy as the best option on diagnosis of CSP despite the large surgical wound, longer hospitalization, and longer recovery time. Laparoscopic excision of the mass of CSP follows the principle of laparotomy, i.e., remove the ectopic gestation tissue and reapproximate the uterine incision safely, conserving the uterus.[103] In experienced hands, endoscopic approach can replace laparotomy in the management of CSP.

Prevention of Ectopic Pregnancy

Sexually transmitted diseases, inflammation, abscess, and rupture of the appendix are common, and are known to cause of fimbrial damage and ectopic pregnancy. Increased awareness and prompt treatment of the above in adolescents will reduce the incidence of tubal damage.[104]

Abdominal Pregnancy

Maternal mortality in abdominal pregnancy is 7.7 times higher than other ectopic pregnancies. Pregnancies have also been reported in upper abdominal organs-liver and spleen.[105,106] Secondary abdominal pregnancies can result from tubal abortion or rupture or less often after uterine rupture with subsequent reimplantation within the abdomen. If hemorrhage is present in the abdomen and pregnancy not found in the pelvis it is imperative to look for pregnancy elsewhere in the abdomen. It is necessary to find chorionic tissue in the abdomen in cases of tubal abortion or ruptured ectopic pregnancy and remove it to prevent secondary chorionic implantation. All this can be carried out laparoscopically. There are reported cases of concurrent appendicitis and ectopic pregnancy.[107] It is good practice to look at appendix routinely more so if the ectopic pregnancies on the right side.

Rudimentary Horn Pregnancy

Rudimentary horn arises as a result of arrested development of one of the two Mullerian ducts. They are found in 75% of bicornuate uteri. Noncommunicating horns occur in 70–90% cases. The overall incidence of a bicornuate uterus with a rudimentary horn is 1 in 5,400.[108] A urogenital evaluation is recommended. Risk of rupture because of poorly developed musculature occurs in 50% of rudimentary horn pregnancies. First trimester ultrasound diagnoses rudimentary horn pregnancy before symptoms occur.[109] Medical treatment before and during laparoscopy can be administered to reduce the size of the horn and reduce intraoperative bleeding.[110-112] Most surgeons used coagulation for excision of the fibrous band that connected the horn. The absence of cervix and communication to the uterus makes the procedure easier with minimal bleeding. The Ipsilateral fallopian tube should be removed to prevent future tubal pregnancy. The excised horn can be removed vaginally[113] or through a suprapubic incision.[114] A rudimentary horn should be removed in symptom free patients as soon as diagnosis is made to avoid potential complications of pregnancy and surgical removal during pregnancy[114] (Fig. 6).

Ovarian Pregnancy

Ovarian pregnancy still represents a diagnostic dilemma. Symptoms and physical findings are similar to those of tubal pregnancy, hemorrhagic corpus luteum, or a ruptured ovarian cyst. Fifty percent of ovarian pregnancy following ovarian hyperstimulation may be diagnosed at an asymptomatic stage.[115]

Spiegelberg criteria for diagnosis:

- Fallopian tube with their fimbriae should be intact and separate from the ovary
- The gestation sac should occupy normal position of ovary
- The gestation should be connected to the uterus by uterine ligament
- Ovarian tissue must be present in the specimen attached to the gestation sac (Spiegelberg 1878).

A modification of the fourth postulate of *Spiegelberg* is the detection of chorionic villi without concurrent detection of an intact ovarian parenchyma for diagnosis. Most ovarian pregnancies rupture in the first trimester (75–90%) with two-thirds occurring during the first 8 weeks. In cases with stimulated ovaries, additional diagnostic problems exist.

Laparoscopy is now the gold standard for the diagnosis of ectopic pregnancy. Definitive surgical treatment can be carried out at the same sitting. In young patients desirous of future pregnancy conservative ovarian surgery is performed, i.e., partial ovariectomy (wedge resection), ovarian cystectomy, or blunt dissection of trophoblast tissue. Medical management is chosen for organ preservation, primary incomplete resection or persisting trophoblast. Fertility in patients treated for an ovarian pregnancy remains unaffected and subsequent pregnancies are invariably intrauterine.

Cervical Pregnancy

Cervical pregnancy is a rare, life threatening type of ectopic pregnancy that constitutes 0.15% of ectopic pregnancies.[116] The incidence is increasing because of increase of *in vitro*

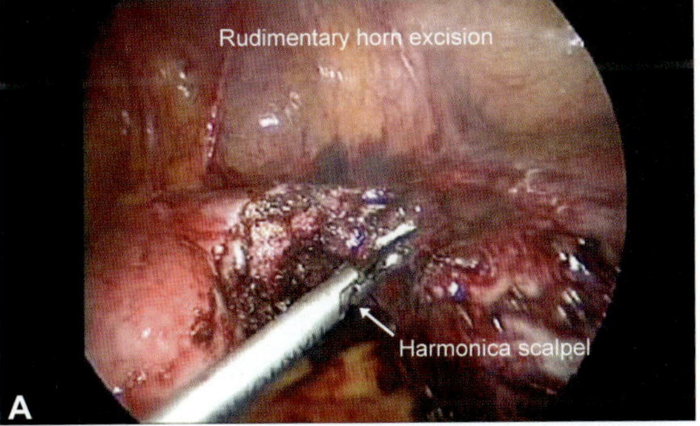

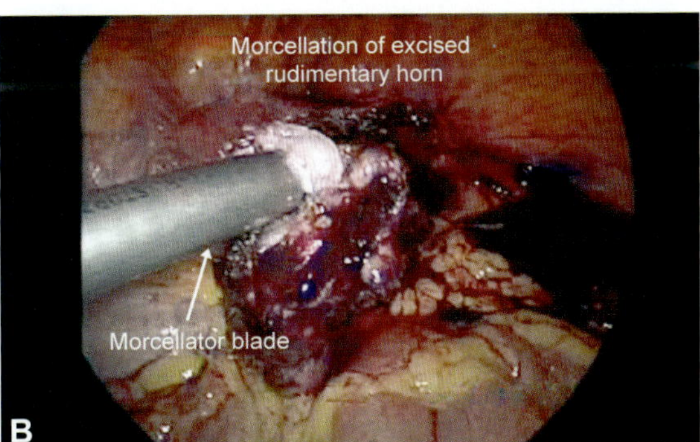

FIGURE 6 Rudimentary horn pregnancy excision. **A,** Rudimentary horn excision; **B,** Morcellation of excised rudimentary horn.

fertilization, cesarean section and curettage. It is commonly diagnosed at first trimester ultrasound. Ultrasound criteria for cervical pregnancy includes—empty uterine cavity, hourglass uterine shape with a ballooned cervical canal, presence of gestational sac or placental tissue within the cervical canal, and closed internal os.[117] Delay in diagnosis and treatment will result in painless, massive bleeding in the endocervical canal requiring multiple transfusions and often hysterectomy. Cervical pregnancy has been managed by various methods. No randomized clinical trials (RCT) have evaluated these treatments and no standard protocol has been established. Conservative fertility preserving treatments include intracervical foley balloon tamponade, cervical cerclage angiographic embolization, large vessel ligation, intra-amniotic potassium chloride, methotrexate injections, and systemic chemotherapy with methotrexate.[117] Novel attempt to treat cervical pregnancy hysteroscopically has been successful. A resectoscope (26 Fr) was used to identify the location of gestation sac, which can be removed with the resectoscope coagulating (current setting 70 W cutting) the bleeders at the implantation site. Vasopressin 0.2 units diluted in saline solution can be injected intracervically prior to the procedure. Since methotrexate is not required after treatment, systemic side effects, such as kidney and liver dysfunction do not occur.

Molar Ectopic Pregnancy

The incidence of hydatidiform molar pregnancy is 1 in 1,000–2,000 pregnancies.[118] Few cases of molar ectopic pregnancy have been reported in the medical literature in the cervix, ovary, and smooth muscle of the uterus.[119-122] Molar cornual ectopic pregnancy is very rare. Signs and symptoms of molar cornual ectopic pregnancy is similar to those of nonmolar ectopic pregnancy, Patients have abnormal vaginal bleeding, expulsion of molar vesicles, uterine enlargement greater than expected for gestation age, absent fetal heart tones, cystic enlargement of the ovaries, hyperemesis, and high levels of hCG for gestational age.[123] Ultrasound findings of multiple echogenic areas within the uterine cavity with or without fetus are reliable for confirmation of diagnosis of molar pregnancy.[124] Earlier treatment consisted of cornual resection or hysterectomy via laparotomy. Currently, they are treated with laparoscopic cornuostomy with systemic methotrexate. Most patients (66%) attain complete remission rapidly after surgical intervention.[119] Postoperative monitoring with serial determination of β-hCG levels is important.[125] Close follow-up is crucial throughout subsequent pregnancies, cesarean section is recommended to avert the possibility of uterine rupture.

Heterotopic Pregnancy

This occurs when there are coexisting intra- and extrauterine pregnancies. Incidence varies widely 1 in 100–1 in 30,000 pregnancies. These pregnancies are associated with diagnostic difficulties. hCG measurements are difficult to interpret because intrauterine pregnancy can cause the hCG concentration to increase appropriately.[126] This often leads to late detection of extrauterine sac. The diagnosis thus remains a diagnostic challenge.[124]

The goal of management is to terminate the extrauterine pregnancy while taking precautions to minimize the possible threat to intrauterine gestations. Laparoscopy is considered the most suitable technique for rapid diagnosis and prompt treatment. General endotracheal anesthesia with adequate monitoring of blood pressure, transcutaneous oxygen saturation, and end tidal CO_2 pressure is required. CO_2 pressure is maintained at less than 12 mmHg. No vaginal manipulation is done. The associated intrauterine pregnancies are at increased risk for spontaneous abortion. In cases of ongoing pregnancy prognosis depends on the time of delivery.[128]

Management of Patients with Ectopic Pregnancy with Massive Hemoperitoneum

The most common site of ectopic with massive hemoperitoneum are interstitial and cornual pregnancy (75%). Ampullary pregnancy is the least frequent (8.1%). If surgical view is not good because of pooled blood, one should identify the site of bleeding while suctioning the pooled blood and hemostasis should be achieved either by coagulation or hemostatic suturing. Then extensive peritoneal lavage should be done. Even in patients with ectopic pregnancy demonstrating massive hemoperitoneum laparoscopic surgery can be performed safely by experienced laparoscopists with the aid of optimal anesthesia, advanced cardiovascular monitoring intraoperative autologous blood transfusion, and postoperative intensive care.[129]

CONCLUSION

Laparoscopic surgery during pregnancy is safe, has multiple advantages over open techniques, can be performed during all gestational ages. It can be performed for surgical as well as obstetric conditions. It is not associated with increased pregnancy complications or long-term fetal sequelae.

REFERENCES

1. Joris JL, Noirot DP, Legrand MJ, et al. Hemodynamic changes during laparoscopic cholecystectomy. Anesth Anal. 1993;76(5):1067-71.
2. Curet MJ, Allen D, Josloff RK, et al. Laparoscopy during pregnancy. Arch Surg. 1996;131:546-50.
3. Steinbrook RA, Brooks DC, Datta S. Laparoscopic cholecystectomy during pregnancy. Review of anesthetic management, surgical considerations. Surg Endosc. 1996;10:511.
4. Sherry Boschert. Low insufflation. Key to laparoscopy in pregnancy, try to avoid surgery in first trimester. Obgyn News. 2003.
5. Visser BC, Glasgow RE, Mulvihil KK, et al. Safety and timing of non obstetric abdominal surgery in pregnancy. Dig Surg. 2001;18(5):409.
6. Rizzo AG. Laparoscopic surgery during pregnancy: long term follow-up. J Laparoendosc Adv Surg Tech A. 2003;13:11-5.
7. Menias CO, Elsayes KM, Peterson CM, et al. CT of pregnancy related complications. Emerg Radiol. 2007;13(6):299-306.
8. Schaefer C, Meister R, Wentzeck R, et al. Fetal outcome after technetium scientifigraphy in early pregnancy. Reprod Toxicol. 2009;28:161-6.
9. Karthikesalingam A MS, Weerakkopdy R, Walsh SR, et al. Radiation exposure during laparoscopic Cholecystectomy with routine Intraoperative cholangiography. Surg Endosc. 2009;23;1845-8.
10. Reedy MB, Galan HL, Richards WE, et al. Laparoscopy during pregnancy. A survey of laparoendoscopic surgeons. J Reprod. Med. 1997;42:33-38.
11. Oelsner G, Stockheim D, Soriano D, et al. Pregnancy outcome after laparoscopy or laparotomy in pregnancy. J Am Assoc Gynecol Laparosc. 2003;10(2):200-4.
12. Fatum M, Rojansky N. Laparoscopic surgery during pregnancy. Obstet Gynecol Surg. 2001;56:50-9.
13. Melnick DM, Wahl WL, Dalton VK. Management of general surgical problems in the pregnant patient. Am J Surg. 2004;187:170-80.
14. Jorgensen JO, Lalak NJ, North L, et al. Venous stasis during laparoscopic Cholecystectomy. Surg Laparosc Endosc. 1994;4:128-33.
15. Risk of and prophylaxis for venous thromboembolism in hospital patients. Thromboembolic risk factors (THRIFT) consensus group. BMJ. 1992;305(6853):567-74.
16. Casele HL. The use of unfractionated heparin and low molecular weight heparins in pregnancy. Clin obs gynecol. 2006;49:895-905.
17. Date RS, Kaushal M, Ramesh A. A review of management of gallstone disease and its complications in pregnancy. Am J Surg. 2008;196:599-608.
18. Society of American Gastrointestinal endoscopic surgeons (SAGES). Guidelines for laparoscopic surgery during pregnancy. Surg Endosc. 1998;12:189-90.
19. Glasgow RE, Visser BC, Harris HW, et al. Changing management of gall stone disease during pregnancy. Surg Endosc. 1998;12:241-6.
20. Scott LD. Gallstone disease and pancreatitis in pregnancy. Gastroenterol Clin North Am. 1992;21(4):803-15.
21. Graham G, Baxi L, Tharakan T. Laparoscopic cholecystectomy during pregnancy: a case series and review of the literature. Obstet Gynecol Surg. 1998;53:566-74.
22. Canis M, Rabischong B, Houlle C, et al. Laparoscopic management of adnexal masses: a gold standard? Curr opin Obstet Gynecol. 2002;14:423-8.
23. Sherard GB 3rd, Hodson CA, Williams HJ, et al. Adnexal masses and pregnancy: a 12-year experience. Am J Obstet Gynecol. 2003;189(2):358-62.
24. Argenta PA, Yeagley TJ, Ott G, et al. Torsion of the uterine adnexa. Pathologic correlations and current management trends. J Reprod Med. 2000;45(10):831-6.

25. Tarraza HM, Moore RD. Gynecologic causes of the acute abdomen and acute abdomen in pregnancy. Surg Clin North Am. 77(6):1371-94.
26. Oelsner G, Bider D, Goldenberg M, et al. Long-term follow-up of the twisted ischemic adnexa managed by detorsion. Fertil Steril. 1993;60(6):976-9.
27. Sharp HT. The acute abdomen during pregnancy. Clin Obstet Gynecol. 2002;45(2):405-13.
28. Tan TC, Devendra K, Tan LK, et al. Tocolytic treatment for the management of preterm labour: a systematic review. Singapore Med J. 2006;47(5):361-6.
29. Kammerer WS. Nonobstetric surgery during pregnancy. Med Clin North Am. 1979;63(6):1157-64.
30. Kort B, Katz VL, Watson WJ. The effect of nonobstetric operation during pregnancy. Surg Gynecol Obs. 1993;177:371-6.
31. Reedy MB, Kallen B, Kuehl TJ. Laparoscopy during pregnancy: a study of five fetal outcome parameters with use of the Swedish Health Registry. Am J Obstet Gynecol. 1997;177(3):673-9.
32. Affleck DG, Handrahan DL, Egger MJ, et al. The laparoscopic management of appendicitis and cholelithiasis during pregnancy. Am J Surg. 1999;178(6):523-9.
33. Barone JE, Bears S, Chen S, et al. Outcome study of cholecystectomy during pregnancy. Am J Surg. 1999;177:232-6.
34. Rollins MD, Chan KJ, Price RR. Laparoscopy for appendicitis and cholelithiasis during pregnancy: a new standard of care. Surg Endosc. 2004;18:237-41.
35. Nezhat FR, Tazuke S, Nezhat CH et al. Laparoscopy during pregnancy. A literature review. JSLS. 1997;1(1):17-27.
36. Muench J, Albrink M, Serafini F, et al. Delay in treatment of biliary disease during pregnancy increases morbidity and can be avoided with safe laparoscopic cholecystectomy. Am Surg. 2001;67(6):539-42.
37. Guidelines for laparoscopic surgery during pregnancy. Surg Endosc. 1998;12(2):189-90.
38. Bhavani-Shankar K, Steinbrook RA, Brooks DC, et al. Arterial to end-tidal carbon dioxide pressure difference during laparoscopic surgery in pregnancy. Anesthesiology. 2000;93:370-3.
39. Printen KJ, Ott RA. Cholecystectomy during pregnancy. Am Surg. 1978;44:432-4.
40. Sengler P, Heinerman PM, Steiner H, et al. Laparoscopic cholecystectomy and interventional endoscopy for gallstone complications during pregnancy. Surg Endosc. 2000;14:267-71.
41. Andreoli M, Sayegh SK, Hoefer R, et al. Laparoscopic cholecystectomy for recurrent gallstone pancreatitis during pregnancy. South Med J. 1996;89:1114-15.
42. Mahmoodian S. Appendicitis complicating pregnancy. South Med J. 1992;85(1):19-24.
43. Cappell MS, Friedel D. Abdominal pain during pregnancy. Gastroenterol Clin North Am. 2003;32:1-58.
44. Tamir IL, Bongard FS, Klein SR. Acute appendicitis in the pregnant patient. Am J Surg. 1990;160(6):571-5.
45. Weingold AB. Appendicitis in pregnancy. Clin Obstet Gynecol. 1983;26(4):801-9.
46. Shalhav AL, Landman J, Afane J, et al. Laparoscopic adrenalectomy for primary hyperaldosteronism during pregnancy. J Laparoendosc Adv Surg Tech A. 2000;10:169-71.
47. Aishima M, Tanaka M, Haraoka M, et al. Retroperitoneal laparoscopic adrenalectomy in a pregnant woman with Cushing's syndrome. J Urol. 2000;164:770-1.
48. Pace DE, Chiasson PM, Schlachta CM, et al. Minimally invasive adrenalectomy for pheochromocytoma during pregnancy. Surg Laparosc Endosc Percutan Tech. 2002;12:122-5.
49. Wolf A, Goretzki PE, Rohrborn A, et al. Pheochromocytoma during pregnancy: laparoscopic and conventional surgical treatment of two cases. Exp Clin Endocrinol Diabetes. 2004;112:98-101.
50. Kim PT, Kreisman SH, Vaughn R, et al. Laparoscopic adrenalectomy for pheochromocytoma in pregnancy. Can J Surg. 2006;49:62-3.
51. Hardwick RH, Slade RR, Smith PA, et al. Laparoscopic plenectomy in pregnancy. J Obstet Gynaecol Can. 1999;27(8):771-4.
52. Allran CF Jr., Weiss CA 3rd, Park AE. Urgent laparoscopic splenectomy in a morbidly obese pregnant woman: case report and literature review. J Laparoendosc Adv Surg Tech A. 2002;12:445-7.
53. Griffiths J, Sia W, Shapiro AM, et al. Laparoscopic splenectomy for the treatment of refractory immune thrombocytopenia in pregnancy. J Obstet Gynaecol Can. 2005;27:771-4.
54. Anglin BV, Rutherford C, Ramus R, et al. Immune thrombocytopenic purpura during pregnancy: laparoscopic treatment. JSLS. 2001;5:63-7.
55. O'Connor JP, Biyani CS, Taylor J, et al. Laparoscopic nephrectomy for renal-cell carcinoma during pregnancy. J Endourol. 2004;18:871-4.
56. Sainsbury DC, Dorkin TJ, MacPhail S, et al. Laparoscopic radical nephrectomy in first-trimester pregnancy. Urology. 2004;64:e1237-8.
57. Sesti F, Pietropoli A, et al Gasless laparoscopic surgery during pregnancy:evaluation of its role and usefulness. Eur J Obstet Gynecol Reprod Biol. 2013;5(13):231-3.
58. Pong Mo Yuen, Allan M, Z Chang. Laparoscopic management of adnexal mass during pregnancy. Acta Obstet Gynecol second. 1997;76:173-6.
59. Leiserowitz GS. Managing ovarian masses during pregnancy. Obstet Gynecol Surv. 2006;61(7):463-70.
60. Albayram F, Hamper UM. Ovarian and adnexal torsion spectrum of sonographic findings and pathologic co-relation. J Ultrasound Med. 2001:20(10):1083-9.
61. Gazarclli S, Mazzuca N. One laparoscopic puncture for treatment of ovarian cysts with adnexal torsion in early pregnancy: A report of two cases. J Reprod Med. 1994;39:985-6.

62. Savaris RF, Cavazzola LT. Ectopic pregnancy: laparoscopic endoscopic single site surgery. Fertil Steril. 2009;92(3):1170.
63. Morice P, Louis-Sylvestre C, Chapron C, et al. Laparoscopy for adnexal torsion in pregnant women. J Reprod Med. 1997;42(7):435-9.
64. Barnhart K, Esposito M, Coutifaris C. An update on the medical treatment of ectopic pregnancy. Obstet Gynecol Clin North Am. 2000:27:653-67.
65. Ehrenberg-Buchner S, Sandadi S, Moawad NS, et al. Ectopic pregnancy: role of laparoscopic treatment. Clin Obstet Gynecol. 2009;52:372-9.
66. Seeber BE, Barnhart KT. Suspected ectopic pregnancy. Obstet Gynecol. 2006;107:379-413.
67. Chang J, Elam-Evans LD, Berg CI, et al. Pregnancy related mortality surveillance United States 1991-1999. MMWR Surveill Summ. 2003;52:1-8.
68. Dorfman SF. Deaths from ectopic pregnancy, United States, 1979 to 1980. Obstet Gynecol. 1983;62:334-8.
69. Yao M, Tulandi T. Current status of surgical and nonsurgical management of ectopic pregnancy. Fertil Steril. 1997;67:421-33.
70. Barnhart KT. Clinical practice: ectopic pregnancy. N Engl J Med. 2009;361:379-87.
71. Shapiro H, Adler DH. Excision of ectopic pregnancy through the laparoscope. Am J Obstet Gynecol. 1973:117:290-1.
72. Korolio D, Sauerland S, Wood Dauphinee, et al. Evaluation of quality of life after laparoscopic surgery: evidence based guidelines of the European Association for Endoscopic surgery. Surg Endosc. 2004:18:879-7.
73. Hajenius PJ, Mol F, Mol BW, et al. Intervention for tubal ectopic pregnancy. Cochrane Database Syst Rey. 2007;CD 000324.
74. Peter Takacs, Nahida Chakhtoura MD. Laparotomy to laparoscopy changing trends in the surgical management of ectopic pregnancy in a tertiary care teaching hospital. J Min Gynae. 2006;13:175-7.
75. Lenus J. Ectopic Pregnancy: an update. Curr Opin Obstet Gynecol. 2000;12:369-75.
76. Kun WM, Tung WK. On the lookout for rarity interstitial/cornual pregnancy. Eur J Emerg Med. 2001;8:147-50.
77. Tulandi T, Al Jaroudi. Interstitial pregnancy: results generated from the Society of Reproductive surgeons registry. Obstet Gynecol. 2004;103:47-50.
78. Barnhart K, Spenderfer S, Cautifaris C. Medical treatment of interstitial pregnancy. A report of three unsuccessful cases. J Reprod Med. 1997;42:521-4.
79. Woodland MB, D Pasquate SE, Molinari JA, et al. Laparoscopic approach to interstitial pregnancy. JAAGL. 1996;3:439-441.
80. Ostrezenski A. A new laparoscopic technique for interstitial pregnancy resection. A case report. J Reprod Med. 1992; 42:159-60.
81. Pansky M, Bokovsky I, Gonal A, et al. Conservative management of interstitial pregnancy using operative laparoscopy. Surg Endoscop. 1995;9:515-6.
82. Tulandi T, Vilas G, Gomel V. Laparoscopic treatment of interstitial pregnancy. Obstet Gynecol. 1995;85:465-7.
83. Morita Y, Tsutsumi O, Momaeda M, et al. Cornual pregnancy successfully treated laparoscopically with fibrin glue hemostasis. Obstet Gynecol. 1997;90(P1-2):685-7.
84. Chan LY, Yuen PM. Successful treatment of ruptured interstitial pregnancy with laparoscopic surgery. A report of 2 cases. J Reprod Med. 2003;48:569-71.
85. Aumkul S. Rupture of gravid uterus after cornual resections.
86. Beemee T, Ceda V, Luciano AA. Surgical management of interstitial pregnancy. JAAGL. 2000;7:387-9.
87. Reneita Ross, Steven R, Lindhain, et al. Cornual gestation: A systematic literature review and two case reports of a novel treatment regimes. J Min Inv Gynaecol. 2006;13:74-8.
88. Katz DL, Barrett P, Sanfilippo JS, et al. Combined hysteroscopy and laparoscopy in the treatment of interstitial pregnancy. Am J Obstet Gynecol. 2003;188:113-4.
89. Minelli L, Stefiano L, Trivelli G, et al. Cornual pregnancy successfully treated by suction curettage and operative hysteroscopy. BJOG. 2003;188:113-4.
90. Tarim E, Ulusan S, Kilicdag E, et al. Angular pregnancy. J Obstet Gynaecol Res. 2004;30:377.
91. Anthony Siow, Selma NG. Laparoscopic management of 4 cases of recurrent cornual ectopic pregnancy and review of literature. J Min Inv Gynaecol. 2011;18:296-302.
92. Ash A, Smith A, Manwell D. Caesarean scar pregnancy. BJOG. 2007;114(3):253-63.
93. Weimen W, Wenping L. Effect of early pregnancy on a previous lower segment caesarean section scar. Int J Gynecol Obstet. 2002;77(3):201-7.
94. Seow KM, Cheng WC, Chuang J, et al. Methotrexate for caesarean scar pregnancy after in vitro fertilization and embryo transfer. A case report. J Reprod Med. 2000;45(9):754-7.
95. Vial Y, Petiguat P, Hohlfeld P. Pregnancy in a caesarean scar. Ultrasound Obstet Gynecol. 2000;16:592-3.
96. Wang YL, Su TH, Chen HS. Laparoscopic management of ectopic pregnancy in a lower segment caesarean section scar: a review and case report. J Minim Invasive Gynecol. 2005;12:73-9.
97. Yan CM. A report of four cases of caesarean scar pregnancy in a period of 12 months. Hong Kong Med J. 2007;13:141-3.
98. Chuang J, Seow KM, Cheng WC, et al. Conservative management of ectopic pregnancy in a caesarean section scar. Br J Obstet Gynecol. 2003;110:869-70.
99. Jurkovic, J Ben Naqi D, Ofilli Yebovi, et al. Efficacy of Shirodhkar cervical sutures in securing hemostasis following surgical evacuation of caesarean scar ectopic pregnancy. 2007;30:95-100.
100. King FT, Huang TL, Chen CW, et al. Caesarean scar ectopic pregnancy. Fertil Steril. 2006;85:1508-9.
101. Wong CJ, Chaos AS, Yuan LT, et al. Endoscopic management of caesarian scar pregnancy. Fertil Steril. 2006;85:494-7.

102. Jurkovic D, Helaby K, Woelfer B, et al. First trimester diagnosis and management of pregnancies implanted into the lower uterine segment caesarean section scar. Ultrasound Obstet Gynecol. 2003;21:220-7.
103. Wang YL, Su TH, Chen HS. Laparoscopic management of an ectopic pregnancy in a lower segment caesarean section scar. A review and case report. J Minim Invasive Gynecol. 2005;12(1): 73-9.
104. Mastroianni L Jr. The fallopian tube and reproductive health. J Pediatric Adolesc Gynecol. 1999;12:121-6.
105. Chui Ak, LOKW, Chai PC, et al. Primary hepatic pregnancy. ANZ J Surg. 2001;71:260-1.
106. Kalof AN, Fuller B, Harmon M. Splenic pregnancy a case report and review of literature. Arch Pathol Lab Med. 2004;128: e146-8.
107. Nwobodo EI. Abdominal pregnancy: a case report avinals of African Medicine. 2004;3:195-6.
108. Jayasinghe Y, Rane A, Stalewski H, et al. The presentation and early diagnosis of the rudimentary uterine horn. Obstet Gynecol. 2005;105:1456-7.
109. Tsafrir A, Rojansky N, Sela HY, et al. First trimester prerupture sonographic diagnosis and confirmation by magnetic resonance imaging. J Ultrasound Med. 2005;24:219-23.
110. Edelman AB, Jensen JT, Lee DM, et al. Successful medical abortion of a pregnancy within a noncommunicating rudimentary uterine horn. Am J Obstet Gynecol. 2003;189:886-7.
111. Cutner A, Saridogan E, Hart R, et al. Laparoscopic management of pregnancies occurring in noncommunicating accessory uterine horns. Eur J Obstet Gynecol Reprod Biol. 2003;15: 106-9.
112. Park JK, Dominguer CE. Combined surgical and medical management of rudimentary uterine horn pregnancy. JSLS. 2007;11:119-22.
113. Dulemba J, Midgett W, Freeman M. Laparoscopic management rudimentary horn pregnancy. J Am Assoc Gynecol Laparosc. 1996;3:627-30.
114. Sonmerger M, Taskin S, Atabekoglu C, et al. Laparoscopic management of rudimentary horn pregnancy: case report and literature review. JSLS. 2006;10:396-9.
115. Marcus SF, Brinsden PR. Primary ovarian pregnancy after in vitro fertilization and embryo transfer, report of seven cases. Fertil Steril. 1993;60:167.
116. Parente JT, Chou Su Levy J, Legatt E. Cervical pregnancy analysis; a review and report of five cases. Obstet Gynecol. 1938;62:79-83.
117. Holfmann HM, Uroll W, Hofler H, et al. Cervical pregnancy: case reports and current concepts in diagnosis and treatment. Arch Gynecol Obstet. 1987;241:63-9.
118. American College of Obstetricians and Gynecologists management of gestational trophoblastic disease. ACOG educational bulletin No. 178. Washington DC: American College of Obstetricians and Gynecologists; 1993.
119. Muto MG, Lage JM, Berkowitz RS, et al. Gestational trophoblastic disease of the fallopian tube. J Reprod Med. 1991;36:57-60.
120. Chera RN. Fallopian hydatidiform mole. A case report Indian Med. 1988;81:26-7.
121. Bhatia K, Bentick B. Intra mural molar pregnancy: a case report. J Reprod Med. 2004;49:689-92.
122. Church E, Hanna L, New F, et al. Ovarian molar pregnancy. J Obstet Gynaecol. 2008;28:660-1.
123. Soper JT, Lewis JL Jr, Hammond CB. Gestational trophoblastic disease. In: Hoskins WJ, Perez CA, Young RC, editors. Principals and practice of gynecologic oncology, 2nd ed. Philadelphia, PA: Lippincott-Raven; 1997. pp. 1039-77.
124. Damario MK.; Rock JA. Ectopic Pregnancy. Te Linde RW, Rock JA, Jones HW, editors. Te Linde's Operative Gynecology, 9th ed. Philadelphia, PA: Lippincott Williams & Wilkins; 2003. pp. 507-36.
125. Genes DR, Laborde O, Berkowitz KS, et al. A clinicopathologic study of 153 cases of complete hydatidiform mole (1980-1990); histologic grading lacks prognostic significance. Obstet Gynecol. 1991;78:402-9.
126. Reece EA, Petrie RH, Sirmans MF, et al. Combined intrauterine gestations: a review. Am J Obstet Gynecol. 1983;146:323-30.
127. Shah Y, Zevallos H, Moody L. Combined intra and extrauterine pregnancy a diagnostic challenge. J Reprod Med. 1980;25: 290-2.
128. Soriano D, Vicus D, Schonman R, et al. Long term outcome after laparoscopic treatment of heterotopic pregnancy;19 cases. J Minim Invasive Gynecol. 2010;17(3):321-4.
129. Akihiro Takeda, Shuchi Manabe, Takashi Mitsui, et al. Management of patients with ectopic pregnancy with massive hemoperitoneum by laparoscopic surgery with intraoperative autologous blood transfusion. J Min Inv Gyneol. 2006;13:43-8.

Sexual Behavior

29
CHAPTER

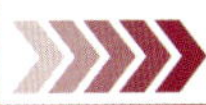

Asmita M Rathore, Reena Rani

INTRODUCTION

Sexuality is a topic with lots of hesitancy and apprehensions on the part of patient, and uncertainty in the mind of doctor. Especially sexual activity during pregnancy and its effect on pregnancy are among one of the grey areas in the literature which need special attention. While pregnancy is itself a state of physical and psychological change, along with cultural, social, religious, and emotional influences, which may affect sexuality and sexual activity, this subject is often neglected as talking about sexuality is difficult for both the doctor and the woman. In a meta-analysis[1] involving 59 studies on sexual activity during pregnancy presented some interesting facts: 68% of young women don't remember their gynecologist talking to them about sexuality in pregnancy. Remaining 27% were given restrictive advice, namely, prescribed interval abstinence before and after birth. Few (10%) were advised alternative coital positions. Only 8–10% of patients stopped intercourse on medical advice to abstain. Frequently, the woman was the first person to begin discussion on the subject but felt uncomfortable raising the subject. During antenatal patient care doctors often come across queries from pregnant women and their partners on whether sex is safe and what negative consequences may result from engaging in sexual activity.

PHYSIOLOGY

Sexual activity for men and women follows four phases known as the sexual response cycle. They are as follows:

1. Excitement phase
2. Plateau phase
3. Orgasmic phase
4. Resolution phase.

The *excitement phase* (also known as the *arousal phase*) is the first stage of the human sexual response cycle. In this phase the individual's blood vessels in the genitals become dilated. It occurs as the result of any erotic physical or mental stimulation, such as kissing, petting, or viewing erotic images that lead to sexual arousal. During the excitement stage, the body prepares for the next phase, i.e., coitus, sexual intercourse, or the plateau phase.

The *plateau phase* is the period of sexual excitement prior to orgasm. This phase is characterized by an increased circulation and heart rate in both sexes, increased sexual pleasure with increased stimulation, and further increased muscle tension. Also, respiratory rate continues to be elevated.

Orgasm is the conclusion of the plateau phase and is experienced by both males and females. It is accompanied by quick cycles of muscle contraction in the lower pelvic muscles, which surround both the anus and the primary sexual organs. Women also experience uterine and vaginal contractions. Orgasms are often associated with other involuntary actions, including vocalizations and muscular spasms in other areas of the body, and a generally euphoric sensation. Heart rate is increased even further.

In men, orgasm is usually associated with ejaculation. Each ejection is associated with a wave of sexual pleasure, especially in the penis and loins. Thereafter, each contraction is associated with a diminishing volume of semen and a milder wave of pleasure. Orgasms in females may play a role in fertilization. The muscular spasms are theorized to aid in the movement of sperm up the vagina into the cervix.

The *resolution phase* (or *refractory period*) occurs after orgasm and allows the muscles to relax, blood pressure to drop, and the body to slow down from its excited state. Men and women may or may not experience a refractory period, and further stimulation may cause a return to the plateau stage. This allows the possibility of multiple orgasms in both sexes. Refractory periods range from person to person, with some being immediate (no refractory) and some being as long as 12–24 hours.

EFFECT OF PREGNANCY ON SEXUAL ACTIVITY

Pregnancy being a progesterone rich state, results in some physical and mental changes that alters female sexuality. In the same context a Canadian study[2] revealed that vaginal intercourse and sexual activity overall decreased throughout pregnancy (P = 0.004 and 0.05, respectively) with the trimester of pregnancy being the only independent predictor. Most women report a decrease in sexual desire (58%). Overall, 49% of women worried that sexual intercourse may harm the pregnancy.

Below are some physiological changes in sexual response cycle during pregnancy:

Sexual excitability is often reduced in women because of discomfort and the fatigue induced by vasodilatation and the low systemic blood pressure. Decreased sexual activity may be attributable to nausea, fear of miscarriage, fear of harming the fetus, lack of interest, discomfort, physical awkwardness, fear of membrane rupture, or fear of infection or fatigue. Woman's self-perception of decreased attractiveness leads to decreased libido and sexual satisfaction.

During *plateau phase*, vulval and vaginal tissue congestion often leads to dyspareunia. In addition reduced cellular immunity and elevated estrogen levels leads to high risk of recurrent and chronic vaginal mycotic infection which exacerbates dyspareunia.

Copious vaginal discharge and involuntary urine leakage during pregnancy negatively affect quality of female sexual life.

Lubrication and *orgasm* are usually heightened. Orgasm in the third trimester may cause discomfort. Coital positions may also require adjustment in the third trimester.

CONCERNS ASSOCIATED WITH SEXUAL INTERCOURSE DURING PREGNANCY

- Miscarriage
- Preterm labor
- Premature rupture of membrane
- Antepartum hemorrhage
- Venous air embolism.

Miscarriage

Sexual intercourse is often considered a risk factor for threatened abortion and early pregnancy loss. But there is no evidence that sexual intercourse causes miscarriage.[3] However, it may be useful to advise women with threatened miscarriage to avoid intercourse until after the bleeding has completely resolved, so if miscarriage does occur, the couple does not feel that they may have triggered or exacerbated events.

Preterm Labor

The risk of preterm labor varies depending on the presence or absence of specific risk factors. These risk factor include previous preterm labor, multiple gestation, and cervical incompetence. Restriction of sexual intercourse is routinely recommended for the prevention and management of threatened preterm labor because of the perceived risk of intercourse as a method of inducing labor.

Proposed Mechanism of Induction of Labor

- Oxytocin is released from the posterior pituitary on nipple and genital stimulation
- Cervical ripening caused by prostaglandins released from mechanical stimulation of the cervix
- Prostaglandins in semen may cause cervical ripening.

But a Cochrane review[4] on sexual intercourse for cervical ripening and induction of labor failed to confirm the role of sexual intercourse as a method of induction of labor and emphasized the need for future clinical trials to investigate sexual intercourse as a method of induction.

Tan et al.[5] in a randomized control trial (RCT) compared 108 term pregnant women who were advised to have sex and compared to 102 control group who were not given this advice. The coitus rate was not that different (60% in the intervention group compared to 40% in the control group). The two groups were similar in the rates of spontaneous onset of labor, caesarean section, and neonatal outcomes.

Mills and coworkers[6] followed 10,981 singleton low-risk pregnancies and found no significant differences in the frequency of preterm labor in women who abstained from sex compared with those having sex. Frequent intercourse was associated with an increased risk of preterm delivery only in the subset of women colonized with *Mycoplasma hominis* or *Trichomonas vaginalis*.[7] Women with low-risk pregnancies who have no symptoms or evidence of lower genital tract infection should be reassured that sex does not increase the risk of preterm delivery.[8]

Evidence to guide recommendations on sexual activity in women who are at an increased risk of preterm labor because of a history of previous preterm labor, multiple gestation, or cervical incompetence are lacking. These women are usually advised to abstain from sex.

Yost and colleagues[9] studied the impact of sexual intercourse on recurrent preterm delivery in women with a previous spontaneous preterm birth at less than 32 weeks' gestation. Frequency of sexual intercourse at the time of study enrolment had no effect on the incidence of recurrent preterm delivery. However, women with a higher number of lifetime sexual partners had an increased risk of preterm delivery. This may be because of an increased incidence of asymptomatic bacterial colonization of the genital tract, leading to subclinical infection, which can induce preterm labor. For this reason, the current guidelines from the Society of Obstetricians and Gynaecologists of Canada (SOGC)[10] recommend that women at increased risk for preterm labor receive screening and treatment for bacterial vaginosis. Similar studies have been done in twin pregnancies and women with cervical incompetence, which showed no significant difference in the frequency of sexual activity among patients who delivered at term compared with those who delivered preterm.[11] In populations at increased risk for preterm labor, there is no evidence to suggest a clear benefit from restricted sexual activity; however, this is a simple intervention that causes no harm and may be a reasonable recommendation until better evidence emerges.

Preterm Premature Rupture of Membrane

Coitus with or without orgasm in late pregnancy is inconsistently associated with preterm rupture of membranes. Ekwo et al.[12] studied women aged 15–45 years in three groups having preterm premature rupture of membranes, term premature rupture of membranes, or preterm delivery without premature rupture of membranes. Only the male superior position was significantly associated with preterm premature rupture of membranes (odds ratio 2.40, 95% confidence interval 1.16–4.97) and preterm delivery without premature rupture of membranes (odds ratio 1.82, confidence interval 1.02–3.25). No sexual activities related significantly to term premature rupture of membranes.

Antepartum Hemorrhage in Placenta Previa

As per vaginum examination is strictly prohibited in patients with placenta previa, it has been theorized that penile contact with the cervix during intercourse can result in a risk of torrential hemorrhage, and as a result, patients with placenta previa are advised to abstain from sexual activity during pregnancy. However, there is a paucity of prospective data to support or refute this recommendation. The torrential hemorrhage described with digital examination of the cervix is more likely due to the flexion of the distal phalanges, allowing the fingers to enter the cervix and come into direct contact with the placenta. Despite limited evidence, it is probably safest to advise patients with placenta previa to abstain from sexual activity to reduce the theoretical risk of catastrophic antepartum hemorrhage.

Venous Air Embolism

Venous air embolism, a rare but potentially life threatening event, has been reported in pregnant and peripartum in patients having orogenital and penile-vaginal sex.[13,14] During pregnancy and the puerperium, there is direct communication from the vagina to the distended uteroplacental vasculature, and air can be forced into the cervical canal by oral insufflation or the piston-like effect of a penis or finger in the vagina. Air introduced into the venous circulation and pulmonary vasculature can result in serious morbidity, in addition to cardiopulmonary arrest and death. Although the true incidence of venous air embolism in pregnancy is unknown, Batman et al.[14] reported 18 deaths caused by venous air embolism out of 20 million pregnancies. Pregnant patients should be advised to avoid orogenital sex with air insufflation because this activity seems to confer an increased risk for venous thromboembolism. Penile-vaginal sex, especially in the rear entry position where the level of the uterus is above the level of the heart, may also increase the risk of embolism.[13]

RESUMPTION OF SEXUAL INTERCOURSE DURING THE POSTNATAL PERIOD

When is it safe to resume sexual activity after childbirth? Sexual dysfunction after child birth is common and should be addressed during postnatal visit along with neonatal health and contraception. In a review of the literature on postpartum sexual dysfunction, 90% of women resumed sex by 3–4 months postpartum, and sex was usually painful for the first 1–2 months but improved with time.[15] A quicker return to intercourse was seen if no perineal trauma was present at delivery.[15,16] In addition, increased rates of painful intercourse and sexual dysfunction have been noted with operative vaginal delivery, with inconsistent results for cesarean deliveries.[15] Painful intercourse other than perineal trauma can result from postpartum vaginal dryness due to the hypoestrogenic state induced by breastfeeding. Rowland et al.[17] showed that breastfeeding women were less likely to have resumed intercourse by the time of their first postpartum visit compared with women who were not breastfeeding.

There are no specific guidelines about when to resume sexual intercourse postpartum. It seems reasonable to advise couples to try intercourse when they are feeling comfortable enough to do so. Women may experience some pain with intercourse, which can be relieved by lubrication, or, if needed, vaginal estrogen, and they should be reassured to expect improvement with time.

ROLE OF HEALTH CARE PROVIDER

Society of Obstetricians and Gynaecologists of Canada provided few recommendations on this topic for health care providers which are discussed below.[18]

- Health care providers should discuss sexuality at the early prenatal visit, before discharge from the hospital postpartum, and at the postnatal check-up
- Healthcare providers should communicate that they are open to discussing sexual concerns; educate patients about normal fluctuations in sexual interest and frequency; discuss the range of noncoital sexual activities if intercourse is difficult, painful, or prohibited for medical reasons; and emphasize the importance of the quality of lovemaking rather than coital frequency for sexual satisfaction
- Healthcare providers should provide advice to support sexual adjustment and deal with challenges to sexual function during pregnancy.

CONCLUSION

Sex is generally considered safe in pregnancy. Abstinence is commonly recommended only for women who are at risk for preterm labor, or antepartum hemorrhage because of placenta previa but its impact on outcome is not known.

It is important that doctors, along with other healthcare workers in the obstetric field, should be able to provide advice regarding the emotional and sexual aspects of pregnancy, including changes that may be expected during this time. Understanding these changes may help to minimize anxiety on behalf of the woman or her partner. It is important that couples be reassured that sexual intercourse will not normally cause complications in pregnancy. The resumption of intercourse postpartum should be dictated by a woman's level of comfort.

REFRENCES

1. Sydow KV. Sexuality during pregnancy and after childbirth: a metacontent analysis of 59 studies. J Psychosom Res .1999;47(1):27-49.
2. Bartellas E, Crane JM, Daley M, et al. Sexuality and sexual activity in pregnancy. BJOG. 2000;107(8):964-8.
3. Moscrop A. Can sex during pregnancy cause a miscarriage? A concise history of not knowing. Br J Gen Pract. 2012;62(597):e308-10.
4. Kavanagh J, Kelly AJ, Thomas J. Sexual intercourse for cervical ripening and induction of labor. Cochrane Database Syst Rev. 2001;(2):CD003093.
5. Tan PC, Yow CM, Omar SZ. Coitus and orgasm at term: effect on spontaneous labour and pregnancy outcome. Singapore Med J. 2009;50(11):1062-7.
6. Mills JL, Harlap S, Harley EE. Should coitus late in pregnancy be discouraged? Lancet. 1981;2(8238):136-8.
7. Read JS, Klebanoff MA. Sexual intercourse during pregnancy and preterm delivery: effects of vaginal microorganisms. The Vaginal Infections and Prematurity Study Group. Am J Obstet Gynecol. 1993;168(2):514-9.
8. Chhabra S, Verma P. Sexual activity and onset of preterm labour. Indian J Matern Child Health. 1991;2(2):54-5.
9. Yost NP, Owen J, Berghella V, et al. Effect of coitus on recurrent preterm birth. Obstet Gynecol. 2006;107(4):793-7.
10. Yudin MH, Money DM. Infectious Diseases Committee. Screening and management of bacterial vaginosis in pregnancy. J Obstet Gynaecol Can. 2008;30(8):702-16.
11. Neilson JP, Mutambira M. Coitus, twin pregnancy, and preterm labor. Am J Obstet Gynecol. 1989;160(2):416-8.
12. Ekwo EE, Gosselink CA, Woolson R, et al. Coitus late in pregnancy: risk of preterm rupture of amniotic sac membranes. Am J Obstet Gynecol. 1993;168(1 Pt 1):22-31.
13. Truhlar A, Cerny V, Dostal P, et al. Out-of-hospital cardiac arrest from air embolism during sexual intercourse: case report and review of the literature. Resuscitation. 2007;73(3):475-84.
14. Batman PA, Thomlinson J, Moore VC, et al. Death due to air embolism during sexual intercourse in the puerperium. Postgrad Med J. 1998;74(876):612-3
15. Hicks TL, Goodall SF, Quattrone EM, et al. Postpartum sexual functioning and method of delivery: summary of the evidence. J Midwifery Womens Health. 2004;49(5):430-6.
16. Radestad I, Olsson A, Nissen E, et al. Tears in the vagina, perineum, sphincter ani, and rectum at first sexual intercourse after childbirth: a nationwide follow-up. Birth. 2008;35(2):98-106.
17. Rowland M, Foxcroft L, Hopman WM, et al. Breastfeeding and sexuality immediately postpartum. Can Fam Physician. 2005;51:1366-7.
18. Lamont J. Female sexual health consensus: clinical guidelines. J Obstet Gynaecol Can. 2012;34(8):769-75.

Vaginal Bleeding

30

CHAPTER

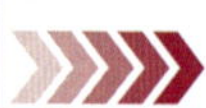

Sadhana Gupta

GENERAL CONSIDERATION

Two out of ten pregnant women have vaginal bleeding in the first trimester. Of these 50% will go on to have normal pregnancies, while the other 50% will have a pregnancy loss. Beside, viable pregnancy with history of vaginal bleeding in first trimester can be associated with subsequent adverse pregnancy outcome. Hence, first trimester vaginal bleeding with or without other symptoms is a matter of concern for pregnant women, and treating doctor and warrants adequate evaluation.

ETIOLOGICAL FACTORS

The causes of first trimester vaginal bleeding may range from physiological implantation bleeding to life threatening ectopic pregnancy. Viable and nonviable intrauterine pregnancy, gestational trophoblastic disease and neoplasm, ectopic pregnancy, and bleeding from genital tract are major causes of bleeding in first trimester. Box 1 summarizes the causes of first trimester vaginal bleeding.

CLINICAL HISTORY TAKING AND EXAMINATION

The clinical approach in history taking and general gynecological examination should be compassionate, orderly, and focused. The following points in history taking should be elicited.

Epidemiological

Age, marital status, occupation, and social status; these facts help in assessing lifestyle risk behavior and direct further management of women.

Box 1: Causes of vaginal bleeding in first trimester

Obstetric causes

- Viable intrauterine pregnancy
  - Implantation bleeding
  - Threatened miscarriage
  - Presence of second nonviable sac
- Early pregnancy failure
  - Spontaneous miscarriage
  - Missed abortion
  - Incomplete miscarriage
  - Induced miscarriage
  - Complete miscarriage
  - Septic miscarriage
- Ectopic pregnancy
- Molar pregnancy

Gynecological causes

- Vaginal trauma and torn vessel in ruptured hymen
- Vaginal and vulvar varicosities
- Cervical lesions—polyp, erosion, and decubitus ulcer
- Cervical carcinoma
- Red degeneration in myoma

Menstrual History

Period of amenorrhea, previous menstrual cycles, and past history of any bleeding disorder.

Obstetric History

History of previous miscarriages: spontaneous or induced, full term and preterm live births, any handicap, congenital, or genetic problem in previous sibling, history of molar pregnancy, treatment for infertility, medically or surgically managed ectopic pregnancy, use of contraceptives like intrauterine contraceptive device or any other method.

Drug Intake

Use of emergency contraceptives, drugs for medical abortion, and postponing menstrual bleeding has increased due to over the counter availability. This history may often not be volunteered by the patient.

Gynecological Causes

History of previous reproductive tract infection, dilatation and curettage, genital prolapse, contact bleeding and vaginal discharge primary, or secondary infertility are important considerations for further evaluation.

Box 2 summarizes the important risk factors for ectopic pregnancy in history taking.

Box 2: Risk factors of ectopic pregnancy

- Any tubal abnormality
- Previous tubal pregnancy
- History of tubal reconstructive surgery
- History of pelvic inflammatory disease
- History of infertility treatment/assisted reproductive technology procedure
- History of intrauterine contraceptive device insertion and tubal sterilization
- Increased age and parity
- Previous cesarean section

CLINICAL EXAMINATION

Properly conducted general and gynecological examination usually gives important clues to diagnosis.

General Condition

Rapid evaluation of vital signs is crucial. Presence of marked pallor, unstable hemodynamic condition warrants prompt start of supportive treatment, and rapid evaluation and management. Presence of hypertension and signs of thyrotoxicosis in early pregnancy should raise the suspicion of molar pregnancy. Fever points to possibility of associated reproductive or urinary tract infection.

Gynecological Examination

It should be gentle and systematic to have maximum information and include following:

- Per abdominal examination: for assessing size of uterus, any tenderness, adnexal mass, and presence of free fluid
- Per speculum examination: for any vulval, vaginal or cervical pathology, presence of products of conception or any molar tissue in cervical canal, dilatation of cervix, and any local site of bleeding
- Bimanual per vaginal examination should be performed gently as over enthusiastic examination can rupture a tubal pregnancy besides causing discomfort to the patient. Size, consistency and axis of uterus, presence or absence of any adnexal mass, bogginess in the posterior pouch, and cervical motion tenderness are important points to be documented. Uterine size that is small for gestational age suggests mistaken dates or nonviable pregnancy, while uterine size larger than dates should raise the doubt of molar or multiple pregnancy.

INVESTIGATIONS

ELISA Urine Test

Rapid enzyme-linked immunosorbent (ELISA) urine test for pregnancy should be performed as it confirms a pregnancy. Weakly positive pregnancy test always raises the suspicion of adverse pregnancy outcome.

Serial Ultrasound Scans

Serial ultrasound scans may be required to confirm the location and viability of a pregnancy.

Complete Blood Count

It is important, as a low hemoglobin points toward internal or external blood loss. However, a fall in hematocrit over several hours is more valuable index of blood loss than a single value. Increased leukocyte count is present in ectopic pregnancy and septic abortion. *Blood group and Rh typing* should always be performed for two reasons:

1. For group and save serum if needed
2. Anti-D immunoglobulin should be administered in Rh negative women with first trimester bleeding, because 5% women can become isoimmunized without it. However, American College of Obstetricians and Gynecologists (ACOG) (1999)[1] and Weissman et al. (2002)[2] question the use of anti-D in threatened abortion because of lack of evidence.

Serial Beta-human Chorionic Gonadotropin

Serial beta-human chorionic gonadotropin (β-hCG) doubles in 48 hours in 90% of intrauterine viable pregnancies.[3] On the other hand, 65% of abnormal pregnancies had disproportionately low serum β-hCG levels for gestational sac size. It has a positive predictive value and specificity of 100%.[4] Very high levels of β-hCG should raise the suspicion of molar pregnancy which should be confirmed by ultrasound scan.

Pattern of slowly rising or falling levels of serum β-hCG are diagnostic of abnormal pregnancy, a blighted ovum, spontaneous abortion, or ectopic pregnancy.

In ectopic pregnancy, the pattern of β-hCG rise can vary a lot. However, empty uterus with a serum β-hCG more than/1,500 IU almost confirms ectopic pregnancy.[5] Importantly Silva et al.[6] caution that one third of women with ectopic pregnancy will have 53% rise of β-hCG in 48 hours. They further reported that there is no single pattern to characterize ectopic pregnancy, and half of them can have increasing β-hCG levels while another half decreasing. *Serial β-hCG level must be interpreted in accordance with clinical and ultrasound examination.*

Serial β-hCG levels are also most important part of follow-up in medically or conservatively managed ectopic pregnancy and molar pregnancy after suction evacuation.

Serum Progesterone

Recently, there has been revived interest in role of serum progesterone levels in evaluation of ectopic pregnancy (ACOG 2008).[7] Levels >25 ng/mL strongly suggests viable intrauterine pregnancy and less than 5 ng/mL suggests a failing pregnancy with 100% sensitivity and 27% specificity.[8]

Other Investigations

Urine routine microscopy and culture, hepatitis B, and human immunodeficiency virus (HIV) status with pre- and post-test counseling should be an integral part of every prenatal care.

IMAGING

Ultrasonogram

Ultrasonogram (USG) is an indispensable tool for evaluation and management of first trimester vaginal bleeding. It is rapid, noninvasive, and easily available. Points to be considered while performing USG examination in evaluation in first trimester vaginal bleeding are discussed below.

Transabdominal Versus Transvaginal Scan

One should combine transabdominal (TAS) and transvaginal (TVS) to avoid missing the obvious. TAS gives a panoramic view of uterus, intra- or extra-uterine pregnancy, any uterine or extrauterine mass, and free fluid in pelvis as well as peritoneal cavity to give an idea of internal blood loss. TAS must be followed by TVS which can detect intrauterine pregnancy at 4–5 weeks gestation with positive cardiac activity at 6 weeks Only TAS can miss both early intra- and extra-uterine pregnancy. Corelation of USG finding with levels of serum β-hCG is very important. An intrauterine pregnancy with β-hCG more than 1,500/mL should be visualized by TVS and with a β-hCG more than 6,000/mL by TAS.

Prognostic Signs of Intrauterine Pregnancy

A circular well defined yolk sac (Fig. 1) suggests good prognosis as compared to large size and irregular yolk sac. Choriodecidual hemorrhage is associated with poor fetal outcome. An embryonic gestation is characterized by absence of embryo from gestational sac more than 18 mm size on TVS and more than 25 mm on TAS. Likewise, an embryo or fetus without cardiac activity denotes missed abortion (Fig. 2). However, two serial scans at an interval of 5–7 days will eliminate the possibility of disturbing a viable pregnancy. In 1995, there was a public enquiry in UK in a case of misdiagnosis of embryonic death on ultrasound and it was recommended that whenever embryonic death is suspected, two TVS separated by a minimum of 7 days should be performed.[9] Identification of a second nonviable sac is sometimes an explanation for vaginal bleeding (Fig. 3).

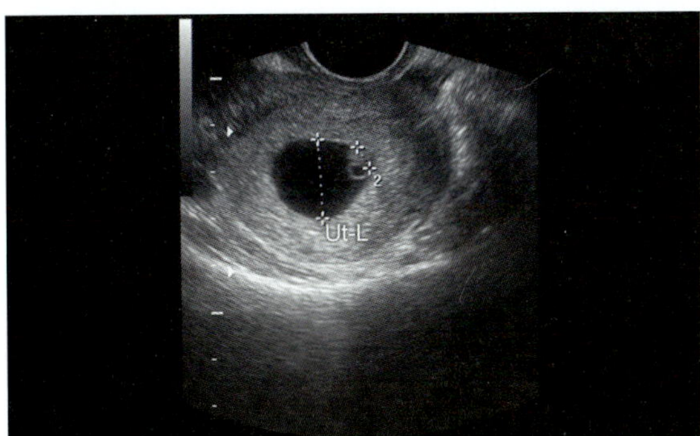

FIGURE 1 Early pregnancy with yolk sac.

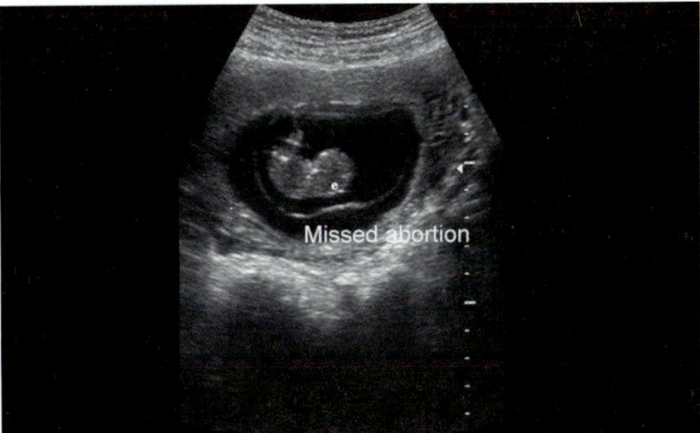

FIGURE 2 Missed abortion.

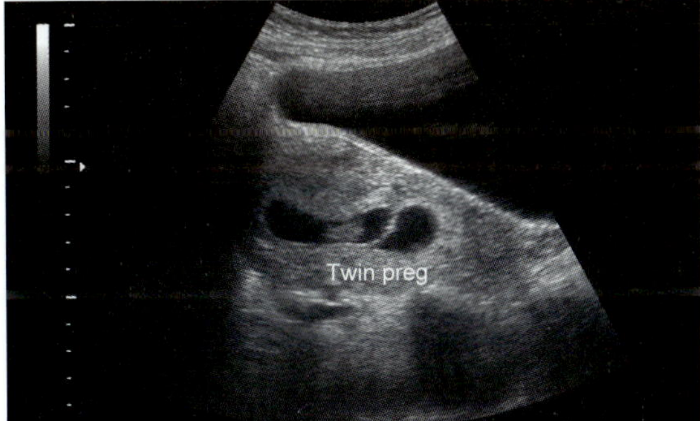

FIGURE 3 Twin gestational sac with nonviable pregnancy in one sac.

A large or irregular gestational sac, eccentric fetal pole, presence of large chorionic bleed and fetal bradycardia (<85 bpm) are poor prognostic signs.

Dysfunctional Uterine Bleeding and Molar Pregnancy

Absent intrauterine pregnancy with negative urine pregnancy test almost confirms dysfunctional uterine bleeding. Typical snow storm appearance with positive urine pregnancy test and very high levels of serum β-hCG is diagnostic of molar pregnancy, however, in partial mole USG picture is more variable and complex and sometimes only confirmed on histopathology (Fig. 4).

Ectopic Pregnancy

In ectopic pregnancy, USG reveals thickened decidualized endometrium or a pseudogestational sac like appearance due to decidual sloughing, which must be differentiated from double ring appearance of normal intrauterine pregnancy (Fig. 5). Empty uterus with adnexal mass and β-hCG levels above discriminatory zone (>1,500 IU) strongly suggest ectopic pregnancy but one should rule out hemorrhagic corpus luteal cyst and inflammatory adnexal mass. Corpus luteal cyst is sometimes very difficult to differentiate from ectopic pregnancy. It gives more spongiform lace-like or reticular pattern as compared to ectopic pregnancy. Ring of fire on color Doppler is peculiar to ectopic pregnancy but sometimes found also in corpus luteal cyst. It is important to note that clear extrauterine yolk sac or embryo is found only in 15–30% of cases Paul (2000).[10] Probe tenderness is also suggestive of ectopic pregnancy and examiner should document it's presence or absence. Presence of free fluid with empty uterus strongly suggests ectopic pregnancy but presence of small and nonechogenic fluid is nonspecific. Presence of intraperitoneal fluid is also not a reliable indicator of rupture, as rupture is present in 21% of patient with no fluid (Frates et al.).[11]

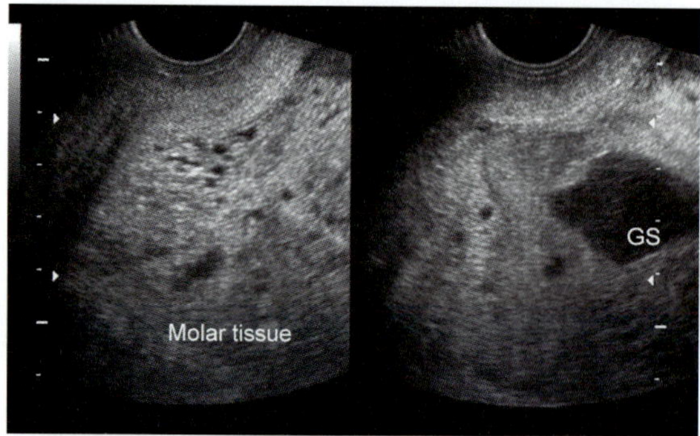

FIGURE 4 Partial molar pregnancy.

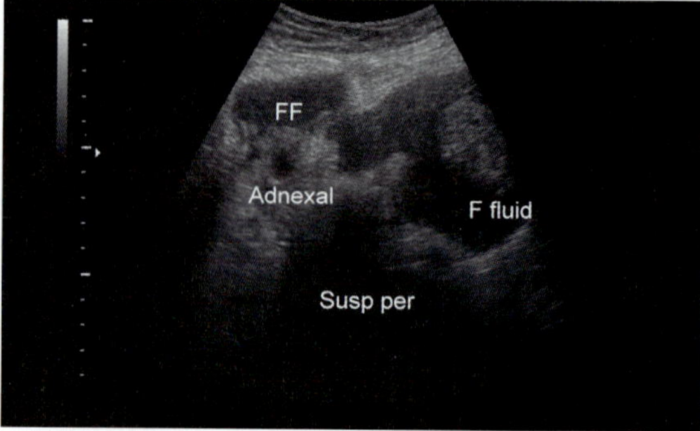

FIGURE 5 Ectopic pregnancy.

Box 3 summarizes differential diagnosis of adnexal mass on ultrasound.

Color Doppler can show high velocity, low impedance flow outside the uterus, but has sensitivity of only 48% (Achiron et al.).[12] Though its presence within the uterus and absence outside the uterus excludes ectopic gestation with specificity of 89%.

Rare situations of heterotopic ectopic and cesarean scar pregnancy should also be kept in mind, especially if there is history of assisted

Box 3: Differential diagnosis of adnexal mass in first trimester

- Ectopic pregnancy
- Hemorrhagic corpus luteal cyst
- Endometriosis
- Pelvic abscess
- Dermoid cyst/ovarian neoplasm
- Fibroid

Box 4: Ultrasound signs of ectopic pregnancy

- Tubal ring probe tenderness on adnexa
- Adnexal mass
- Free fluid in pelvis
- Interstitial line in interstitial pregnancy (thin echogenic line from endometrial canal up to cornual sac or hemorrhagic mass)
- Cesarean scar pregnancy (low gestational sac, local thinning of myometrium with prominent vascularity)

reproductive technology (ART) procedure and cesarean section, respectively. One should be very careful to look for these conditions which have inherent risk of potential catastrophic hemorrhage. Box 4 highlights the USG features of ectopic pregnancy.

Magnetic Resonance Imaging

Magnetic resonance imaging (MRI) is usually not required but sometimes useful in diagnosing pregnancy at unusual sites like cervical pregnancy, interstitial pregnancy, and cesarean scar pregnancy.

Other Investigations

Dilatation and Curettage

It is rarely performed as a diagnostic procedure, however, it may prove useful, as it can confirm or exclude intrauterine pregnancy in case of undesired or nonviable pregnancy. On histological examination if chorionic villi are recovered, the diagnosis of an intrauterine pregnancy is confirmed. On the other hand if only decidua is obtained, ectopic pregnancy is a strong diagnosis.

Culdocentesis

With advent of endovaginal ultrasound and accurate serum β-hCG values, culdocentesis is seldom performed. It still has a role for the patient with a positive pregnancy test, no intrauterine sac and free fluid in the cul de sac, in differential diagnosis of pelvic abscess or when facility of transvaginal scan, and/or β-hCG is not available. Aspiration of nonclotting blood suggest hemoperitoneum from ectopic pregnancy, aspiration of pus confirms pelvic abscess while bloody aspirates which subsequently clots indicates puncture of adjacent pelvic vessels.

Laparoscopy

The need for laparoscopy for diagnosis of ectopic pregnancy has declined with increasing use of high resolution ultrasound. However, in difficult situations it can be used with option of definitive surgical treatment of ectopic pregnancy at the same time.

MANAGEMENT

Following the above clinical approach in cases of first trimester vaginal bleeding, we can have following management approach:

- *Dysfunctional uterine bleeding*: History of amenorrhea, uterus and adnexa normal on clinical examination, urine pregnancy test negative, USG shows no intrauterine pregnancy, no adnexal mass, may be corpus luteal or follicular cyst or polycystic ovaries, and β-hCG below discriminatory level.

  This condition is managed by hormone therapy for withdrawal bleeding and observation in next cycles. However, one should be cautious of very early implantation and repeat scan is recommended if withdrawal does not occur
- *Intrauterine viable pregnancy*: Confirmed by serial clinical and ultrasound examination. Hormonal levels are usually not required.

  Management is routine prenatal care and follow-up

- *Intrauterine nonviable pregnancy*: Confirmed by serial clinical, hormonal, and transvaginal ultrasound examinations.

  Management is expectant, medical, or surgical termination of pregnancy with counseling for further pregnancy
- *Molar pregnancy*: Symptom and signs of molar pregnancy, urine pregnancy test positive, very high β-hCG levels, and snow storm appearance in uterus.

  Management is suction evacuation with all due precautions required in molar pregnancy and counseling for follow-up
- *Ectopic pregnancy*: Clinical history and examination suggestive of ectopic pregnancy, serial abnormal rise or fall of β-hCG levels, empty uterine cavity with adnexal mass and free fluid in pelvis.

  Management will be directed by hemodynamic condition of women, presence or absence of intact extrauterine pregnancy, adnexal mass and free fluid, serial β-hCG levels, and compliance of patient. Options are medical and surgical. Surgical approach may be tube conserving or salpingectomy, route may be laparoscopic or laparotomy according to resources available.

Clinical and management approach in different scenarios of first trimester vaginal bleeding is summarized in algorithms 1 and 2.

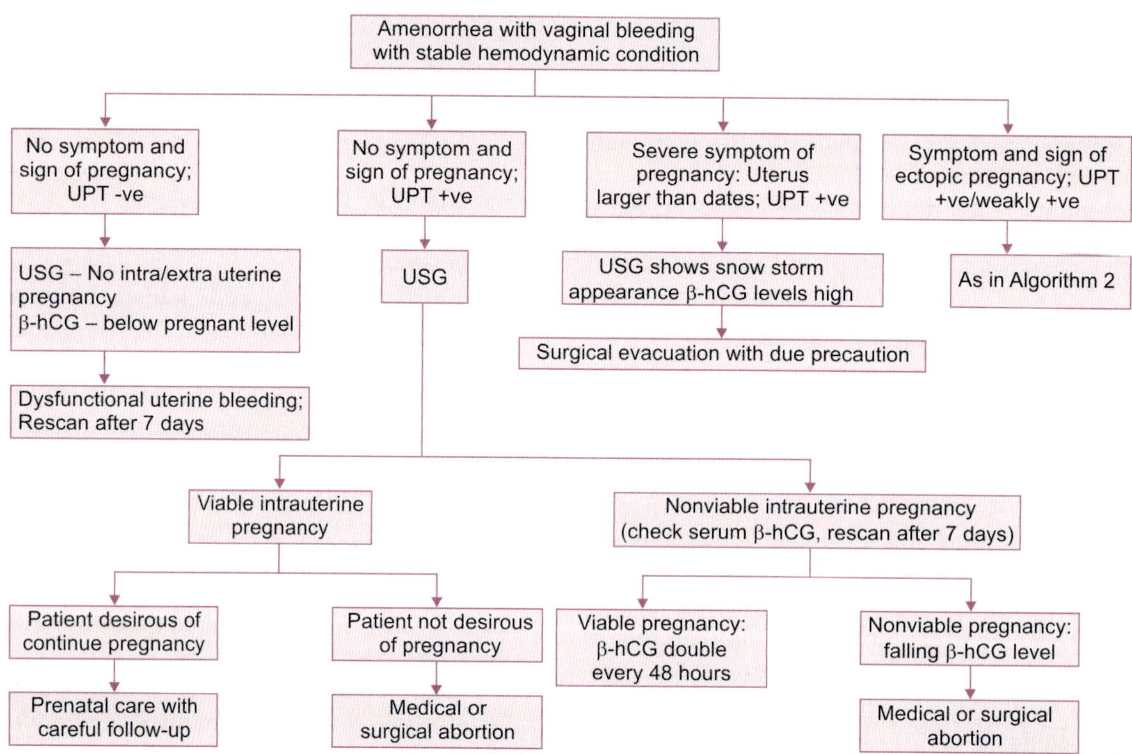

ALGORITHM 1 Clinical and management approach to first trimester vaginal bleeding.

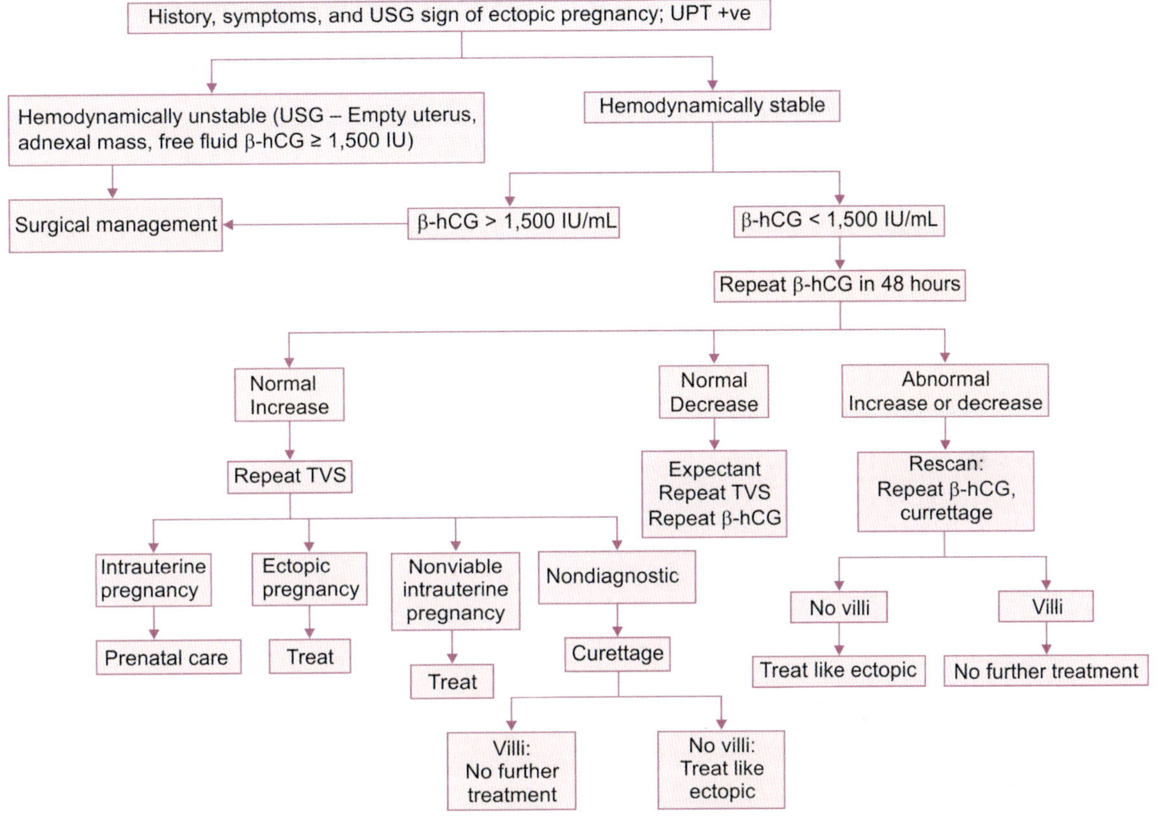

USG, ultrasonogram; UPT, urine pregnancy test; β-hCG, beta-human chorionic gonadotropin; TVS, transvaginal.

ALGORITHM 2 Mangement approach to first trimester vaginal bleeding in ectopic pregnancy.

CONCLUSION

First trimester vaginal bleeding is a very common outpatient complaint and emergency admission as well. It can be caused by wide range of obstetrical and nonobstetrical causes and thus requires thorough evaluation of patient.

Step wise and serial evaluation using multimodality approach is the crux of management. Proper interpretation of investigations like ultrasound, β-hCG, and appropriately guided course of management saves patients from worry and anxiety of uncertainty and also their time and money. Above all, it provides optimum outcome not only for present condition but also future reproductive health.

REFERENCES

1. Weissman AM, Dawson JD, Rijhsinghani A, et al. Non-evidenced based use of Rho(D) immunoglobulin for treatment of abortion by family practice and obstetric faculty physician. J Reprod Med. 2002;47(11):909-12.
2. ACOG. Prevention of Rh D alloimmunization. Practice Bulletin No 4. 1999.
3. Kadar N, Romero R. Observation on the log human chorionic gonadotropin time relationship in early pregnancy and its practical implications. Am J Obstet Gynecol. 1987;157(1): 73-8.

4. Nyberg DA, Filly RA, Filho DL, et al. Abnormal pregnancy: early diagnosis by US and serum chorionic gonadotropin levels. Radiology. 1986;158(2):393-6.
5. Barnhart KT, Sammel MD, Rinaudo PF, et al. Symptomatic patients with an early viable intrauterine pregnancy: HCG curves redefined. Obstet Gynecol. 2004;104(1):50-5.
6. Silva C, Sammel MD, Zhou L, et al. Human chorionic gonadotropin profile for women with ectopic pregnancy. Obstet Gynecol. 2006;107(3):605-10.
7. ACOG. Medical Management of ectopic pregnancy. Practice Bulletin no. 94. 2008.
8. Buckley RG, King KJ, Disney JD, et al. Serum progesterone testing to predict ectopic pregnancy in symptomatic first trimester patients. Am Emerg Med. 2000;36(2):95-100.
9. Hately W, Case J, Campbell S. Establishing the death of an embryo by ultrasound: report of a public enquiry with recommendation. Ultrasound Obstet Gynecol. 1995;5(5):353-7.
10. Paul M, Schaff E, Nichols M. The role of clinical assessment, human chorionic gonadotropin assay and ultrasonography in medical abortion pracice. Am J Obstet Gynecol. 2000;183(2 Suppl):S34-43.
11. Frates MC, Brown DL, Doubilet PM, et al. Tubal rupture in patients with ectopic pregnancy: Diagnosis with transvaginal US. Radiology. 1994;191(3):769-72.
12. Achiron R, Goldenberg M, Lipitz S, et al. Transvaginal Doppler sonography for detecting ectopic pregnancy: is it really necessary? Isr J Med Sci. 1994;30(11):820-5.

Sepsis

31

CHAPTER

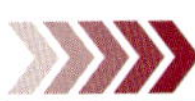

Neela Mukhopadhaya, Kusum G Kapoor, Pragya M Choudhary

INTRODUCTION

Sepsis is among the leading causes of preventable maternal deaths not only in the developing countries but also in the developed world. The current estimated maternal mortality ratio in India is 301 per 100,000 live births.[1] This translates into about 80,000 pregnant women or new mothers dying annually often from preventable causes.

The CMACE (Centre of Maternal and Child Enquiries) released the "Saving mothers" lives 2006-2008[2] report which reviewed maternal deaths during the 2006-2008 triennium, in which sepsis accounted for 26 direct deaths and 3 "late direct" deaths making it the leading cause of direct maternal deaths in the United Kingdom (UK). Group A streptococcal infection was largely responsible for sepsis related maternal deaths in the UK. *Causes of maternal deaths in India are similar to those elsewhere and includes*:

- Hemorrhage or bleeding (38%)
- Sepsis (11%)
- Hypertensive disorders in pregnancy (5%)
- Obstructed labor (5%)
- Abortion (8%)
- Other conditions (35%).

Unsafe abortion is one of the very important causes of sepsis in the first trimester. Seventy-five million unwanted pregnancies occur annually worldwide, out of which approximately 50 million unwanted pregnancies are terminated and some 20 million of these are unsafe abortions performed by unskilled persons, in an environment lacking minimal medical standards. This leads to 68,000 maternal deaths[3] and over 5 million disability adjusted life years lost.[4] Fifty-five percent of unsafe abortions occur in Asia, and India has some of the persistently high maternal mortality rates in the world.[5,6] Poor data collection mechanisms, and the stigma and legal issues surrounding unsafe abortion mean the impact of unsafe abortion on maternal mortality rates in India is likely underestimated.

DEFINITION

Sepsis is defined as a systemic inflammatory response to infection and severe sepsis has an associated organ dysfunction. Septic shock is defined as sepsis with hypotension that is refractory to fluid resuscitation.

Sepsis is considered to be present if infection is highly suspected or proven and two or more of the *systemic inflammatory response syndrome* criteria are met (Table 1).[7]

Applying these criteria to pregnant patients is problematic due to physiological changes associated with pregnancy. White blood cell counts increase throughout pregnancy and

TABLE 1: Criteria for systemic inflammatory response syndrome

Heart rate	>90 beats/minute
Body temperature	<36°C (96.8° F) or >38°C (100.4° F)
Hyperventilation (high respiratory rate)	>20 breaths per minute or on blood gas, a $PaCO_2$ less than 32 mmHg
White blood cell count	<4,000 cells/mm^3 or >12,000 cells/mm^3 (<4×10^9 or >12×10^9 cells/liter) or >10% band forms (immature white blood cells)

maternal temperature may increase during neuraxial labor analgesia.[6] The pathophysiology of sepsis is discussed in figure 1.

CAUSATIVE ORGANISMS

The organisms causing sepsis can be *endogenous* or *exogenous*. Endogenous organisms are the normal inhabitants present in and around the reproductive region which attack on alteration of environment or due to lowering of resistance in the case of trauma. Exogenous on the other hand are those organisms which are being introduced into the site from external source by processes like repeated vaginal examinations and instrumentation. The microbiology of sepsis in pregnant patients is distinct from that of nonpregnant patients. The common etiologic agent for sepsis in pregnancy is endotoxin producing Gram-negative rods whereas that in nonpregnant patients is Gram-positive bacteria.[6]

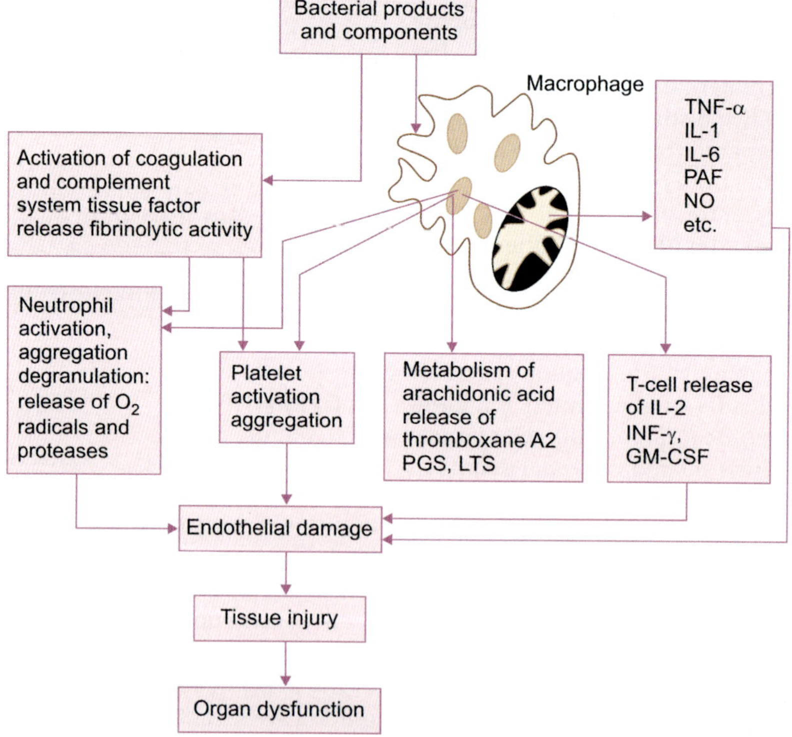

TNF-α, tumor necrosis factor alpha; IL-1, interleukin-1; IL-6, interleukin-6; PAF, platelet-activating factor; NO, nitric oxide; PGS, prostaglandins; LTS, leukotrienes; INF-γ, interferon gamma; GM-CSF, granulocyte macrophage colony stimulatingn factor.

FIGURE 1 Pathophysiology of sepsis.

In many cases, the etiology is polymicrobial with *Escherichia coli, Enterococci,* and *Klebsiella* species; *staphylococcus aureus* and Beta hemolytic Streptococci being the most frequently recovered organisms in pregnant patients with sepsis.[7]

CAUSES OF SEPSIS IN THE FIRST TRIMESTER

- Cellulitis
- Cholangitis
- Cystitis
- Pyelonephritis (most common cause of septic shock)
- Renal calculi
- Enterocolitis
- Malaria
- Mastitis
- Meningitis
- Pneumonia
- Septic abortion
- Necrotizing fasciitis
- Septic pelvic thrombophlebitis.

CLINICAL FEATURES

Patient oriented factors also contribute significantly to the mortality due to septic abortion and these relate to women inducing termination of pregnancy (TOP) themselves or by untrained people. There is also considerable delay in seeking help due to ignorance, inaccessible health services, and fear of retribution from the hospital.[8]

The clinical severity of sepsis will depend on the maternal pre-existing general condition:

- Patient's general resistance
    - General health condition
    - Presence of anemia and malnutrition
- Other focuses of infection
- Organism and their virulence.

Symptoms[9]

- History of surgical TOP
- Abdominal pain
- Pregnancy with an intrauterine device (IUD)
- Prolonged bleeding in pregnancy
- Feeling unwell with flu-like symptoms (malaise)
- Chills or sweats.

Signs

- Pyrexia
- Tachycardia
- Foul-smelling vaginal discharge
- Distended abdomen
- Rebound tenderness
- Mild hypotension
- Oliguria
- Signs of renal failure
    - Proteinuria, is a measure of renal injury
    - Pyuria, is a sign of infection

Besides this, also look for:

- Foreign material in the vagina
- Purulent vaginal discharge
- Signs of local pelvic infection, uterine tenderness, positive cervical excitation, or adnexal tenderness
- Upper respiratory tract infection
- Urinary tract infection including renal angle tenderness.

RISK ASSESSMENT FOR SEPSIS

Low Risk

- First trimester abortion
- Mild to moderate fever (36.5–38.5°C or 99.5–101.5°F)
- No evidence of intra-abdominal injury
- Stable vital signs.

High Risk

- Second trimester abortion
- High fever (38.5°C or 101.5°F and greater) or subnormal temperature
- Any evidence of intra-abdominal injury

- Distended abdomen, decreased bowel sounds, rigid abdomen, rebound tenderness, nausea, and vomiting
- Any evidence of shock: Low blood pressure (systolic <90 mmHg), anxiety, confusion, unconsciousness, pallor (inner eyelids, around the mouth, and palms), rapid, weak pulse (rate 110/min or more), and rapid breathing (respiration 30/minute or greater).

SIGNS OF CRITICAL ILLNESS[9]

Physiological

Signs of Sympathetic Activation

Tachycardia, hypertension, pallor, clamminess, and peripheral shutdown.

Signs of Systemic Inflammation

Fever or hypothermia, tachycardia, and increased respiratory rate.

Sign of Organ Hypoperfusion

Cold peripheries, hypoxemia, confusion, hypotension, and oliguria.

Biochemical

Metabolic Acidosis

- Increased lactate levels more than 2 mmol/L
- High or low white cell count
- Low platelet count
- Raised urea and creatinine concentration
- Raised C-reactive protein concentration.

Common Sequence of Organ Failure (Fig. 2)[10]

- Primary involvement
  - Heart and circulation
- Secondary involvement
  - Kidneys

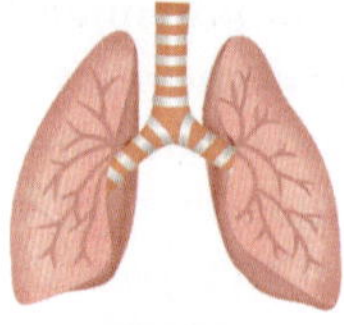

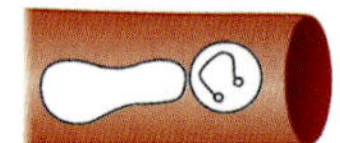

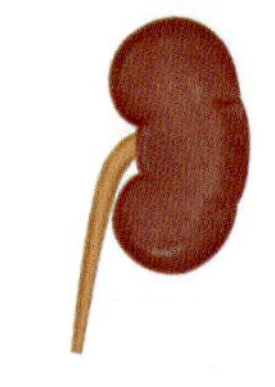

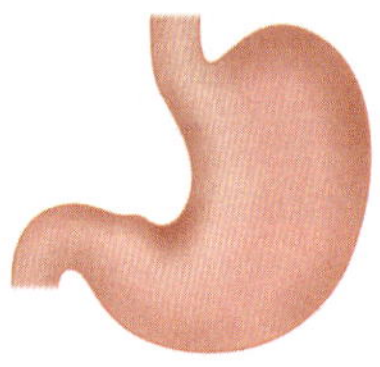

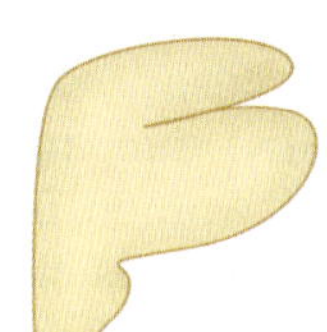

ARDS, acute respiratory distress syndromes.

FIGURE 2 Effects of sepsis on individual organs.

  - Respiratory system
  - Brain
- Tertiary involvement
  - Liver
  - Hemostatic system.

With the concentration of protein C and antithrombin III bring reduced in sepsis, the net effect is a procoagulant state. Pregnancy is in itself a hypercoagulable state; hence, the situation is exacerbated. The formation of emboli in the microvasculature is thought to lead to microcirculatory dysfunction and ultimately organ failure.

INVESTIGATIONS

Blood

- Hemoglobin or hematocrit
- Complete blood count for measure of infection
- Platelet count, if less, points to coagulopathy
- C-reactive protein blood cultures
- Renal function test
- Coagulation test
- Liver function test
- Peripheral smear for toxic granules and shift to the left of neutrophils.

Urine

- Mid-stream sample of urine for culture and sensitivity
- Urine output.

Vaginal or wound swab

Examination of the chest

- Auscultation
- Chest X-ray if indicated.

Abdominal X-ray

- Identify air or fluid in the bowel
- Signs of pelvic abscess or collection
- Clostridial infection—gas may be seen in the tissues
- Presence of an IUD may be confirmed
- Upright abdominal X-ray films will show air under the diaphragm from uterine or bowel perforation.

Ultrasound

- For fluid, abscesses, and collection in the peritoneal cavity
- For retained products.

Computed tomography scan

- To differentiate gas in tissue planes
- To delineate the parametrial infection.

PRINCIPLES OF MANAGEMENT

- Restore circulating volume to ensure adequate organ perfusion and correct acidosis
- Institute empiric antimicrobial therapy
- Surgically debride infected tissue; curette infected uterine contents and drain abscesses
- Monitor effects of therapy on vital functions and provide supportive care for organ system dysfunction.

TREATMENT

Fluids: Start intravenous (IV) crystalloids immediately. Colloids are indicated where there is severe hypotension. Medical advice from a physician should be sought if the renal functions are deranged or if renal failure is thought to be imminent.

Antibiotics: Intravenous preferred. If IV is not available, intramuscular (IM) or oral is acceptable. Start antibiotics immediately. Give broad spectrum antibiotics which are effective against Gram-negative bacteria, Gram-positive bacteria, anaerobic organisms, and *Chlamydia*. The current practice is to administer gentamycin (5 mg/kg body weight/day), metronidazole 500 mg three times a day IV and ampicillin 500 mg four times a day IV or any first generation cephalosporins until patient is apyrexial and then switch to an oral preparation.

Tetanus toxoid: Intramuscular, if there is a possibility that the woman was exposed to tetanus, and there is any uncertainty of her vaccination history, then give her tetanus toxoid and tetanus antitoxin.

Pain control: Oral or IV paracetamol as indicated. Anti-inflammatory drug, such as nonsteroidal anti-inflammatory drugs are useful in cases with significant inflammation or abscesses.

Thromboprophylaxis: Sepsis in pregnancy is a procoagulant state and hence, low molecular weight heparin by subcutaneous injection and thromboembolic stockings must be used.

Organ system support: Organ system support in the form of intubation to support lung function or dialysis to support kidney function can be provided in the intensive care unit.

Surgery: Laparotomy to drain pelvic abscesses or computed tomography guided aspiration of pus may be required to expedite recovery. Surgery to remove the source of infection, such as amputation of extremities may have to be done in rare cases to save some patient's lives.

SURVIVING SEPSIS CAMPAIGN GUIDELINES FOR MANAGEMENT OF SEPSIS AND SEPTIC SHOCK 2008[11]

This guideline provides:

- Early goal—directed resuscitation of the septic patient during the first 6 hours after recognition (1C)
- Blood cultures before antibiotic therapy (1C)
- Imaging studies performed promptly to confirm potential source of infection (1C)
- Administration of broad spectrum antibiotic therapy within 1 hour of diagnosis of septic shock (1B) and severe sepsis without septic shock (1D)
- Reassessment of antibiotic therapy with microbiology and clinical data to narrow coverage when appropriate (1C)
- A usual 7–10 days of antibiotic therapy guided by clinical response (1D)
- Source control with attention to the balance of risks and benefits of the chosen method (1C)
- Administration of either crystalloid or colloid fluid resuscitation (1B)
- Fluid challenge to restore mean circulating filling pressure (1C)
- Reduction in rate of fluid administration with rising filling pressures and no improvement in tissue perfusion (1D)
- Vasopressor preference for norepinephrine or dopamine to maintain an initial target of mean arterial pressure more than or equal 65 mmHg (1C).

PROGNOSIS OR OUTCOME WITH SEPSIS

The factors which determine the prognosis or outcome of patients with sepsis include severity or stage of sepsis and underlying health status of the patient. The mortality rate for patients with sepsis and ongoing sign of organ failure at the time of diagnosis is 15–30% whereas patients with severe sepsis or septic shock have a mortality rate of about 40–60% (Table 2).[2]

PREVENTION OF SEPSIS

A multidisciplinary approach is needed to prevent sepsis. This includes the obstetrician, the operating theatre nurse, and all paramedical theatre staff. Prevention of infection is one of the most important methods to reduce the incidence of sepsis. Prevention of infection can be done by good hygiene, hand washing, and avoiding any potential source of infection. All invasive procedures performed should utilize adequately autoclaved instruments and proper

TABLE 2: Final and contributory causes of maternal deaths in pregnancy related sepsis[8]

Organ system	*No.*	*Percent*
Hypovolemic shock	-	-
Septic shock	30	73.2%
Respiratory failure	07	17.1%
Cardiac failure	04	09.8%
Renal failure	01	02.4%
Liver failure	-	-
Cerebral complication	-	-
Metabolic complication	01	02.4%
Disseminated intravascular coagulation	03	07.3%
Multi-organ failure	10	24.4%
Immune system failure	06	14.6%
Unknown	01	02.4%

A patient can have more than one final and/or contributory cause of deaths.

aseptic techniques. TOP should be covered with prophylactic broad spectrum antibiotic cover, for Gram-negative and anaerobic organisms, for at least 48 hours.

Vaccinating for chicken pox, hepatitis A and B, influenza, meningitis, and pneumonia, and administering childhood vaccines can go a long way in prevention of sepsis. Early treatment for bacterial infection is especially important in high-risk patients, such as those who have suppressed immune system, those with cancer, diabetes, and HIV infection.

CONCLUSION

Sepsis during pregnancy presents a continuing challenge as it is often difficult to recognize and manage. In order to save lives, better training, structured approach, easy recognition, good care in both community, and hospital settings is needed. However, some deaths will always be unavoidable.[2]

Sepsis in the first trimester can be as life threatening as sepsis in the second or third trimester. Crucial to management of sepsis is early recognition, prompt investigation, and rigorous treatment particularly immediate IV antibiotic treatment and early involvement of senior obstetricians, anesthetists, and critical care consultants.[2]

"Since Group A Streptococcal infection, the single largest contributor to maternal deaths due to genital tract sepsis in this triennium, is predominantly a community acquired infection, the importance of antenatal education programs to raise awareness of good personal and perineal hygiene cannot be overstated." (*Centre for maternal and child Enquiries, UK*).[2] Directing women to safe clinics for TOP services by public advertising campaigns and making every woman aware of their rights would considerably decrease mortality due to septic abortion.

More clinical guidelines on the recognition and management of sepsis in pregnancy should be developed and implemented as a matter of priority.

REFERENCES

1. India SRS Sample Registration System; 2003.
2. Cantwell R, Clutton-Brock T, Cooper G, et al. Saving Mothers Lives: Reviewing maternal deaths to make motherhood safer: 2006-2008. The Eighth Report of the Confidential Enquiries into Maternal Deaths in the United Kingdom. BJOG. 2011;118 Suppl 1:1-203.
3. Grimes DA, Benson J, Singh S, et al. Unsafe abortion: the preventable pandemic. Lancet. 2006;368(9550):1908-19.
4. Singh S. Hospital admission resulting from unsafe abortion: estimates from 13 developing countries. Lancet. 2006; 368(9550):1187-92.
5. Mavalankar DV, Roseneld A. Maternal mortality in resource-poor settings: policy barriers to care. Am J Public Health. 2005;95(2):200-3.
6. Varkey P, Balakrishna PP, Prasad JH, et al. The reality of unsafe abortion in a rural community in South India. Reproductive Health Matters. 2000;8(16):83-91.
7. Galvagno SM Jr, Camann W. Sepsis and acute renal failure in pregnancy. Anesth Analg. 2009;108(2):572-5.
8. Saving Mothers 2005-2007: Fourth Report on Confidential Enquiries into Maternal Deaths in South Africa Expanded Executive Summary By NCCEMD.
9. WHO. Clinical Management of Abortion complications: A practical guide. Chapter 6; pp 41-45. Accessed on 14th Sept 2013.
10. Mackenzie I, Lever A. Management of sepsis. BMJ. 2007; 335(7626):929-32.
11. Dellinger RP, Levy MM, Carlet JM. Surviving Sepsis Campaign: international guidelines for management of severe sepsis and septic shock: 2008. Intensive Care Med. 2008;34(1): 17-60.

Termination of Pregnancy

32
CHAPTER

Kiran Kurtkoti

INTRODUCTION

Termination of pregnancy implies induced termination. The term "miscarriage" is used if it occurs spontaneously before 20 weeks of pregnancy.

- Medical termination of pregnancy (MTP) is legally allowed up to 20 weeks in India
- Spontaneous miscarriage is defined as loss of a fetus before the twentieth week of pregnancy or less than 500 g in weight.

Various presentations of spontaneous miscarriage are:

- Blighted ovum: A fertilized ovum that does not develop or whose development ceases at an early stage, before 6 or 7 weeks of gestation is termed as blighted ovum. On ultrasound examination of a blighted ovum, only the gestational sac with a yolk sac can be seen. There is usually no fetal pole visible in the gestational sac. A blighted ovum is a form of early spontaneous miscarriage. More than 50% of these are due to chromosome abnormalities in the developing embryo
- Missed miscarriage: When cardiac activity in a previously live pregnancy disappears and there is gradual resolution of pregnancy symptoms. They may present with dark colored bleeding or spotting. On ultrasound examination, a fetal pole is visible but the cardiac activity is absent
- Complete miscarriage: When all products of conception are expelled spontaneously
- Incomplete abortion: When some products of conception are expelled spontaneously but some may be partially retained leading to bleeding.

INDIAN STATISTICS FOR TERMINATION OF PREGNANCY

According to the Consortium on National Consensus for Medical terminations in India, the available statistics are grossly inadequate as hospitals keep records of only legal and reported abortions. In table 1 number of abortions reported includes legal reported induced abortions.

TABLE 1: Number of abortions reported

Year	1972	1975	1980	1985	1990	1995	2000
Number of abortions reported	24,300	214,197	388,405	583,704	581,215	570,914	723,142

METHODS

Surgical Procedures

There are a number of options for surgical termination of pregnancy.

Vacuum Aspiration

Vacuum aspiration (VA) is the preferred surgical technique for abortion up to 12 completed weeks of pregnancy. Complete abortion rates between 95% and 100% are reported. Electric and manual vacuum technologies appear to be equally effective.

Vacuum aspiration involves the evacuation of the contents of the uterus through a plastic or metal cannula, attached to a vacuum source. With manual VA (MVA), the vacuum is created using a hand-held, hand-activated, plastic 60 mL aspirator (also called a syringe). Available aspirators accommodate different sizes of plastic cannulae, ranging from 4 to at least 12 mm in diameter. In very early pregnancy, the cannula may be inserted without prior dilatation of the cervix. Usually, however, dilatation is required using mechanical or osmotic dilators. Priming with prostaglandin alone or a combination of mifepristone and misoprostol is preferred prior to surgical evacuation. VA is a very safe procedure with less than 0.1% of the women experiencing serious complications requiring hospitalization.

Dilatation and Curettage

Dilatation and curettage (D&C), involves dilating the cervix with mechanical dilators or pharmacological agents and then using a sharp metal curette to scrape the walls of the uterus. D&C is less safe than VA and considerably more painful for women. The rates of major complications are two to three times higher with D&C than with VA. These complications include increased blood loss, (VA being quicker is associated with less blood loss than D&C) increased risk of uterine perforation and increased risk of incomplete evacuation. Long-term complications like endometritis, Asherman's syndrome, cervical incompetence, and secondary subfertility are higher after D&C.

Dilatation and Evacuation

Dilatation and evacuation is a safe and most effective surgical technique. It requires preparing the cervix with a prostaglandin such as misoprostol, laminaria, or similar hydrophilic dilator. Some studies have used nitric oxide donors for cervical priming.[1] After dilating the cervix, the uterus is evacuated using ovum forceps. This is most suitable for retained products of conception either after spontaneous miscarriage or surgical termination of pregnancy.

Complications of Surgical Medical Termination of Pregnancy

In spite of training of doctors, and increased operative and anesthesia safety, complications arising during MTP remain a cause of concern. The various causes for this high rate of complications in spite of legislation to legalize termination are:

- Inadequate availability of services
- Improper evaluation of pregnancy
- Inadequately trained medical personnel
- High number of cases
- Casual approach of practitioners toward the procedure
- Women not able to access existing MTP services
- Ignorance and lack of awareness of availability of MTP services.

Complications of MTP are classified in to three categories

1. Immediate complications
2. Delayed complications
3. Late complications.

Immediate Complications

Anesthesia complications: Systemic toxic reaction: Though very rare it is the most serious complication of local anesthesia. This occurs because of inadvertent intravenous administration of the drug and can be prevented by confirmation that the needle in not in the blood vessel. Patient usually complains of paresthesia, drowsiness, vertigo, blurred vision, and twitching. There may be convulsions, vomiting, or diarrhea. Breathing may become rapid and shallow, and cyanosis might occur.

Hypersensitivity and allergic reaction to local anesthesia: Sensitivity is not related to dosage and can occur even after a sensitivity test. It may occur immediately or several hours after the procedure and is manifested by urticaria, bronchospasm, joint pains, swelling of eyelids, etc.

Complications during surgical MTP procedure:

- *Hemorrhage*: This can result from:
  - Retained products of conception
  - Trauma or damage to the cervix
  - Uterine perforation (rarely).

  Depending on the cause, appropriate treatment may include re-evacuation of the uterus and administration of uterotonic drugs to stop the bleeding, intravenous fluid replacement, and in severe cases, blood transfusion is required. If perforation is suspected, immediate laparoscopy or exploratory laparotomy is indicated. Blood transfusion incidence varies from 0.05 per 100 to 4.9 per 100 abortions and quantity of blood lost varies from 100 mL to 1,000 mL. The incidence increases for abortions performed later in pregnancy. Every service-delivery site must be able to stabilize and treat or refer women with hemorrhage as quickly as possible.
- *Perforation of the uterus*: It is an uncommon but serious complication and may have grave consequences. MTP is a blind procedure and the pregnant uterus being soft is prone to perforation, which can occur while passing the dilator, curette, or cannula. The risk of perforation is higher in certain cases like nullipara whose cervix is not sufficiently soft thereby, difficulty in dilating the os may result in false passage, acutely anteverted or retroverted uterus, repeated termination of pregnancy, fibroid uterus or septum distorting the uterine cavity, previous uterine surgery (caesarean section), and multiparity.

  Perforation can be avoided by:
  - Proper assessment of the size and position of the uterus
  - Straightening the cervical canal by traction on vulsellum while inserting the instruments into the uterine cavity
  - Cervical ripening by 400 µg misoprostol 4 hours prior to the procedure
  - Performing the procedure under ultrasound guidance, in cases of difficult dilatation.
- *Cervical injury*: Most common is superficial laceration caused by the tenaculum. At the extreme are the cervicovaginal fistula and the longitudinal laceration ascending to the level of uterine vessels. To reduce the risk, it is advisable to use misoprostol to ripen the cervix. Use of local anesthesia and slow dilatation of cervix are recommended
  - *Acute hematometra*: Acute hematometra, also known as *postabortal syndrome* or the *redo syndrome*, is an important complication of suction curettage. The cause is unknown. Women with this condition develop severe cramping within 2 hours of abortion. Vaginal bleeding is less than expected. The uterus is large and markedly tender. Treatment consists of prompt repeat curettage, usually without anesthesia or dilatation, and evacuation of both liquid blood and clots with administration of oxytocics. This leads to rapid resolution of symptoms
- *Broken plastic cannula*: Occasionally, the tip of the plastic cannula breaks off and remains in the uterus. If this happens, use a fresh cannula to complete the procedure. Do not keep exploring the cavity. The detached tip can be left in place and will usually be expelled spontaneously. Ultrasound guided removal or

hysteroscopy guided removal may be required later

- *Syncope*: This is usually due to parasympathetic reaction to painful stimuli or due to early ambulation after MTP. It may also be due to undetected excessive bleeding or perforation. Preoperative counseling, gentle handling during surgery, and postoperative rest will minimize this complication.

Delayed Complications

Incomplete evacuation: It is the most common complication. Patient presents with excessive or prolonged bleeding per vaginum, fever or pain abdomen, and enlarged uterus with an open or closed internal os. Treatment is by re-evacuation under antibiotic cover.

Continuation of pregnancy: Sometimes there may be failure to terminate pregnancy. This can occur due to many reasons:

- In early gestation, since the conceptus is very small, it may be lying near the cornua and may fail to get evacuated
- Suction of cervical canal only rather than the uterine cavity. This may occur inadvertently in:
  - Distortion of the uterine cavity due to presence of fibroids
  - Failure to assess the size and position of uterus
  - Difficulty in dilatation resulting in formation of false passage
- Use of small size cannulae where the openings are too small
- Ineffective suction pump system leading to inadequate generation of vacuum
- Presence of uterine anomalies like bicornuate uterus with a noncommunicating horn carrying the pregnancy.

Infection: Infection is a risk of all intrauterine procedures. The symptoms generally appear on the second or third day after the procedure but can be delayed for up to 10 days. Infection should be prevented by taking aseptic precautions while performing the procedure, ensuring that all the instruments used are properly sterilized and a "no touch technique" is observed. Treatment is with antibiotics; and re-evacuation if there is evidence of retained products they are evacuated by a senior member under antibiotic cover. Cases of peritonitis or septic shock should be managed in the intensive care unit (ICU).

Late Complications

Cervical injury: Permanent structural damage to cervix may result from forceful mechanical dilatation beyond 10 mm. This may lead to cervical incompetence, mid-trimester pregnancy losses, and preterm births.

Chronic pelvic inflammation: Chronic pelvic inflammation following MTP may result in secondary infertility, ectopic pregnancy, and menstrual disorders.

Asherman's syndrome/uterine synechiae: It may occur due to vigorous curettage and/or presence of infection. It may lead to secondary amenorrhea and infertility.

Obstetric complications: Complications may occur during future pregnancies, e.g., placenta praevia, adherent placenta, and uterine rupture due to previous undiagnosed perforation.

Psychosomatic symptoms: Long-term depression may be seen, especially if the termination has been carried out for medical reasons or has been enforced by the woman's husband or family members.

Rh sensitization: Rh sensitization chances increase with advancing gestational age at the time of termination. Hence, blood group should be known prior to performing MTP. Anti-D immunoglobulin 250 IU should be administered to Rh negative patients after MTP.

Septic abortion: Septic abortion, is associated with infection and complicated by fever, endometritis, and parametritis. It remains one of the most serious threats to the health of women throughout the world. Morbidity and mortality from septic abortion are infrequent in countries where induced abortion is legal but are widespread in the many developing countries where it is either illegal or inaccessible.

Treatment: Most women with septic abortion respond rapidly to uterine evacuation and broad spectrum antibiotics. Adequate intravenous infusions to maintain fluid and electrolyte balance, and modification of antibiotics according to blood and discharge culture reports is recommended. Laparotomy for pelvic abscess or foreign body in the abdomen may be required in serious patients. Septic shock if developed needs to be treated aggressively, in an ICU.

Medical Abortion

Medical abortion requires active patient participation and offers several advantages over suction curettage. There is success without surgery or anesthesia, it is similar to a "natural abortion", and a more private and proactive patient experience.[2]

Medical abortion was first approved in France in 1988, followed by approvals in the UK (1991), and Sweden (1992). Medical abortion was approved in India in 2002. The use of mifepristone and misoprostol is approved for use up to 63 days after the missed period. This is conditional to the provider following the MTP act in its entirety including filling Form C and Form I. Drug regimens are shown in box 1.

Complications of Medical Abortion

The mifepristone-misoprostol combination is effective in 92–97% cases and 1–2% may fail to abort. Two to three percent have incomplete abortion for which surgical methods are to be used. 0.1–0.2% may have profuse bleeding requiring blood transfusion.

Box 1: Regimens for medical abortion[3]

Up to 49 days

- Day 1: Mifepristone 200 mg orally (injection anti-D to Rh-negative patient)
- Day 3: 800 µg misoprostol per vaginum/buccal/sublingual. 400 µg—oral (WHO 2012)
- Day 14: Follow-up visit to assess for completion of abortion preferably clinically or by ultrasound

Regime from 49 days to 63 days

- Day 1: Mifepristone 200 mg orally (Injection anti-D to Rh-negative patient)
- Day 3: 800 µg of misoprostol vaginal preferred/sublingual/buccal. No oral route (WHO 2012)
- Day 14: Follow-up visit to assess for completion of abortion clinically or preferably by ultrasound

Persistent Gestational Sac

If the woman has not expelled the pregnancy by the time of her follow-up visit and the pregnancy is nonviable, she can be offered the following:

- Expectant management: This means that she will wait for the pregnancy to be expelled naturally. With time, this usually occurs without further intervention
- Administer an additional dose of misoprostol to women who have persistent nonviable gestational sacs
- If the woman prefers not to make return visits or is experiencing uncomfortable symptoms, such as heavy bleeding, VA to remove the products is preferred.

Continuing Pregnancy

Presence of cardiac activity 2 weeks after misoprostol dose indicates failure of medical abortion. Surgical termination is recommended in these cases, because if the pregnancy continues, there is a risk of fetal malformation.

Hemorrhage

Women tend to bleed or spot longer after medical abortion than after abortion using VA. Studies indicate an average duration of bleeding with medical abortion of 9–16 days, though only a minority of women may have some bleeding for extended periods of time.[4] Providers must have clearly documented procedures for assessing and managing abnormally heavy bleeding (>2 pads per hour for >2 hours). Acute hemorrhage associated with medical abortion is likely to require VA along with fluid replacement and, in some instances, blood transfusion.

Infection

Infection of the uterus is rarely associated with medical abortion. If product of conception are retained and the woman displays signs and symptoms of uterine infection, uterine evacuation with VA should be performed under cover of broad-spectrum antibiotics.

Undiagnosed Ectopic Pregnancy

Ectopic pregnancy may go undiagnosed when a woman seeking a medical abortion undergoes clinical assessment before the procedure or an ultrasound before 6 weeks. Ectopic pregnancy was diagnosed infrequently following medical abortion procedures, occurring in 0.02% women. One should remember, if the patient does not start bleeding within 6–8 hours after the misoprostol dose then a suspicion of ectopic pregnancy must be made and appropriate diagnosis should be established.

Termination of pregnancy can be done by both, surgical and medical methods. Medical method has several advantages over surgical methods. It is advisable to counsel patients about both methods and allow her to make an informed choice. Medical methods are to be preferred as they are noninvasive. Proper documentation and reporting is mandatory after both methods. Complications can occur with both methods and must be dealt with accordingly. Follow-up visit should emphasize the need for follow on contraception.

REFERENCES

1. Promsonthi P, Preechapornprasert D, Chanrachakul B. Nitric oxide donors for cervical ripening in first-trimester surgical abortion. Cochrane Database Syst Rev. 2009;(4):CD007444.
2. Woldetsadik MA, Sendekie TY, White MT, et al. Client preferences and acceptability for medical abortion and MVA as early pregnancy termination method in northwest Ethiopia. Reprod Health. 2011;8:19.
3. WHO. Guidelines for Medical Abortion. 2012
4. Say L, Kulier R, Gülmezoglu M, et al. Medical versus surgical methods for first trimester termination of pregnancy. Cochrane Database syst Rev. 2002;(4);CD003037.

Medico Legal Aspects Termination of Pregancy

33

CHAPTER

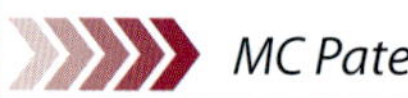

MC Patel

INTRODUCTION

Medical termination of pregnancy (MTP) is a very common procedure, which normally is uneventful but whenever there is complication, of a serious nature, it may put life of the pregnant woman at risk. A woman's death resulting as a consequence of a termination of pregnancy is unacceptable to any family, and if it occurs, is bound to land the physician in the court of law, either in civil or criminal or both.[1]

In India practice of termination of pregnancy is legally governed by "The medical termination of pregnancy act, 1971" and Indian Panel Code section 312–318.[2] Let us understand the provisions of this act to practice MTP safely and litigation free.

WHO CAN TERMINATE FIRST TRIMESTER PREGNANCY?

Section 2(D) of the Act

- Medical practitioner, with a recognised medical degree, registered in a state medical register having experience in the practice of gynecology and obstetrics for a period of not less than 3 years
- Medical practitioner, registered in a state medical register
  - If he has completed 6 months of house surgery in gynecology and obstetrics
  - If he has experience at a hospital for a period of not less than 1 year in the practice of obstetrics and gynecology
  - If he has assisted a registered medical practitioner (RMP) in the performance of 25 cases of MTP of which at least five have been performed independently, in a hospital or training institute, established or maintained, approved for this purpose by the government

Note: This training would enable the RMP to do only first trimester terminations.

- Medical practitioner, registered in a state medical register and who holds a post graduate degree or diploma in gynecology and obstetrics, and has the experience or training gained during the course of such degree or diploma.
- A RMP is one who has a recognized medical qualification under section 2 clause h of Indian Medical Council act1956,and his/her name is in the state medical register
- Person other than allopathic doctor can never be eligible for practicing MTP.

INDICATIONS FOR MEDICAL TERMINATION OF PREGNANCY

Any one of the following indications under the act is acceptable

- Risk to the life of the pregnant woman or of grave injury to her physical or mental health
- Risk to child born, of physical or mental abnormalities leading to serious handicap
- Pregnancy caused by rape-a grave injury to the mental health of the woman
- Pregnancy due to failure of contraception method by male or female—unwanted child presumed—a grave injury to the mental health of the woman.

In deciding the risk of injury to health of the pregnant woman her actual or reasonable foreseeable environment may be taken into account.

CONSENT

- Section 3(4) of the act[2]
- To take consent on form C is mandatory
- It should be an informed consent
- It should be written consent
- Who can give consent?
    - Any major female who is mentally sound
    - In case of minor and mentally ill, a guardian can give consent.

OPINION

- Opinion of the RMP is to be put on the record
- The number of opinion will vary according to the stage of pregnancy
- In 1st trimester, termination opinion of one RMP is sufficient.

Note: Prescribing mifepristone is regarded as procedure of MTP, and all rules and regulations of this act will apply.

PLACE WHERE FIRST TRIMESTER PREGNANCY CAN BE TERMINATED

Under Section 4 of the MTP Act and the rules, place of termination can be:

- A hospital established or maintained by the government[2]
- A place approved by government or a district level committee.

Conditions Which Need to be Satisfied

Termination of pregnancy should be performed under safe and hygienic conditions.

The following facilities are provided therein namely:

- A gynecological examination/labor table
- Instruments for performing abdominal or gynecological surgery
- Resuscitation and sterilization equipments
- Drugs and parental fluid
- Back-up facilities for treatment of shock
- Facilities for transportation.

Registration of Center

Registration is done after:

- Application in Form A is submitted to chief district medical officer (CDMO) with necessary documents
- On inspection and verification if he is satisfied, CDMO will recommend the approval of the place to the district level committee
- District level committee may after considering the application and the recommendations of the CDMO approve such a place and issue a certificate of approval in Form B.

The certificate of approval (Form B) is to be displayed at a conspicuous place easily visible to persons visiting the place.

Suspension or Cancellation of Registration

- This may happen after CDMO prepares a report enumerating the defect and deficiency found at the approved place
- Report is than be placed before district level committee. Committee, which if satisfied, cancels or suspends the registration
- Opportunity must be given to the owner of the place to make a representation before cancellation. Suspension commences from the date of communication.

RECORD KEEPING

Absolute confidentiality of records is to be maintained.

Under the MTP act rules and regulations it is mandatory to keep the following records:

- Consent form in Form C
- Opinion of RMP in Form I
- Maintenance of admission register in Form III
- Monthly reporting to CDMO in Form II.

How to Maintain Record (custody of Forms)

- Form C (consent) and Form I (opinion recorded under section 3 or section 5 and intimation of termination of pregnancy) should be placed in an envelope and envelope is sealed by RMP
- On the envelope shall be noted the serial number assigned to the woman and name of the RMP(s) by whom pregnancy is terminated and such an envelope shall be marked "SECRET"
- Envelopes shall be sent to the head of the hospital or approved place within 3 hours from the termination of pregnancy by the RMP who terminates any pregnancy and he will certify such termination in Form I
- They should be kept in safe custody by the head of the hospital or at an approved place
- Every head of the hospital or owner of the approved place is obligated under the MTP rules to send the record to the CDMO as a monthly statement of the MTP cases performed in the hospital in Form II.

Maintenance of Admission Register (Form III)

- Admission register is a secret document. Information therein is to be kept strictly confidential[3]
- It is to be kept in the custody of the head of the hospital or owner of the approved place
- It is not to be opened to inspection except in some special circumstances
  - When a working/employed woman applies for a certificate for the purpose of obtaining leave
  - Under authority of law
- No entry of the name of the pregnant woman can be made in case sheet, operation theatre register, follow up card, or any other documents
- References to the pregnant woman in such places other than the admission register is to be made by serial number assigned to the woman
- The entries in the admission register shall be made serially and a fresh serial number shall be started at the commencement of each calendar year and the serial number of the particular year shall be distinguished from the serial number of other years by mentioning the year against the serial number, i.e., serial number 6 of 2010 and serial number 6 of 2011 shall be mentioned as 6/2010 and 6/2011.

Reporting and Record Maintenance in Emergency

In Case of MTP done to Save the Life of Woman (Under Section-5)

Where pregnancy is not terminated in an approved place or hospital

- Envelop should be sent to the CDMO by registered post on the same day or on the next working day
- Envelop marked secret shall contain the name and address of the RMP who did termination
- In Form I leave blank column pertaining to the hospital or the approved place and the serial number assigned to the pregnant woman in the admission register.

If pregnancy is terminated in an approved place
- Procedure will be the same as provided in regulation 6 (1) (as shown in previous para of custody of Forms).

Preservation of Record

- Admission register should be preserved for a period of 5 years from the end of the calendar year it relates to
- In case of litigation, records are to be preserved till final disposal of litigation.

Offences and Penalties

- Termination of pregnancy by any person at unapproved place or termination of pregnancy by any person other than RMP will be liable for imprisonment not less than 2 years and may extend up to 7 years
- Any contravention of the requirement of record keeping will invite a fine which may extend to 1,000 rupees.

WORDS OF CAUTION

- Rule out ectopic pregnancy
- If patient is Rh negative, treat her accordingly with anti D immunoglobulin
- If it is partial or complete molar pregnancy, manage accordingly post operatively
- Take valid consent
- Practice MTP at registered place only
- Comply with the provisions of MTP act 1971
- Use of medical abortion with mifepristone and misoprostol also needs complying with all these provisions of MTP act.

It is essential to comply with the provisions of MTP act. This will result in litigation free practice.

REFERENCES

1. Hirve SS. Abortion law, policy and services in India: a critical review. Reprod Health Matters. 2004;12(24 Suppl):114-21.
2. The Medical Termination Of Pregnancy Act; 1971.
3. Duggal R, Ramachandran V. The abortion assessment project—India: key findings and recommendations. Reprod Health Matters. 2004;12(24 Suppl):122-9.
4. Yadav M, Kumar A. Medical Termination of Pregnancy (Amendment) Act, 2002. An Answer to Mother's Health & 'Female Foeticide. JIAFM. 2005:27(1).

Annexures

PRACTICAL TIPS *for* ULTRASOUND

Ajay V Valia

Transvaginal Ultrasound

- First Trimester is the period from conception to the 13th menstrual week. The embryonic period is the duration of dynamic growth of organ systems which is from 0–10 weeks
- There is a risk of 40% implanted zygotes miscarrying.

Annexure 1

Indications

- Confirmation of pregnancy
- Location of pregnancy – intrauterine or extrauterine
- Number - single or multiple
- Dating of pregnancy - Size versus dates discrepancy
- Viability
- Vaginal bleeding
- Abdominal or pelvic pain: rule out ectopic pregnancy/torsion/heterotopic pregnancy/ ovarian cyst
- To recognize pelvic mass; ovarian tumor, uterine myoma; uterine anomaly – bicornuate
- Congenital anomaly detection
- Cervix—incomplete os
- Corpus luteum function.

Annexure 2

Gestational Sac

- The sac is identified by transabdominal ultrasound (TAS) as early as 5 weeks', and by transvaginal sonography (TVS) as early as 4 weeks'. At day 32; sac size is 2 mm.
- "Intradecidual Sign"
- Thickening of endometrial stripe. The decidual reaction is not specific for intrauterine pregnancy and can be mimicked by
    - Ectopic pregnancy
        - Endometrial polyp

Ultrasound Appearance (TVS) of 4 Weeks Gestational Sac

- The sac appearance at 4+0-4+6 weeks is shown in figure 1. TVS on day 4+3 following last menstrual period will show chorionic sac in the uterus, visible in the endometrium lateral of the midline.
- Ectopic pseudo sac in the midline can be seen
- Beta-human chorionic gonadotropin is in the range of 500–1,000 mIU/mL.

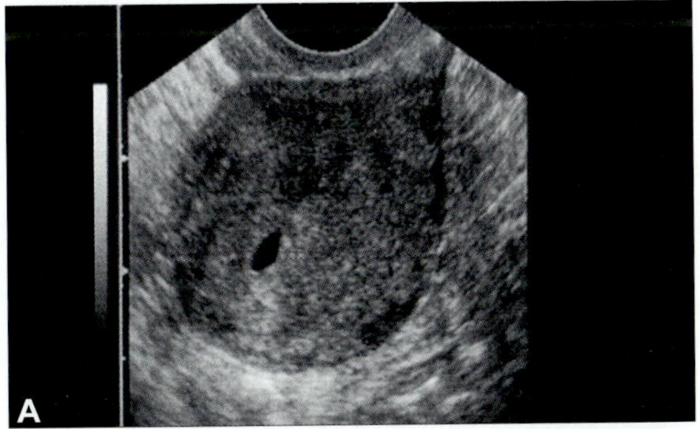

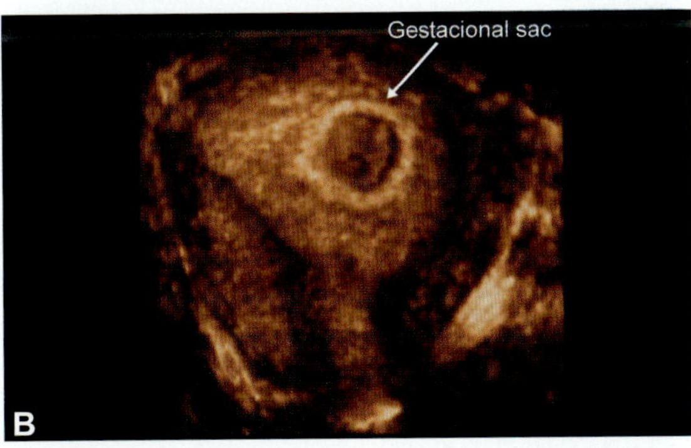

FIGURE 1 Transvaginal sonography at 4 weeks following last menstrual period.

Ultrasound Appearance (TVS) of 5 Weeks Gestational Sac

- The sac is round or oval with smooth contours containing fluid
- It has an echogenic border > 2 mm thick which is called 'choriodecidual reaction'. The sac is visualized as round echo-free/hypoechoic/black area surrounded by a thick white echogenic ring (Figure 2)
- The gestational sac measures 5–7 mm at (5+1) - (5+2) weeks
- The yolk sac appears at (5+1) - (5+2) weeks
- On Color Doppler, arcuate artery, radial and spiral arterioles are visible
- The embryo and fetal heart appears at 5+6 weeks (Figure 3)

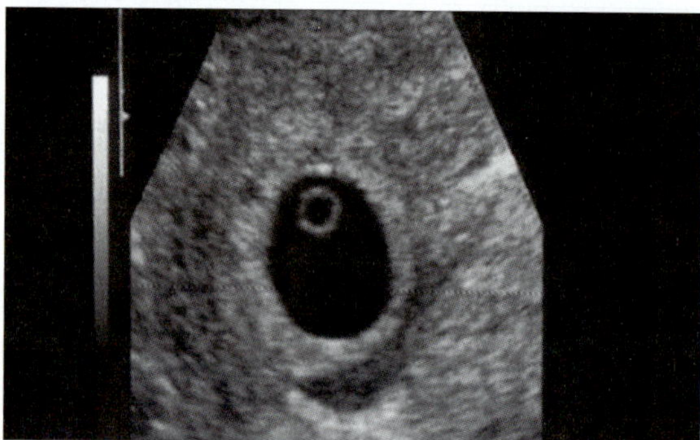

FIGURE 2 TVS of 5 weeks gestational sac and yolk sac.

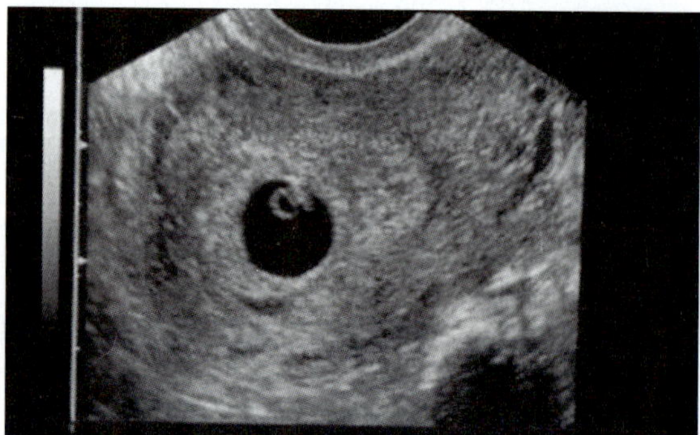

FIGURE 3 Ultrasound appearance (TVS) of 6 weeks embryo and yolk sac.

Double Decidual Sign

- It is seen within the endometrium in approximately 85% of normal pregnancies (Figure 4 A to C)
- It is made by three layers of decidua
  - Decidua vera which lines endometrial cavity
  - Decidua capsularis which covers the gestational sac
  - Decidua basilis which helps in the formation of placenta at the insertion site

Gestation Sac measurement

- The gestational sac is an echo-free space containing the fluid, embryo, and extraembryonic structures (Figure 5)
- The sac is measured inside the hyperechoic rim, including only the echo-free space
- The gestational sac is imaged first in the longitudinal plane, obtaining long axis and anteroposterior measurements perpendicular to each other. Then, in the transverse plane at the level of the anteroposterior measurement, the width measurement is obtained (Figure 6). The three measurements are averaged to obtain the mean sac diameter (MSD)
- The accuracy for dating is found to be ±1 week
- MSD increases at 1.2 mm/day.

Abnormal Gestational Scan

One major and three minor criteria:

Major Criteria

1. No embryo seen in the sac when
   - MSD > 25 mm on TAS
   - MSD ≥ 16 mm on TVS (Figure 7)
2. Abnormal sac position and shape
   - Increase in MSD ≤ 0.7 mm /day (Normal increase is 1.2 mm/day/MSD)
3. No yolk sac seen when
   - MSD > 20 mm on TAS
   - MSD ≥ 8 mm on TVS (Figure 8).

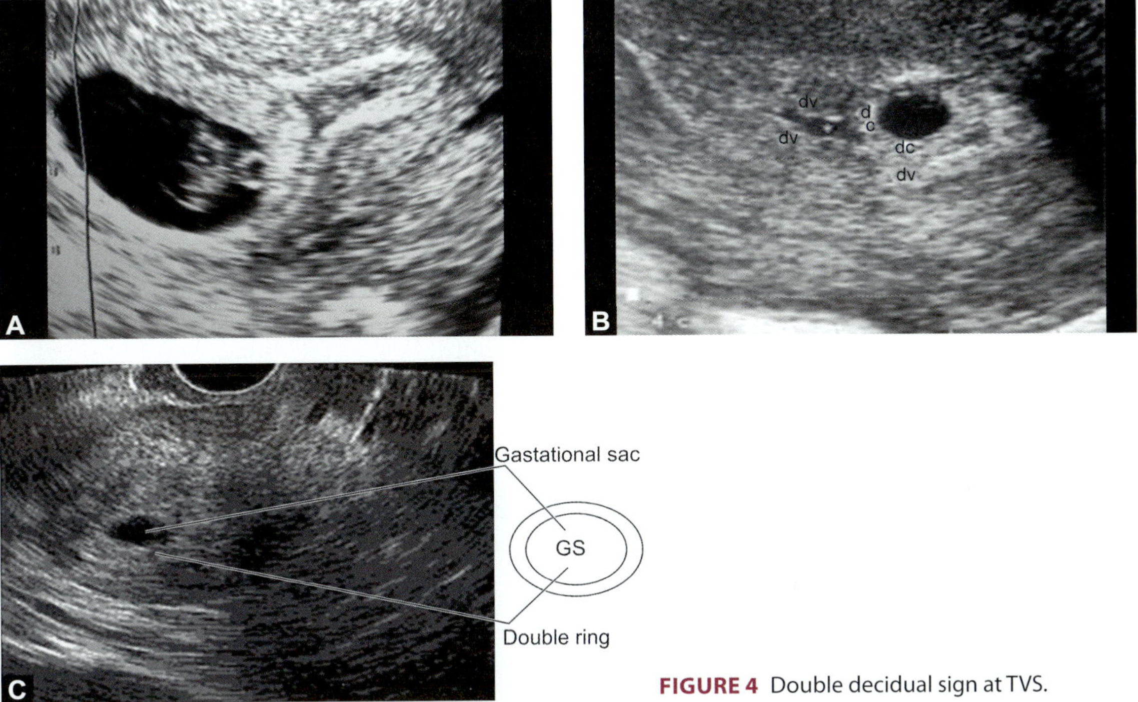

FIGURE 4 Double decidual sign at TVS.

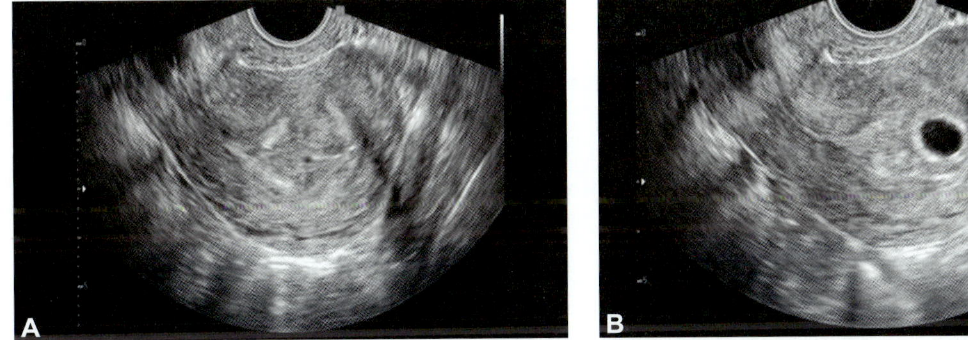

FIGURE 5 Early pregnancy scan (TVS) showing gestational sac.

Minor Criteria

1. Irregular shape
2. Thin choriodecidual reaction (< 3 mm)
3. Weak decidual echogenecity
4. No double decidual sign
5. Sac position too low in the uterine cavity (Figure 9)
6. Absent yolk sac and/or yolk sac > 10 mm or calcified (Figure 8)
7. Amnion is abnormally thickened and expanded
8. Early Growth retardation; MSD minus CRL = ≤ 4 mm
9. Embryo – absent FH rate motion at ≥ 6.5 weeks or 6 mm

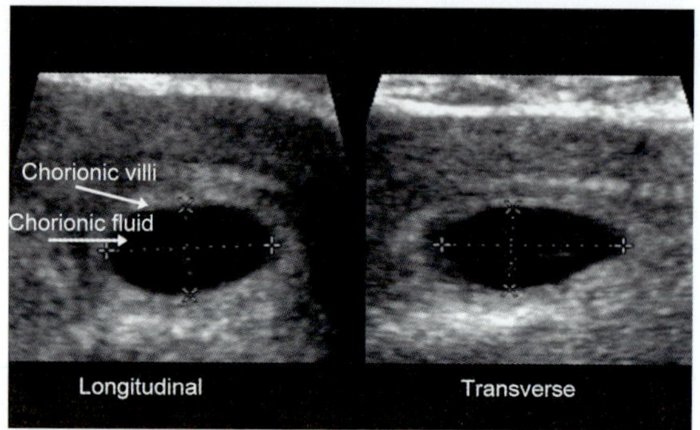

FIGURE 6 Measurement of mean sac diameter.

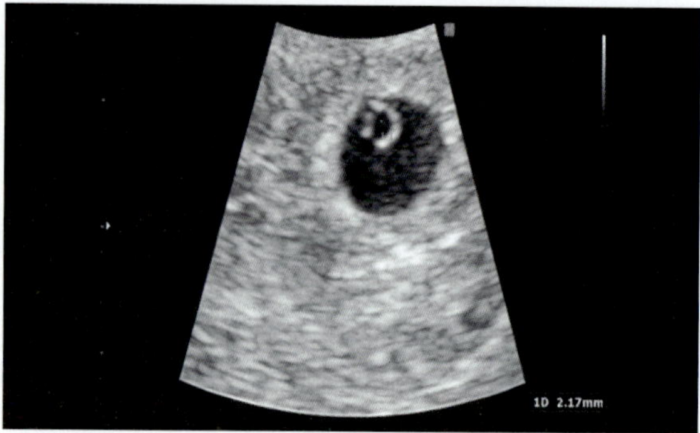

FIGURE 7 No embryo seen at TVS.

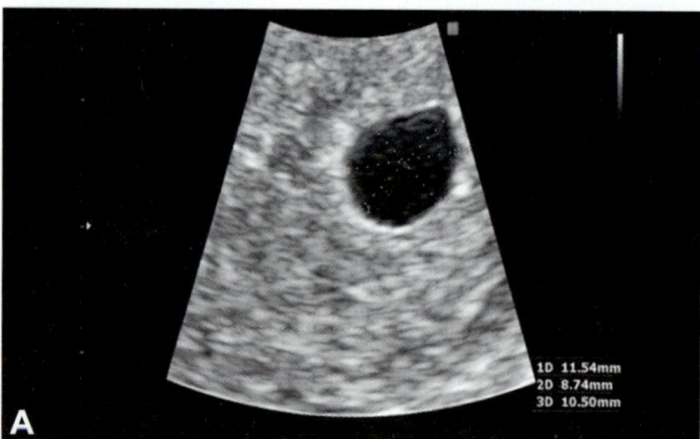

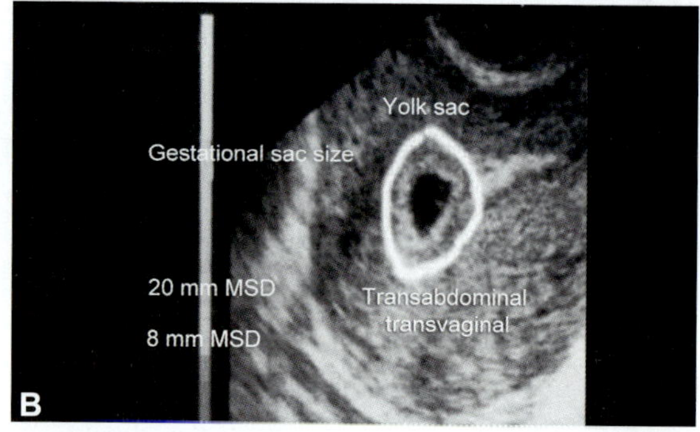

FIGURE 8 No yolk sac seen at TVS.

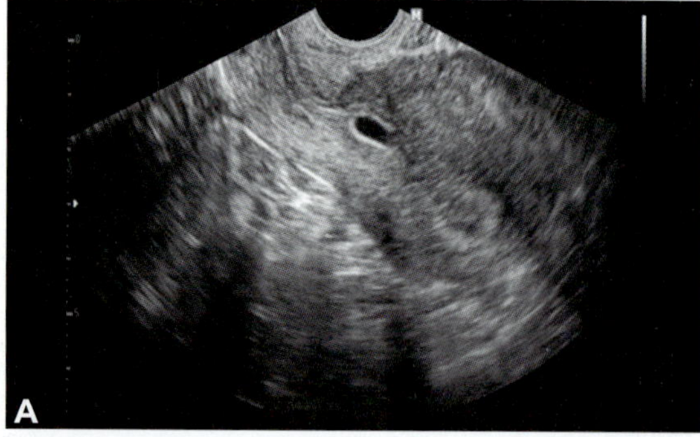

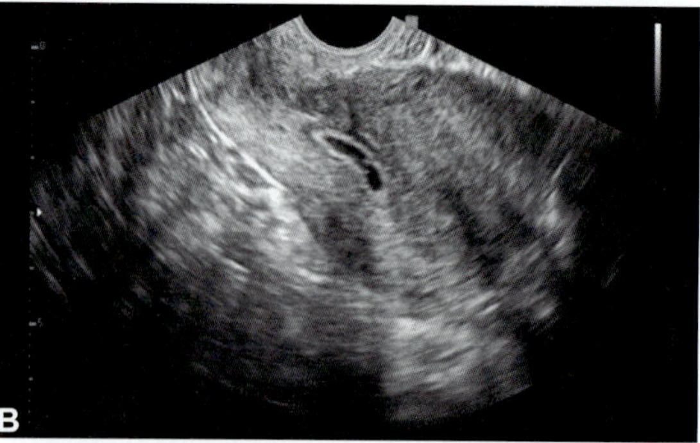

FIGURE 9 Low implantation sac seen at TVS.

Annexure 3

Yolk Sac

- Earliest structure seen within the gestational sac (Figure 1)
- Two to six mm spherical, cystic structure (Figures 2 and 3)
- Floats between amnion and chorion
- Functions as the earliest site of blood cell formation

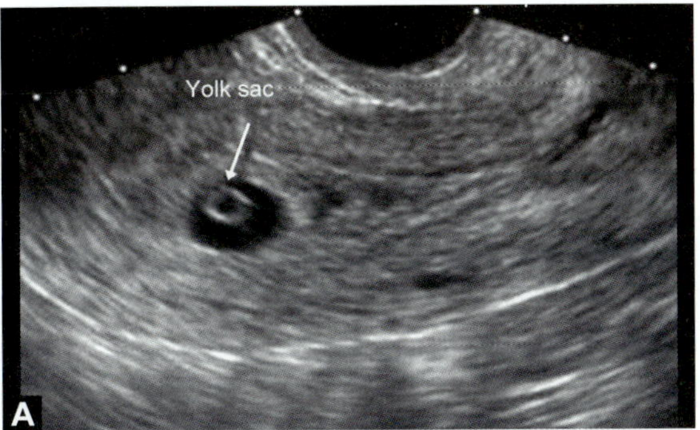

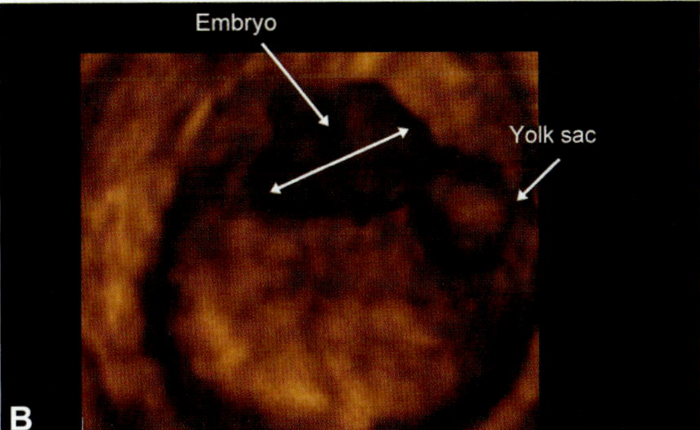

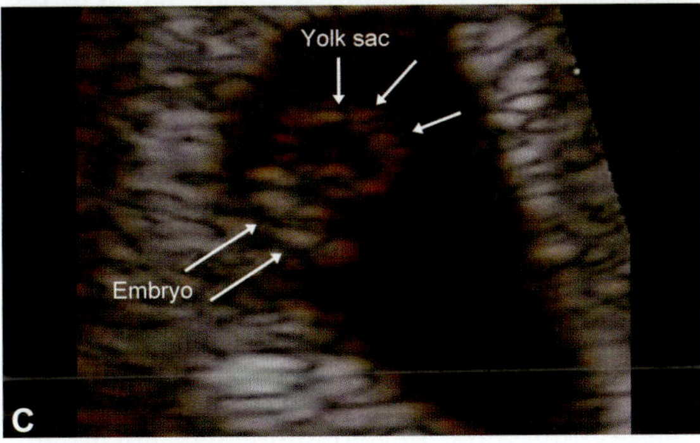

FIGURE 1 Normal yolk sac appearance at TVS.

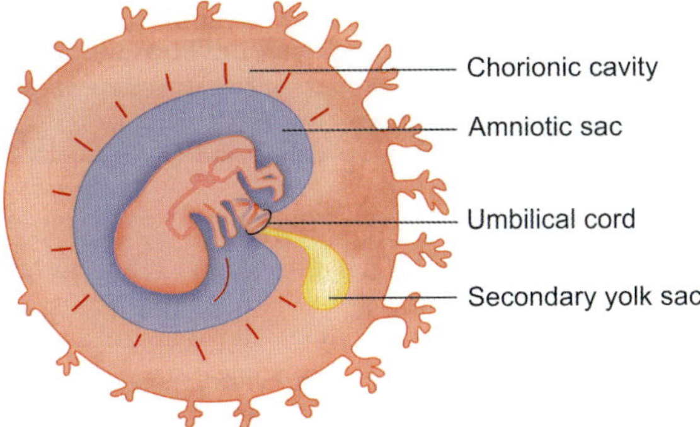

FIGURE 2 Secondary yolk sac.

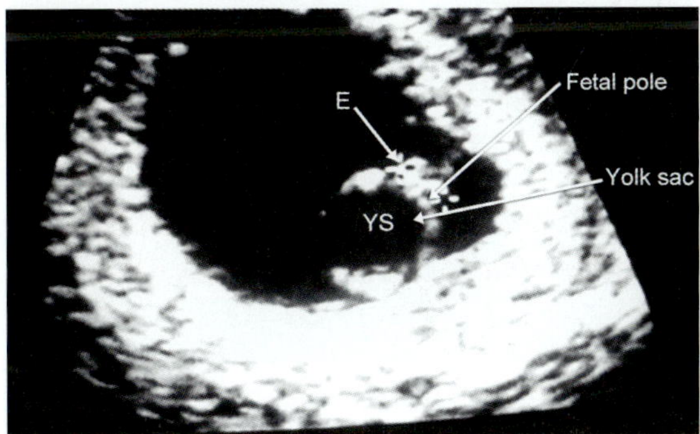

FIGURE 3 Early yolk sac showing embryo, fetal pole and yolk sac.

- Connects itself to embryonic midgut - vitelline duct (Figure 4)
- The yolk sac is attached to the embryo by the body stalk and floats freely in the extraembryonal coelom, until 10th week (Figures 5 and 6).

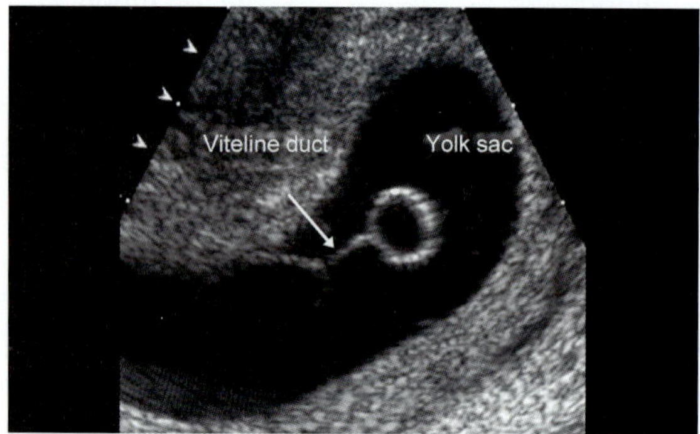

FIGURE 4 Yolk sac connected to the vitelline duct.

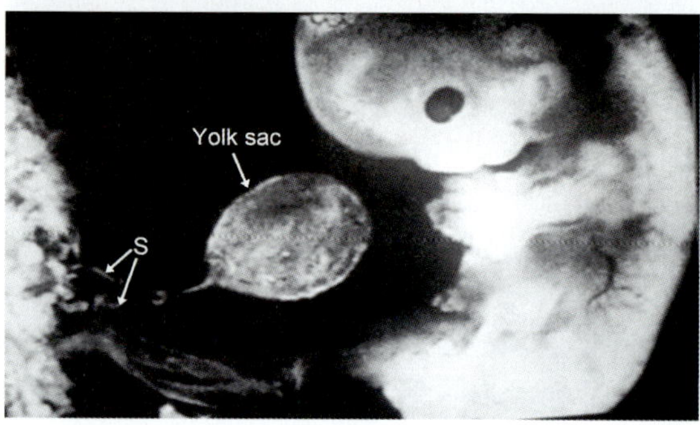

FIGURE 5 Endoscopic appearance of yolk sac.

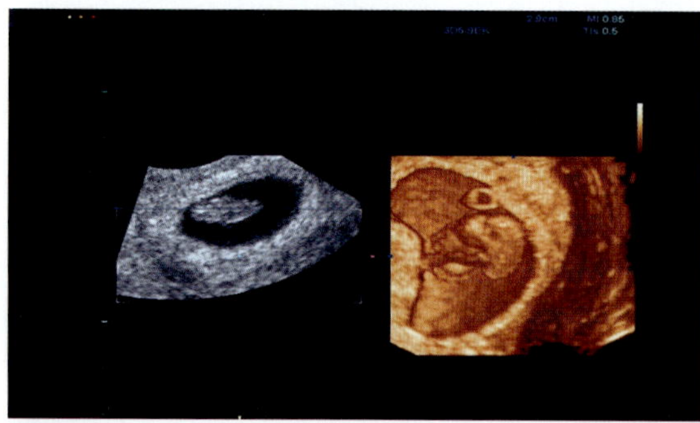

FIGURE 6 2D and 3 D appearance of yolk sac and fetal pole.

Yolk Sac Measurement (Table 1)

- In measuring yolk sac inner to inner diameter is to be measured.
- The walls of yolk sac are not to be included in the measurement.
- Yolk sac diameter refers to mean inner diameter of yolk sac.
- A yolk sac diameter more than 5.5 mm between 5 to 10 weeks of menstrual age is associated with poor outcome.
- A gestational sac with a MSD of more than 8 mm without a yolk sac indicates non-viability.
- Yolk sac may be visible earliest, when mean sac diameter of gestational sac is 8 mm.
- Yolk sac should be visible when gestational sac is 13 mm or more
- Yolk sac if not seen, when gestational sac is more than 20 mm signifies a case of blighted ovum.
- The yolk sac is a definitive evidence of a true gestational sac.
- Presence of yolk sac confirms intrauterine pregnancy
- Presence of yolk sac however does not guarantee a normal outcome of pregnancy
- After 7 weeks, the size of yolk sac is static
- After 12–14 weeks, yolk sac is not seen
- Yolk sac equals to 0.1 mm/mm increase in MSD up to 5 mm in size
- Once yolk sac is seen, it may be assumed that the embryonal development will ensue and appearance of blighted ovum is excluded.

TABLE 1: Events at early pregnancy on ultrasound

Weeks	*Yolk sac*	*CRL/fetal echo*	*FHM*	*GS*
5	3–4 mm	-	-	8 mm
6	4–5 mm	4–5 mm	+	
7	4–5 mm	7–8 mm	+	
8	5 mm	10–11 mm	+	

CRL, crown rump length; FHM, fetal heart monitoring; GS, gestational sac.

Yolk Sac Findings Implying Poor Outcome

- An enlarged yolk sac, greater than 6 mm
- Too small/too large
- Fragmented/Irregular
- Solid/Calcified.

Annexure 4

Assigning Gestational Age and Crown Rump Length Measurement

- Crown rump length (CRL) is the most accurate measurement for determining gestational age if measured correctly
- It measures the embryo or embryonic pole with transabdominal sonography (TAS) between 6–14 weeks and transvaginal sonography (TVS) between 5–14 weeks
- When gestational age from CRL differs by more than 14 days from gestation by last menstrual period (LMP), use CRL for assigning gestational age (algorithm 1)
- The fetus should be in sagittal plane at rest and assuming its natural curvature (Figure 1)
- Exclude extremites and yolk sac

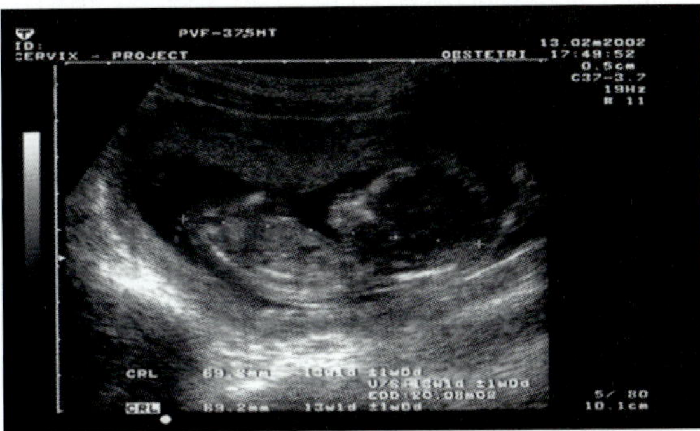

FIGURE 1 CRL is measured with the fetus in its natural curvature.

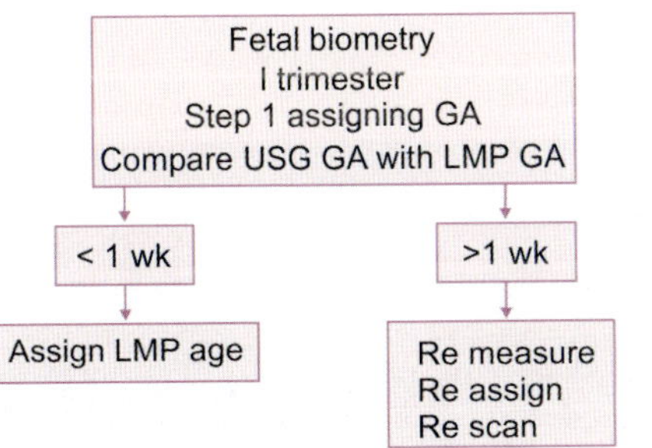

LMP, last menstrual period; USG, ultrasonography; GA, gestational age.

ALGORITHM 1 Assigning gestational age.

- CRL is measured along the longest axis of the fetus
- Measurement of the fetal length from the tip of the cephalic pole to the tip of the caudal pole is done by 3 methods:
  - Single line between calipers
  - Two measurements and add
  - Trace with trackball.

Pitfalls

- Fetal Position – excessive flexion or hyperextension underestimates the CRL

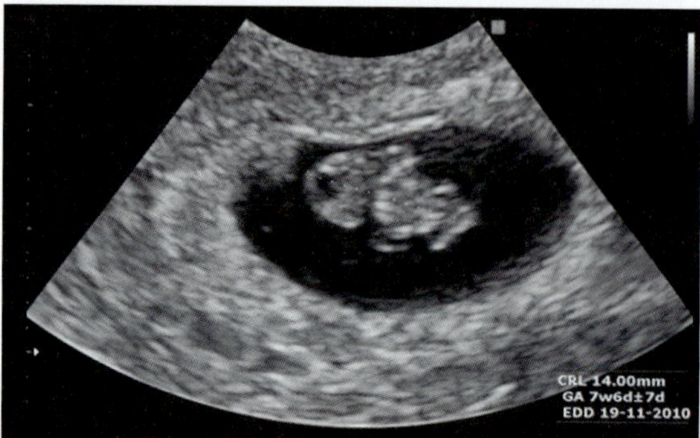

FIGURE 2 Inclusion of yolk sac in CRL measurement.

- Poor measurement plane and improper section i.e. oblique
- Inclusion of yolk sac in CRL measurement in early pregnancy (Figure 2)
- Faulty measurements can make a gestation error of upto 10days
- The embryo is measured along its longest axis to obtain the CRL measurement accurately date pregnancy between 7 and 13 weeks' gestation (Figure 3 A and B)
- At 5 to 6 weeks' distinct landmarks cannot be identified but heart motion can be detected centrally (Figure 4)
- As the pregnancy continues, the head can be easily identified from the rest of the body
- After 12 weeks' gestation excessive curvature of the fetus leads to erroneous shortening of CRL measurement
- Gestational age assessment by CRL was extremely accurate, approaching ±3 to 4 days Subsequent studies have suggested that the CRL is somewhat less accurate; however, the accuracy is still within ±5 to 7 days
- Variations in the measurement of CRL can be attributed to differences in fetal growth patterns. Such differences are related to factors similar to those that influence birth weight curves, including maternal age and parity, prepregnancy maternal weight, geographic location, and population characteristics.

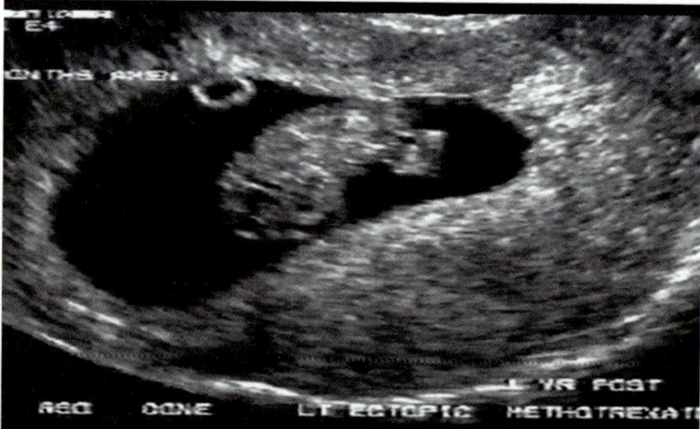

FIGURE 4 Gestational sac with yolk sac and fetal pole at 6 weeks.

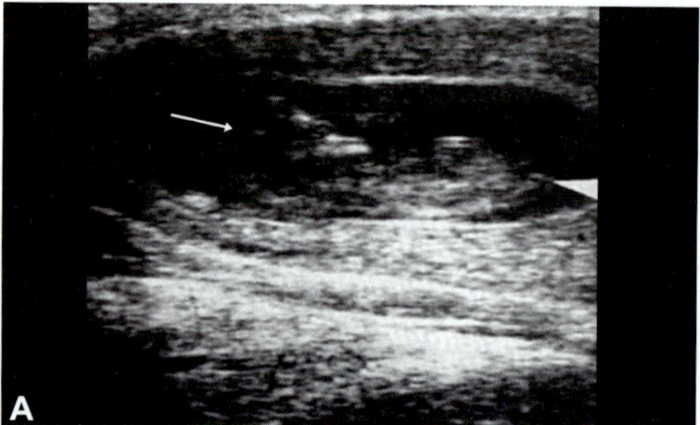

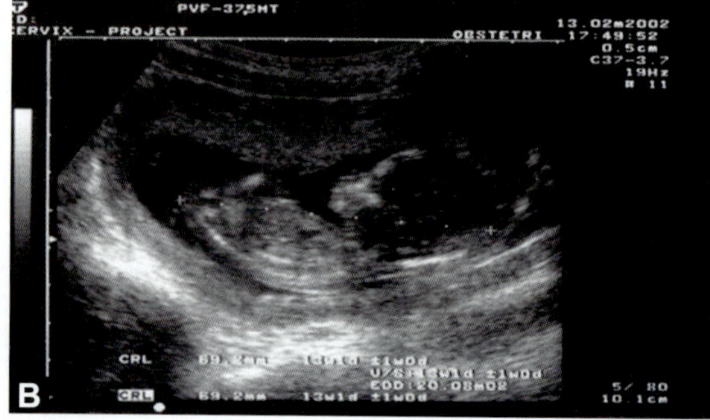

FIGURE 3 A AND B CRL = 9.1–15.9 mm, week 7, Days 13–49.

CRL and Pregnancy Outcome

The possibility of early pregnancy loss is very high and can be related to fetal biometry*

- CRL is < 5 mm - possibility of pregnancy loss is approximately 8%
- CRL 6–10 mm - possibility of pregnancy loss is approximately 3–4%
- CRL > 10 mm - possibility of pregnancy loss is approximately ≤ 1%
- Sixty one percent of women that miscarry had CRL at least 2 standard deviation (SD) below expected

TABLE 1: Clinical predictors of gestational age

Parameter	*Estimated range for 95% of cases*
In vitro fertilization	±1 day
Ovulation induction	±4–6 days
LH surge indicator	±4–6 days
Basal body temperature	±4–6 days
Certain menstrual history	±2 weeks
Bimanual examination (first trimester)	±2 weeks
First fetal heart tones by Doppler	±2 weeks
"Quickening"	±2–4 weeks
First fetal heart tones by auscultation	±2–4 weeks
Fundal height measurement between 18 and 32 weeks' gestation	±4 weeks
Fundal height measurement after 32 weeks' gestation	±4–6 weeks

Assigning Gestational Age

- Last normal menstrual period (Algorithm 1)
- Clinical parameters (Date of positive urine pregnancy test, serum beta HCG levels, or date of embryo transfer in *in vitro* fertilization; Table 1)
- Crown rump length (Table 2)
  - CRL (cms) + 6.5 = Gestational age in weeks
  - CRL (mm) + 42 = Gestational age in days ± 3–5 days

Guideline for Fixing Gestational Age

- Fixing a gestational age as early as possible is the first and most important step for the diagnosis of growth disorders
- When menstrual dates fall outside the confidence limits of ultrasound assessment, assignment of dates should be based on ultrasound assessment of gestational age.

TABLE 2: Determination of gestational age

Gestational age (weeks)	*Sac size (mm)*	*CRL (mm)*
4	3	
5	6	
6	14	
7	27	8
8	29	15
9	33	21
10		31
11		41
12		51
13		71

CRL, crown rump length.

*Kurjak A, Kupesic S, Carrera JM, Ahmed B. Ultrasound Evaluation of Abnormal Early Pregnancy. *Donald School Journal of Ultrasound in Obstetrics and Gynecology*. 2008;2(2):87-105.

- When menstrual dates are unknown, assignment of dates should be based on ultrasound assessment of gestational age.
- Follow up of gestational sac with no fetal pole is depicted in algorithm 2 and follow up of gestational sac after appearance of fetal pole is depicted in algorithm 3.

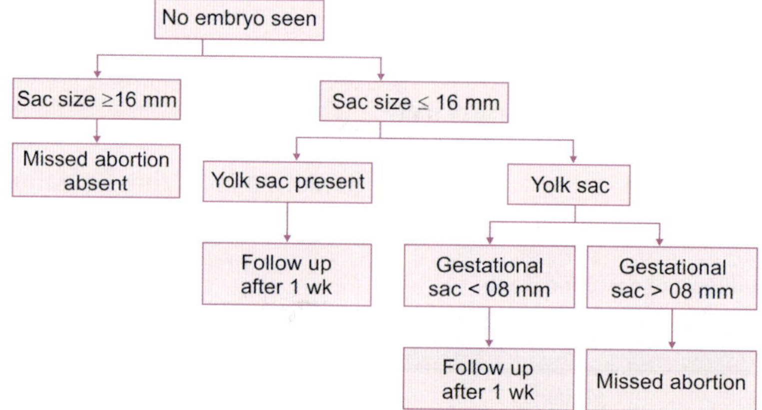

ALGORITHM 2 Follow up of gestational sac with no fetal pole.

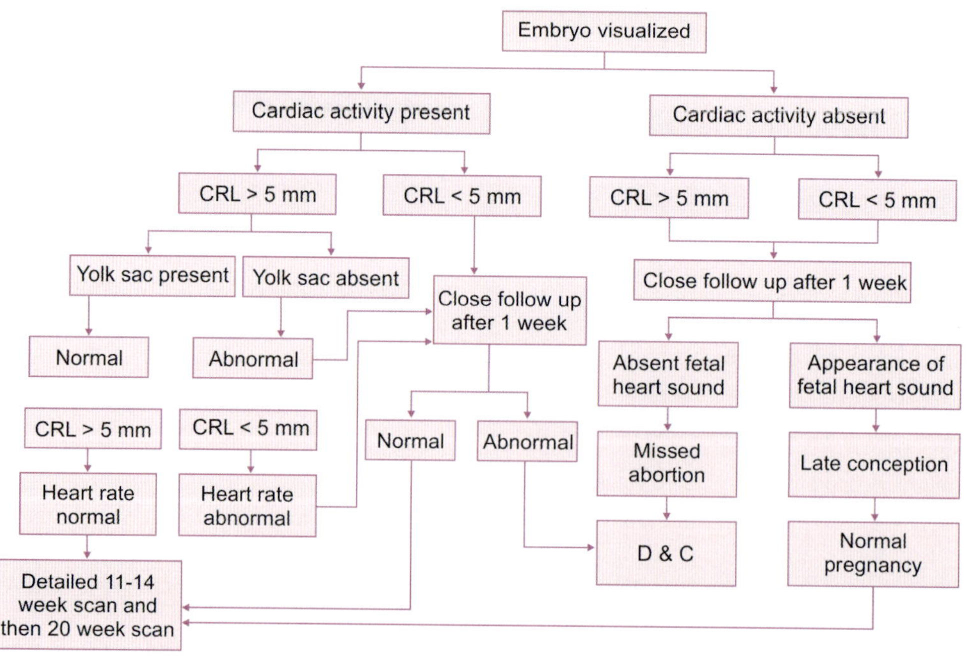

D & C, dilatation and curettage; CRL, crown rump length.

ALGORITHM 3 Follow up of gestational sac with a fetal pole.

Pregnancy Dating with First Trimester Ultrasound

The only utility for "routine" ultrasound as determined by the RADIUS study*

- Early dating is the most accurate (± 5–7 days or 8%)
- Better defines timing for later testing and interventions
  - Triple/quadruple test
  - Tocolysis/steroid administration
- Reduces the incidence of induction for postdates

Measurements

- Mean Sac Diameter (MSD) should be measured in 3 dimensions. It may be all that is visible at the discriminatory zone; intrauterine best confirmed with some fetal element, such as a yolk sac
- Embryonic CRL measurement with fetal cardiac activity is the best measurement for dating purposes.

Typical Measurements

There are tables for determining gestational age based on:

- Gestational Sac Measurement
- CRL
- Biparietal diameter (BPD), head circumference (HC), femur length (FL) and abdominal circumference (AC)

TABLE 3: Ultrasound predictors of gestational age

Parameter	*Estimated range for 95% of cases*
Gestational sac mean diameter	± 1 week
Crown-rump length	± 5–7 days
BPD, 12–26 weeks	± 10–11 days
HC, 12–26 weeks	± 10–14 days
AC, 12–26 weeks	± 10–14 days
FL, 12–26 weeks	± 10–20 days
BPD, 27–42 weeks	± 2–3 weeks
HC, 27–42 weeks	± 2–3 weeks
AC, 27–42 weeks	± 2–3 weeks
FL, 27–42 weeks	± 2–3 weeks

BPD, biparietal diameter; HC, head circumference; FL, femur length; AC, abdominal circumference.

All the ultrasound machines contain software which performs these calculations. The measurements will trigger the gestational age determination (Table 3).

Placenta

- Normal placenta is first seen on ultrasound at 8 weeks as focal thickening and at the periphery of gestational sac.
- At 12 weeks it appears disk like, finely granular, homogenous with smooth chorionic covering.

Grading of placenta begins at the end of first trimester.

*Ewigman BG, Crane JP, Frigoletto FD, LeFevre ML, Bain RP, McNellis D. Effect of prenatal ultrasound screening on perinatal outcome. RADIUS Study Group. *N Engl J Med.* 1993 Sep 16;329(12):821-7.

Annexure 5

Fetal Heart Rate

Fetal heart rate should be done using M- Mode as far as possible particularly in the first trimester (Figure 1).

Predictive Value of Fetal Heart rate

Table 1 shows discriminatory signs of viability.

No Cardiac Activity

Presence of fetal pole greater than 6.5 mm with no cardiac activity signifies a nonviable pregnancy (Figure 2).

Poor Prognostic Signs in First Trimester Ultrasound

- Yolk sac abnormal (irregular, large, free floating and calcified)

TABLE 1: Discriminatory signs of viability

Gestational age	*Fetal heart rate*
5–6 weeks	93/min
6–7 weeks	100/min
7–8 weeks	130/min
8 weeks	143/min

- Slow fetal heart rate (ie HR <85 bmp at 6–8 weeks is associated with 0% survival)
- Oligoamniotic sac (MSD-CRL <5 mm)
- Fetal tachycardia/bradycardia - Fetal tachycardia (Figure 3) is more commonly seen in trisomy 13, Turner's syndrome and fetal bradycardia is often seen in trisomy 18
- Miscarriage rate in women with large (> 40% of gestational sac volume) subchorionic hematoma and first trimester bleeding is high
- Follow-up ultrasound in one week.

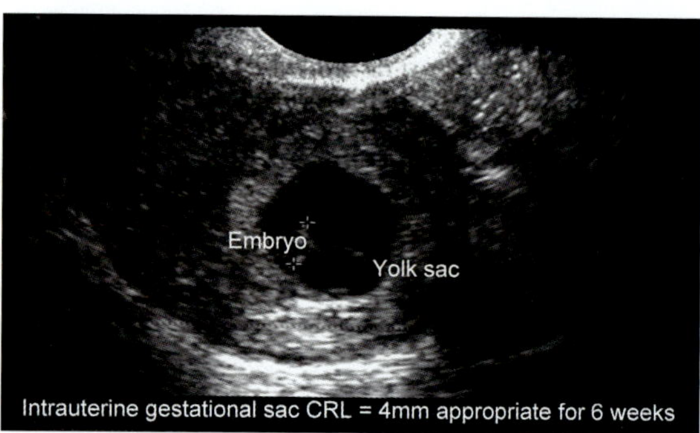

FIGURE 2 A nonviable pregnancy with fetal pole > 6.5 mm.

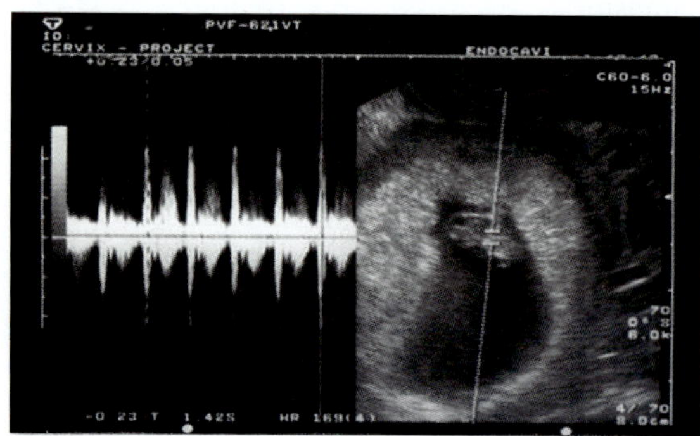

FIGURE 1 Viable intrauterine pregnancy showing embryo and fetal heart rate.

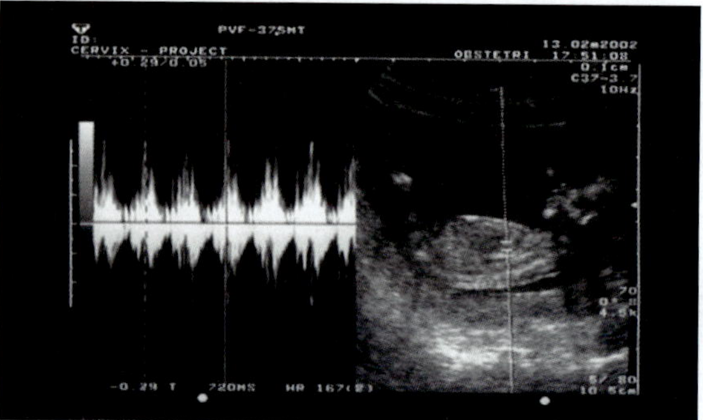

FIGURE 3 Ultrasound showing fetal tachycardia.

Annexure 6

Multiple Pregnancy

There is an increased incidence of perinatal morbidity and mortality in multifetal pregnancy as compared to singleton pregnancy. Multifetal pregnancy need to be reduced to twin pregnancy for a favourable outcome. Increased morbidity may be due to

- Prematurity
- Polyhydramnios
- Congenital anomolies
- Discordant growth
- Umbilical cord accidents.

How Many Embryos/Fetus?

- Before telling the exact number of fetuses one should examine with transvaginal sonography (TVS) and transabdominal sonography (TAS) in different angles and position (Figure 1 &2). One may also use 3-D to avoid making mistakes. Wide angle TVS probe is preferable and ideal time of scan is 8 – 10 weeks.
- When the diagnosis is not obvious the clues to the diagnosis are mainly the findings of :
  - Abnormal position between different organs; eg. heart and head in discordant orientation (heart pointing to the head)
  - Too many limb organs
  - Organs that change position too rapidly; eg. after seeing a heart in the lower left quadrant another in the upper right will be seen.

Zygosity

There are two types of twins

- 70% — fraternal - dizygotic; two different ova. Dizygotic are usually dichorionic and diamniotic; maybe with fused placenta or different placentas
- 30% — identical - monozygotic; splitting of a single embryo. The type of monozygotic twinning depends on the day of embryonic split (Figures 3, 4, 5)
  - 1–4 days: Dichorionic/Diamniotic (DC/DA)
  - 4–7 days: Monochorionic/Diamniotic (MC/DA)
  - After 7 days: Monochorionic/Monoamniotic (MC/MA)
  - High incidence of perinatal mortality in monozygotic twins may be due to intraplacental vascular communications

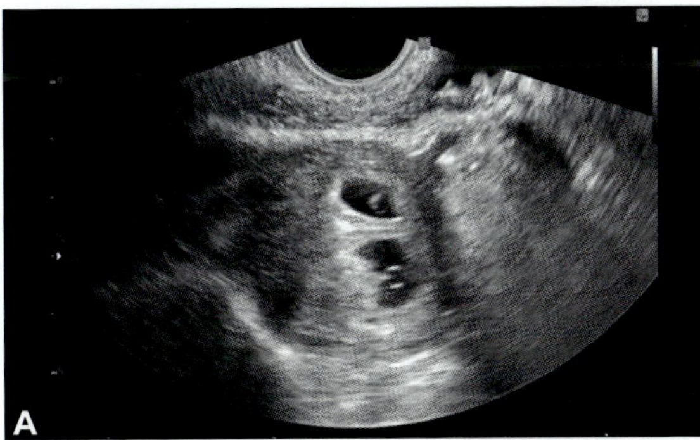

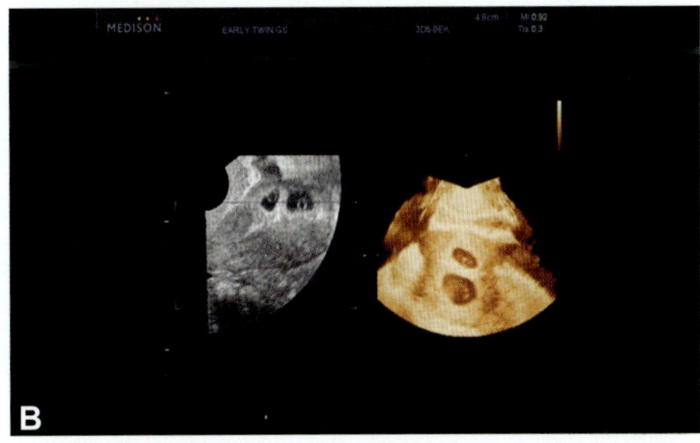

FIGURE 1 TVS showing twin pregnancy.

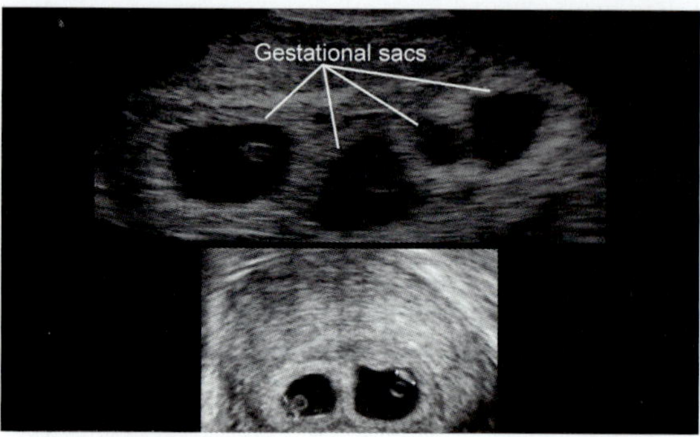

FIGURE 2 Multiple gestational sacs.

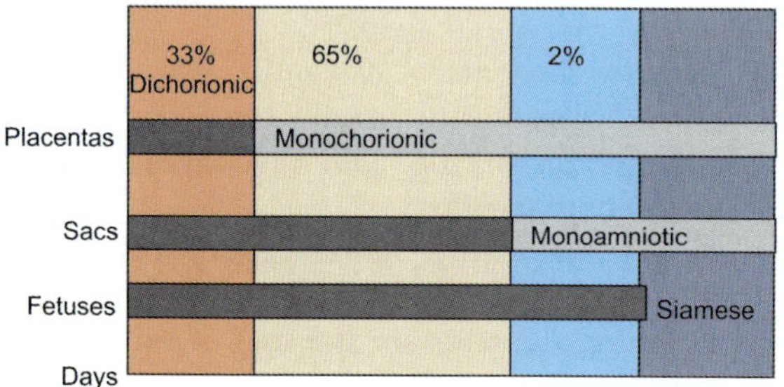

FIGURE 3 Types of monozygotic twinning.

- ○ High chances of malformations may be caused by process of monozygotic twinning
- ○ Deformities caused by overcrowding
- ○ Twin to twin transfusion –15–30%. The small donor twin – stuck twin - shows intrauterine growth retardation (IUGR), oligohydramnios and pinned to the side while other shows polyhydramnios, cardiomegaly, hydrops, enlarged bladder etc.

Conjoined Twins

- The incidence is 1 in 50,000. Thoracophagus (two bodies fused from the upper thorax to lower belly) is the most common. Others include
  - ○ Xiphophagus (two bodies fused in the xiphoid cartilage)
  - ○ Omphalophagus (Two bodies fused at the lower chest)

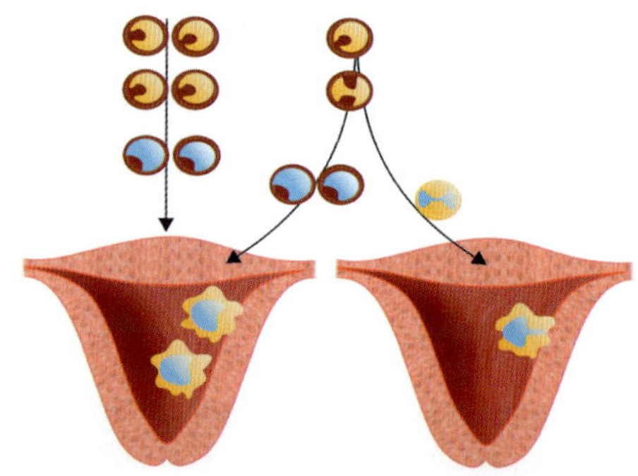

Dichorionic - Diamniotic

Monochorionic - Diamniotic

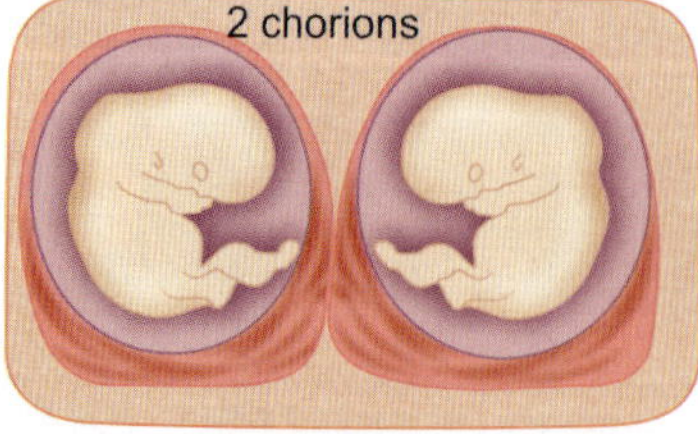

2 placentas

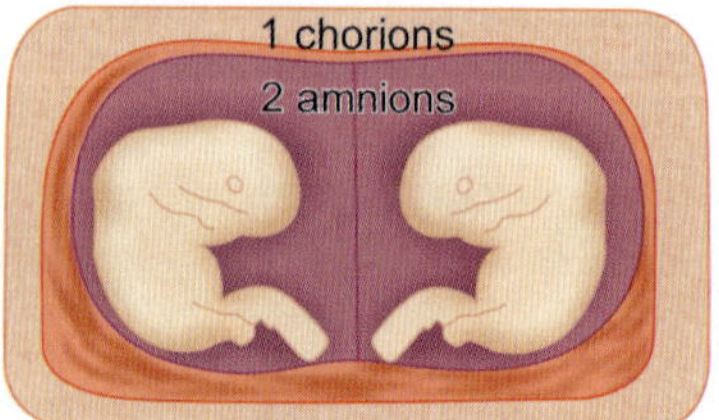

Single placenta

FIGURE 4 Type of twins.

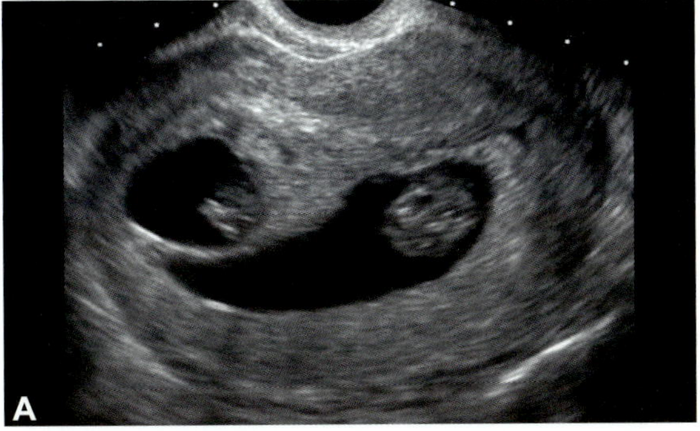

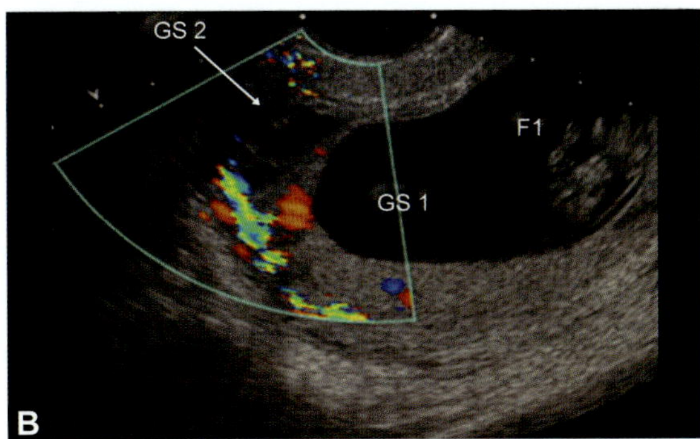

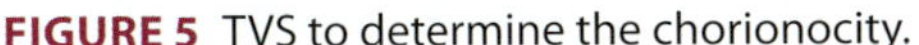
FIGURE 5 TVS to determine the chorionocity.

    - Pyophagus (two bodies joined at the pelvis)
    - Ischiophagus (fused lower half of the two bodies, with spines conjoined end-to-end at a 180° angle)
    - Craniophagus (fused skulls, but separate bodies)
- Joining is suspected when dividing membrane is not seen
- They move together, have a peculiar position with hyperextended head and intertwined limbs
- There are associated defects, especially complex heart anomalies

Serial ultrasonography is required to identify conjoined twin where same organ in the different twins remain in same correlation.

Discordant Twins

Twins are labelled discordant when there is approximately 25% difference in the biometry of two twins.

Vanishing Twins

- The second gestational sac is usually a blighted ovum or anembryonic sac and roughly 70% of twin gestations diagnosed early in the pregnancy result in singleton pregnancy at the time of delivery.
- With the advent of high resolution gray scale equipment, it becomes obvious that in most cases the second sac was not a true gestational sac but a normal phenomenon representing either blood in the endometrial canal related to implantation hemorrhage or a prominent hypoechogenic decidua vera.
- Twin gestational sacs with live embryo have indeed been recorded with subsequent resorption of one of the embryos, but this is a rare phenomenon.

Demise of Co-twin

- Twin embryonic syndrome is caused by passage of thromboplastic material into the circulation of the surviving co-twin in a monochorionic twin pregnancy resulting in DIC.
- Serial ultrasound after death of one twin is helpful to monitor a well-being mainly when the live twin cannot be delivered because of prematurity.

Chorionic Peak Sign

It is also called the twin peak sign is the presence of projecting zone of tissue, similar echotexture of placenta, triangular cross section, wider at chorionic surface of the placenta extending into and tapering to a point within the intertwin

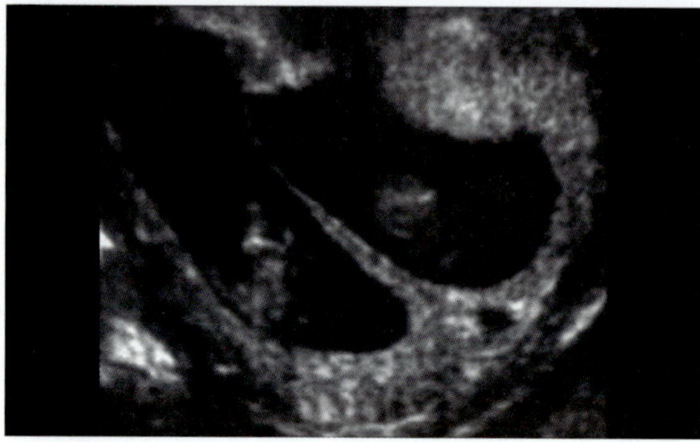

FIGURE 6 Twin Peak Lambda Sign.

membrane (Figure 6). This is seen in dichorionic pregnancy because there is a potential interchorionic space between the layers of twin membrane. The incidence of this sign exceeds 50%.

Triplet Pregnancy

Ultrasound appearance of triplet pregnancy is shown in figure 7.

Selective Reduction in Multiple Fetal Pregnancy

- Associated with high morbidity and mortality and perinatal mortality
- Common after infertility management and *in vitro* fertilization (IVF)
- Ideal timing : 8weeks and more
- Route used : TVS with/without TAS
- 2 ml KCl in 1:1 dilution. The needle is placed in the heart or chest, needle used is 20 gauge. The solution is then injected rapidly in 2ml increments until cardiac asystole is confirmed sonographically
- Cardiac puncture with air embolization - 20 gauge needle is guided into the fetal heart and air injected rapidly through a sterile Millipore filter into the cardiac cavity
- Complications of the procedure are
- Infection- amnionitis, miscarriage,
- bleeding,
- miscarriage
- premature labour
- DIC
- problems of monochorionic placentation
- damage to other gestational sacs
- technical failure.

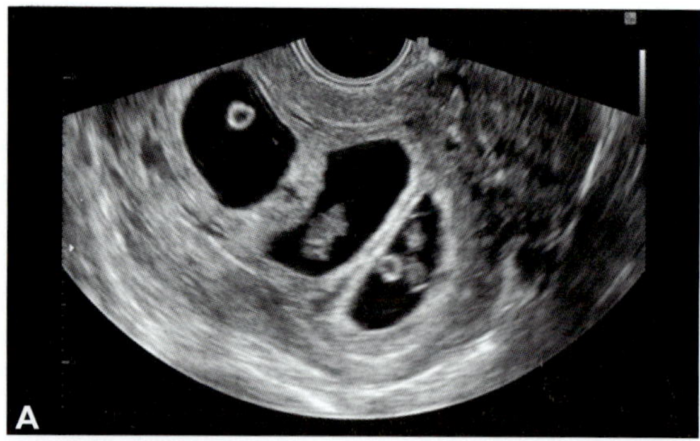

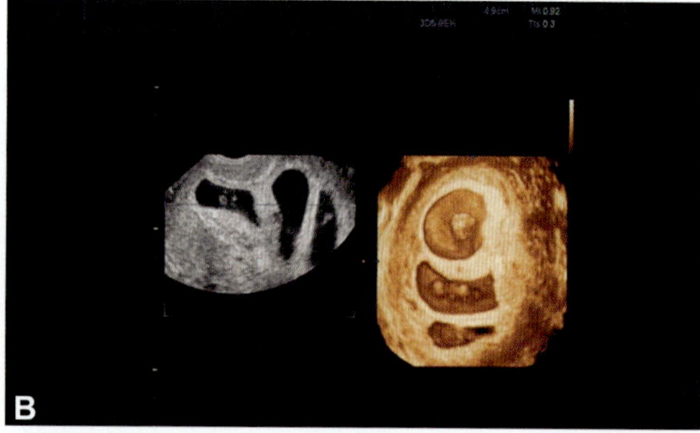

FIGURE 7 Triplet pregnancy.

Annexure 7

First Trimester Bleeding Per Vaginum

Early Pregnancy Failure

- Failure of appropriate interval growth by u/s of embryo
- Fetal pole/yolk sac should be seen by the time the MSD is 20 mm (not as accurate as fetal cardiac activity)
- Fetal cardiac activity should be seen by the time the CRL is 4mm. If not, may repeat the ultrasound in one week.

Causes of Bleeding in Early Pregnancy (Figure 1)

- Physiological bleed
    - About 20% to 50% experience bleeding in 1st week of pregnancy due to anchoring of choriodecidua as it burrows into decidualized endometrium
    - About 20–30% of these progress to threatened abortion with retrochorionic hemorrhage

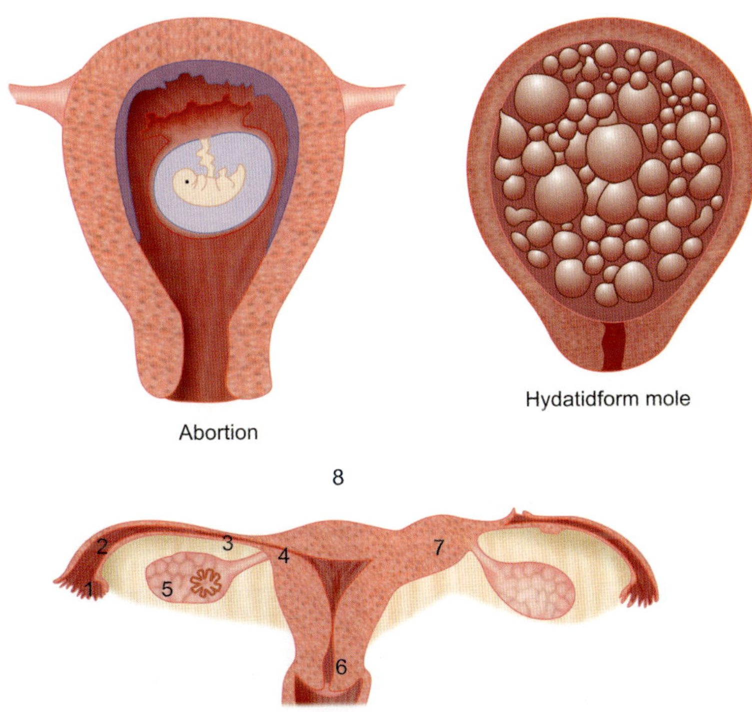

FIGURE 1 Causes of bleeding in early pregnancy.
1. Infundibular (ostial); 2. Tubal (ampullary); 3. Tubal (isthmal); 4. Interstitial; 5. Ovarian; 6. Cervical; 7. Peritoneal; 8. Abdominal.

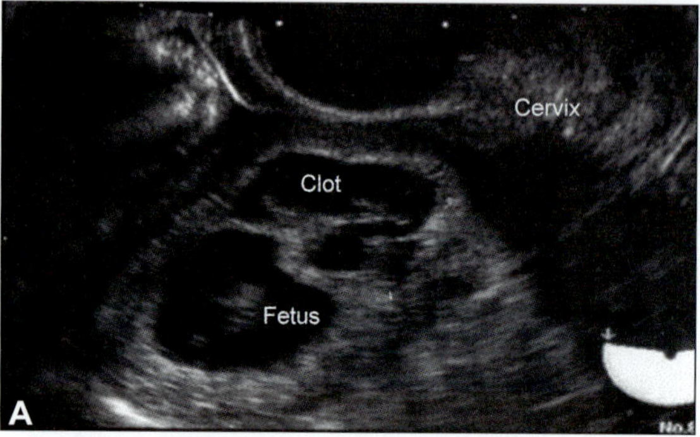

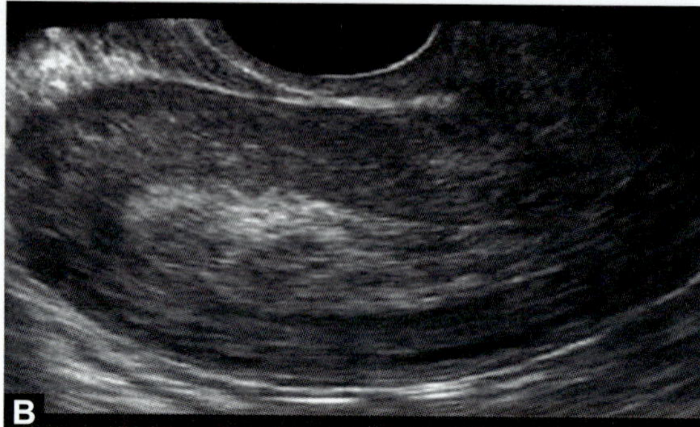

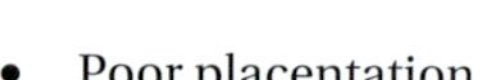
FIGURE 2 TVS showing subchorionic bleed.

- Poor placentation
- Miscarriage
- Ectopic pregnancy (*See* Chapter 16: Ectopic Pregnancy)
- Gestational trophoblastic disease (*See* Chapter 17: Gestational Trophoblastic Disease)
- Cervical lesions (erosion and/or polyp) (*See* Chapter 23: Associated Gynecological conditions)
- Unknown

Empty Gestational Sac

- When no embryo is visualized within the gestational sac, there are three possibilities:
- Very early pregnancy
- Non-viable intrauterine pregnancy
- Anembryonic/blighted ovum
  - Where the embryo never developed
  - Embryo has died

Factors Affecting Prognosis

- Location of the subchorionic bleed is most important.
  - Bleeding under cord insertion (retro-placental) has more chances of fetal abnormalities as compared to sub-chorionic hemorrhage separating membranes opposite to the cord insertion site (Figure 2)
  - Supracervical has better prognosis and is easily drained
  - High chances of miscarriage with fundal haematoma
- Size
  - Pregnancy failure is more common when retrochorionic hemorrhage is more than two-third size of gestational sac
  - Retrochorionic haemorrhage appears as a hypoechoic area surrounding the gestational sac. When the volume is ≤ 25% of gestational sac or ≤ 60 ml, it is likely that pregnancy will progress normally.

Color Doppler in First Trimester Bleeding

Several studies (have shown a gradual increase in velocity and diastolic flow in chorio-decidual (spiral) arteries in early pregnancy (Figure 3). However actual doppler indices do not discriminate between viable and non viable pregnancy.

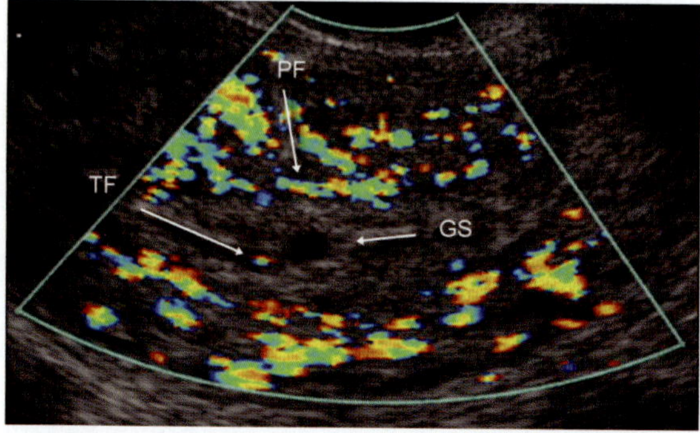

FIGURE 3 Blood flow around the gestational sac.

Annexure 8

Corpus Luteal Cysts

- Most common cystic pelvic masses pregnancy (Figure 1)
- Regress by 16–18 weeks gestational age
- Hemorrhage may be seen in the cyst which may enlarge in size up to 10–15 cm with internal echoes and septations
- Develop at ovulation site
- Thin walled cysts
- Project eccentrically from ovary
- Clotted blood within corpus luteal cyst may simulate embryo.

Differential Diagnosis

The differential diagnosis between corpus luteal cyst and ectopic pregnancy may be difficult. However, if cystic mass arises from the ovary, it is more likely to be a corpus luteal cyst. If the cystic mass is separate from the ovary, it may be an ectopic pregnancy.

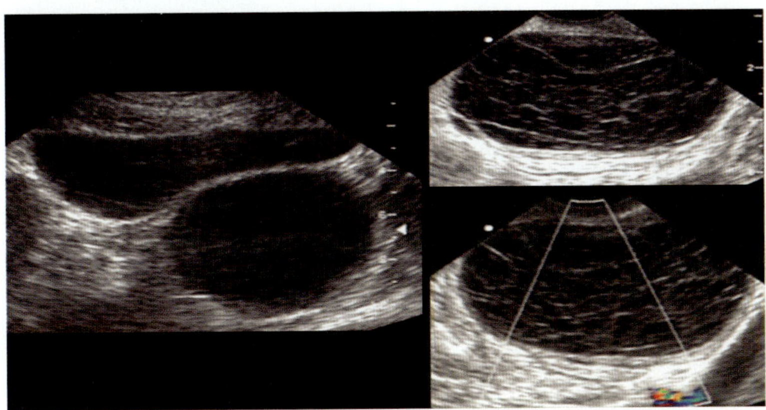

FIGURE 1 Corpus luteal cyst.

Annexure 9

Cervical Measurements

Screening for Cervical Incompetence

Cervical incompetence may be congenital, secondary to cervical lacerations or as a result of excessive dilatation during previous abortion or curettage. Patients at high risk of cervical incompetence require regular screening by transvaginal ultrasound (TVS). It is performed after emptying the bladder. Introduce the probe upto 2 to 3 cm and study the entire length of the cervix in sagittal and coronal plane (Figure 1 and 2).

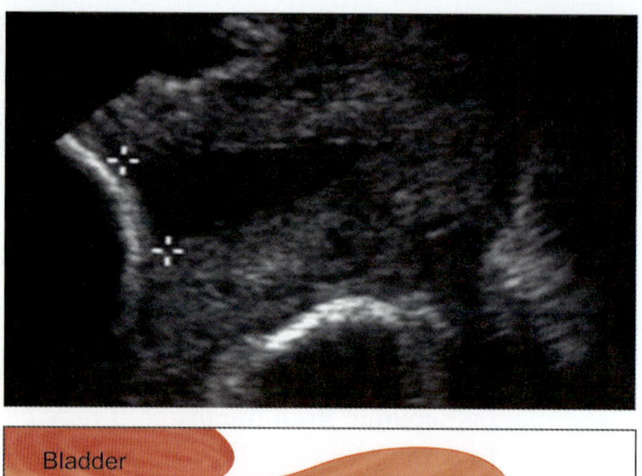

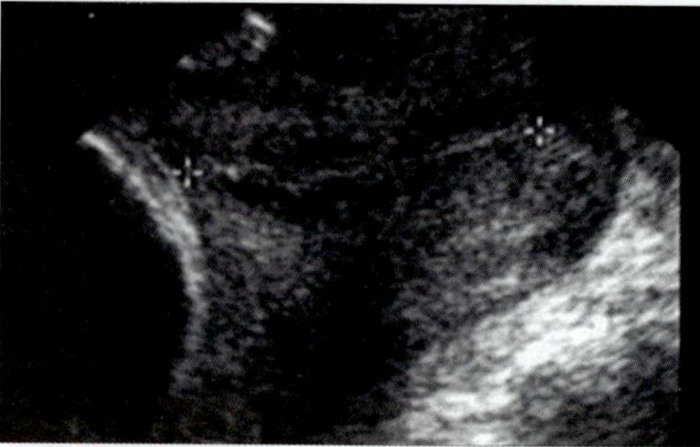

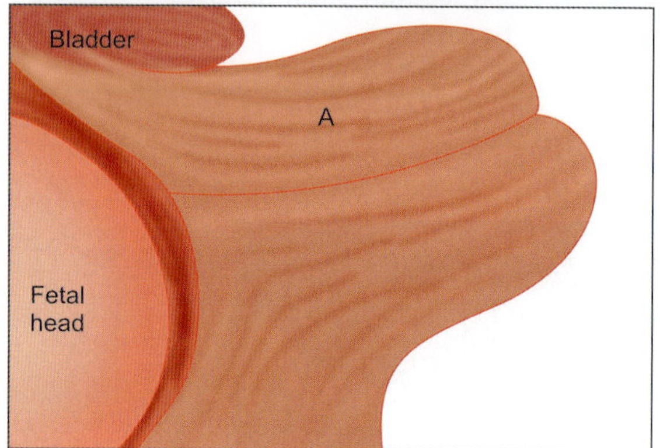

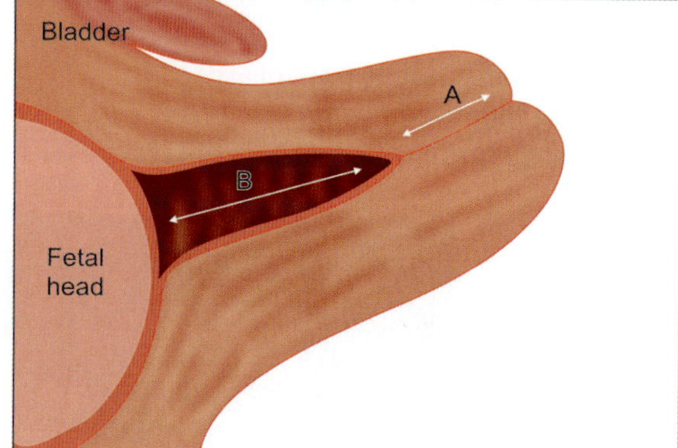

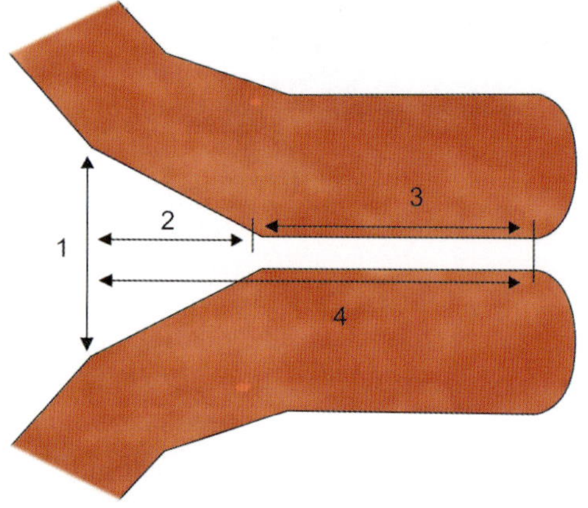

FIGURE 1 Schematic and ultrasound appearance of normal and incompetent cervical canal.
1. Width of internal cervical os; 2. Length of dilated segment of cervix; 3. Length of closed segment of cervix; 4. Total length of cervix.

- Look for integrity of internal os, configuration of lower segment and cervical canal
- Funneling of upper cervical canal should be carefully looked for herniation of membranes and fetal part to be noted
- Normal cervical length is 2.5–4 cm throughout gestation
- Cervical incompetence is defined as dilation of cervical canal > 8 mm

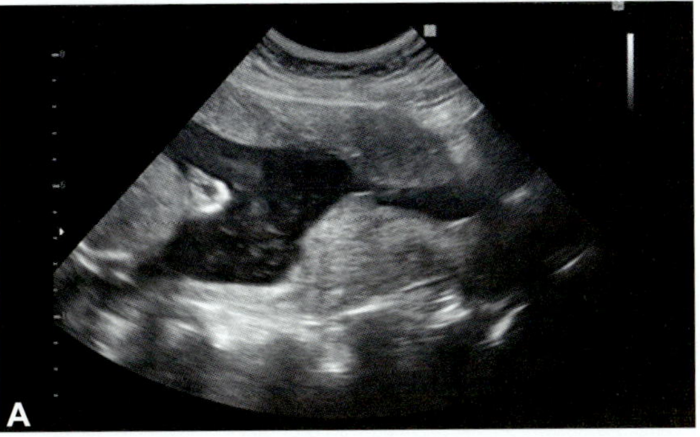

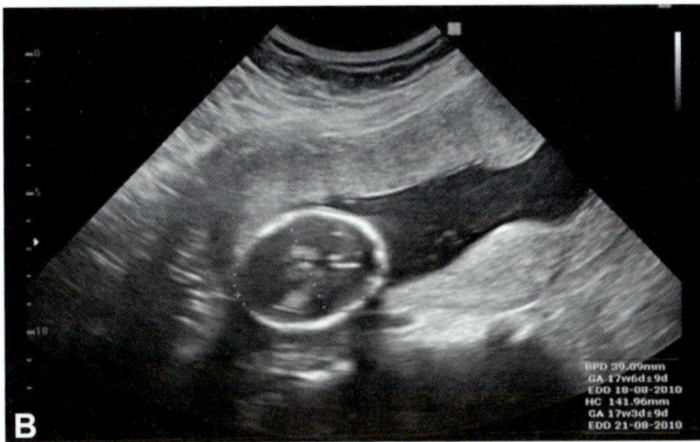

FIGURE 2 Ultrasound (TVS) appearance of cervical incompetence.

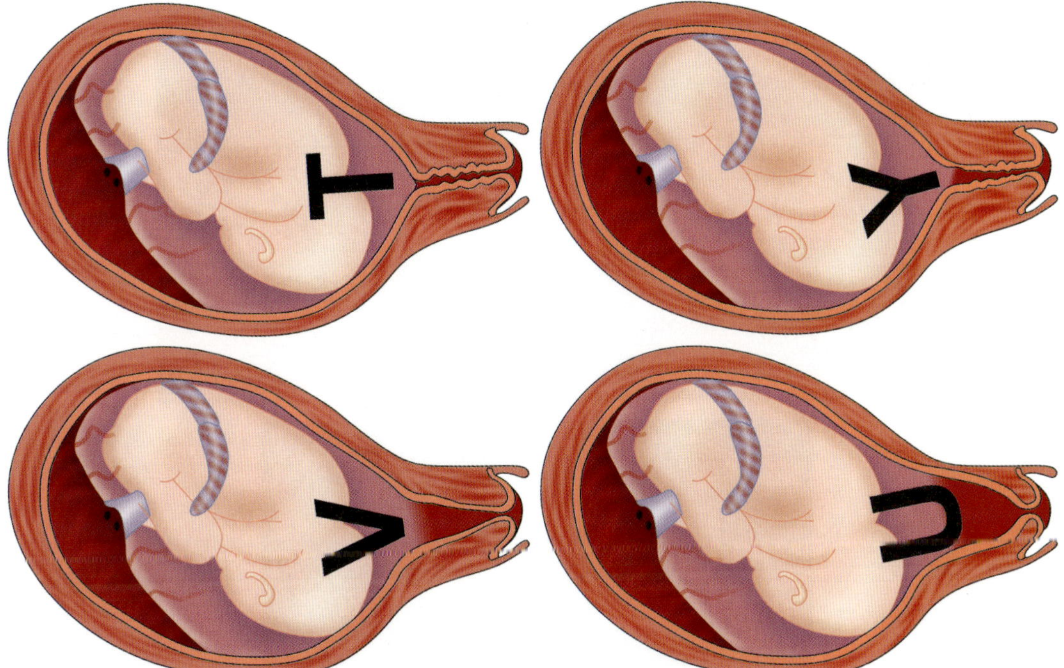

FIGURE 3 Schematic representation of cervical dilatation with uterine pressure

- Relative risk of preterm delivery increases as cervical length decreases below 3 cm cervical length.

Dynamic Cervical Incompetence

- These are the cases where degree of dilatation of cervical canal varies with uterine tension (Figure 3)
- The competence of the internal os as can be tested provocatively while doing TVS by pressing gently on the abdominal wall by free hand
- Dilatation of internal os signifies cervical incompetence.

Cervical Cerclage

It can be visualized as echogenic linear structures with acoustic shadow (Figures 4).

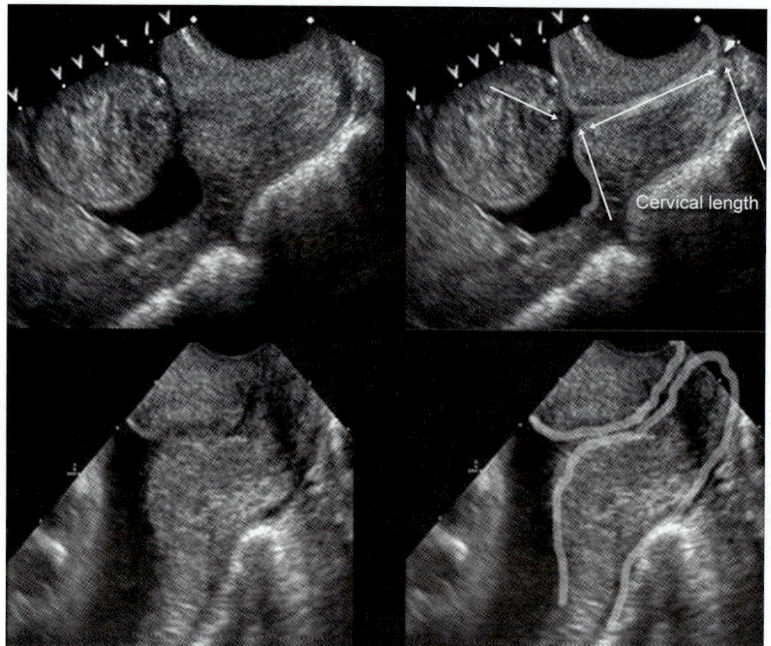

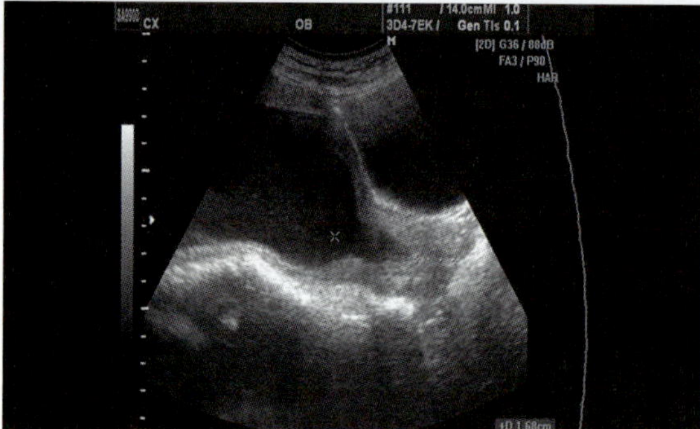

FIGURE 4 Ultrasound (TVS) appearance of cervical cerclage.

Annexure 10

Amniotic Sheet

- Seen in uterine synechia
- Membranous structures project in uterine cavity as sheets arising from folding of membranes which occurs over an intrauterine adhesion
- No fetal deformities are associated
- Risk Factors
  - Prior history of dilatation and curettage
  - Therapeutic abortion
- Ultrasound appearance (Figure 1)
  - Bulbous-free edge
  - Thinner midportion
  - Thickened base.

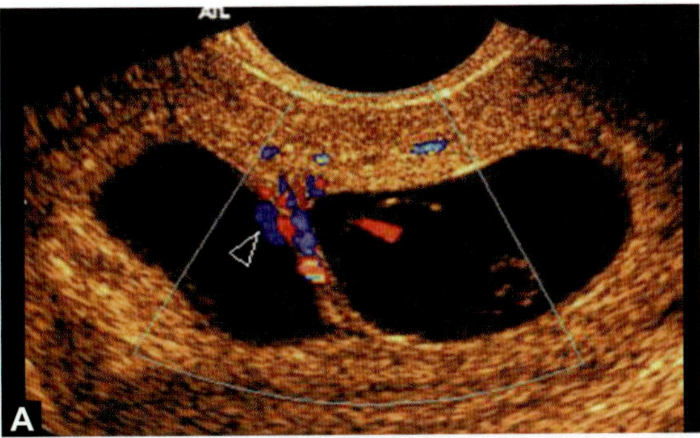

FIGURE 1 Ultrasound appearance (TVS) of amniotic sheet.

Annexure 11

Vesicular Mole

Gestational trophoblastic disease occurs in 1 in 1000–2000 pregnancies on ultrasound. There are two types (Figure 1):

- Complete - Diploid
- Partial (aka Triploidy).

Ultrasound Appearance (Figures 2–6)

- Placental edema
- Trophoblastic proliferation
  - Grape-like appearance
  - Swollen villi/vesicular.

Hyaditiform Moles: Complete

- Complete mole occurs in 70% of cases
  - Entire placenta
  - No fetus
  - Diploid karyotype.
- Ultrasound shows snowstorm appearance with multiple echogenic foci of vesicles (Figure 7).

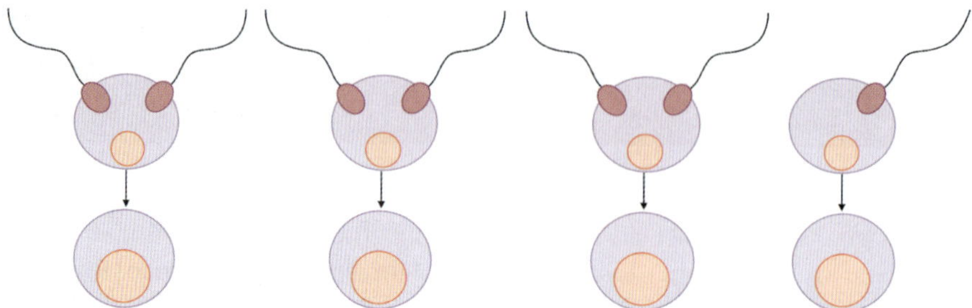

FIGURE 1 Types of gestational trophoblastic disease

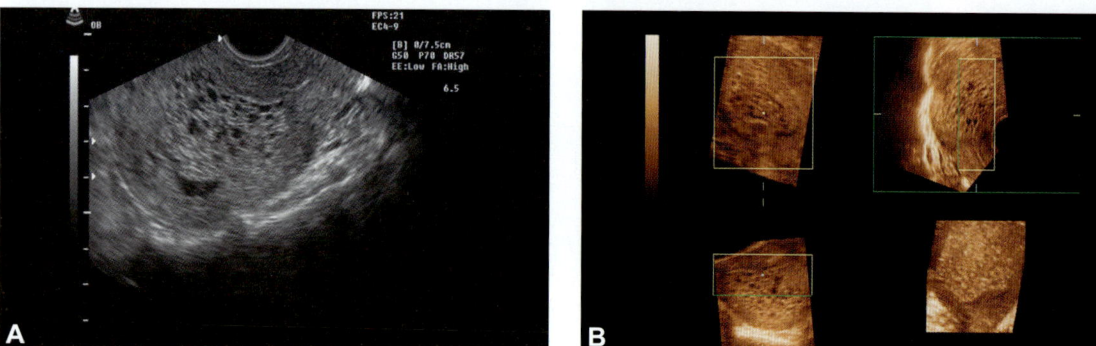

FIGURE 2 Ultrasound appearance (TVS) of gestational trophoblastic disease.

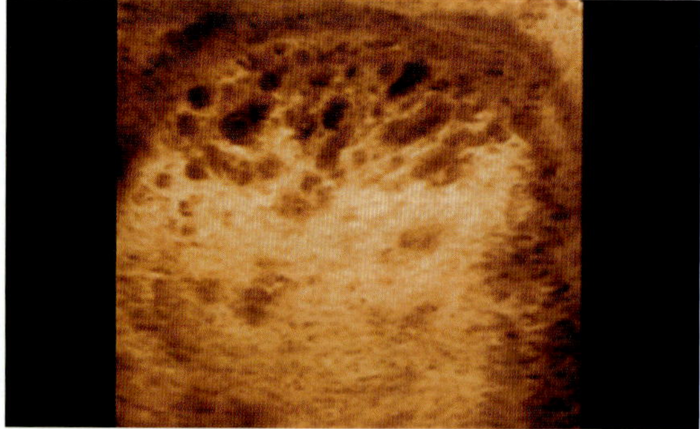

FIGURE 3 Ultrasound appearance (TVS) of gestational trophoblastic disease.

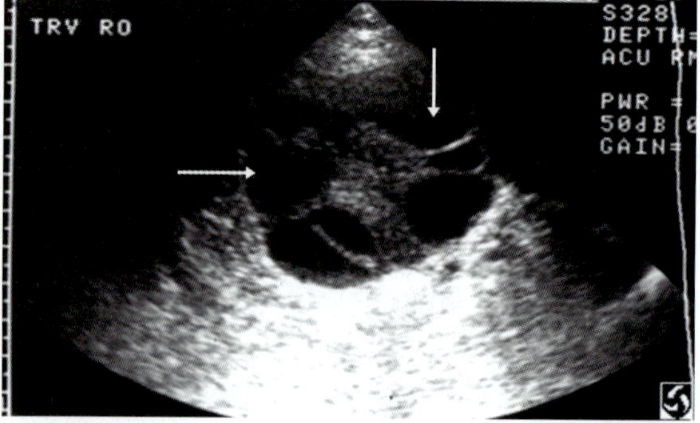

FIGURE 4 Ultrasound appearance (TVS) of gestational trophoblastic disease

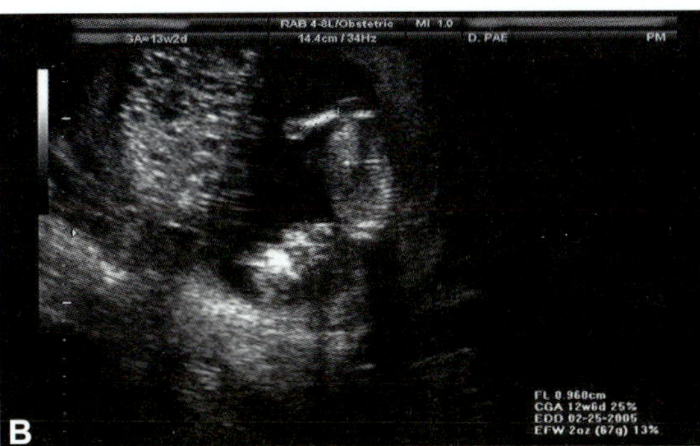

FIGURE 5 Ultrasound appearance (TVS) of gestational trophoblastic disease.

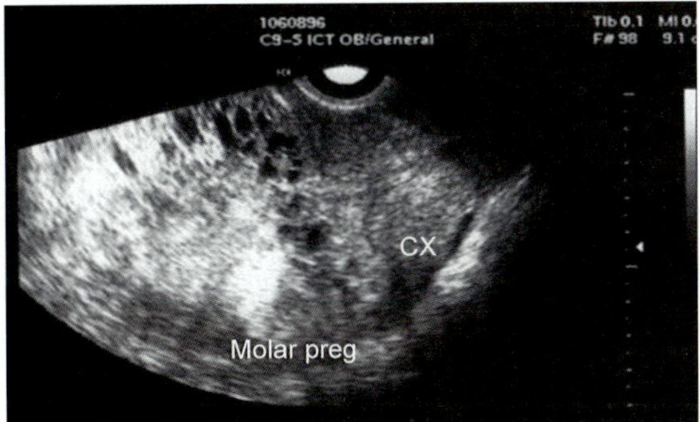

FIGURE 6 Ultrasound appearance (TVS) of gestational trophoblastic disease.

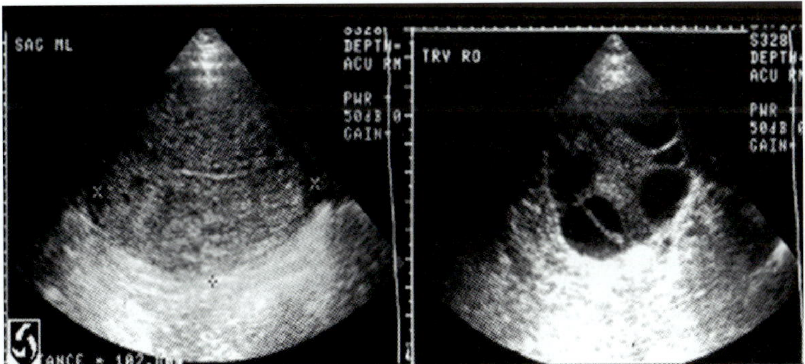

FIGURE 7 Snowstorm appearance on complete hyaditiform mole.

Annexure 12

Ectopic Pregnancy

The classical clinical triad of pain, vaginal bleeding and palpable adnexal mass is seen in about 45% patients. Usually the presentation is of classical ruptured ectopic in 60%; 25% with chronic ectopic and only 15% present before rupture.

Sites of Ectopic Pregnancy (Figure 1)

- Tubal (>95%)
  - Ampulla (70%)
  - Isthmic (12%)
  - Fimbrial (11.1%)
- Ovarian (3.2%)
- Interstitial (2.4%)
- Abdominal (1.3%)

Sonographic Findings by Transvaginal Sonography (Figure 2 and 3)

Intrauterine findings
- Empty uterus/thickened endometrium
- Central hypoechogenic area
- A sac like structure (pseudogestational sac)

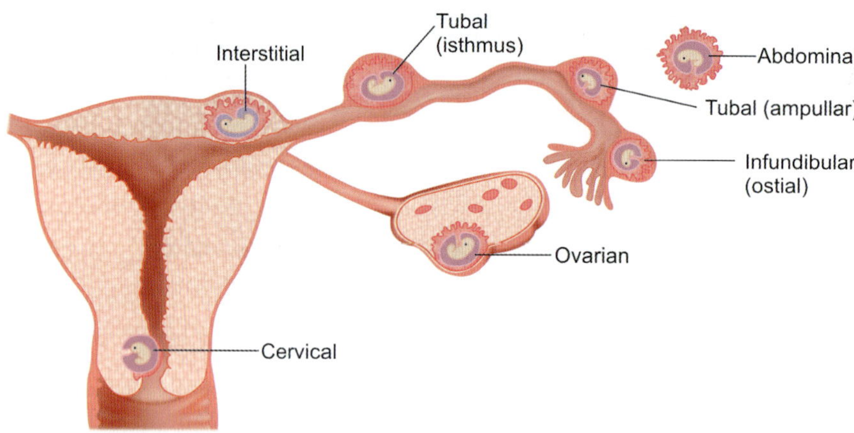

FIGURE 1 Sites of ectopic pregnancy.

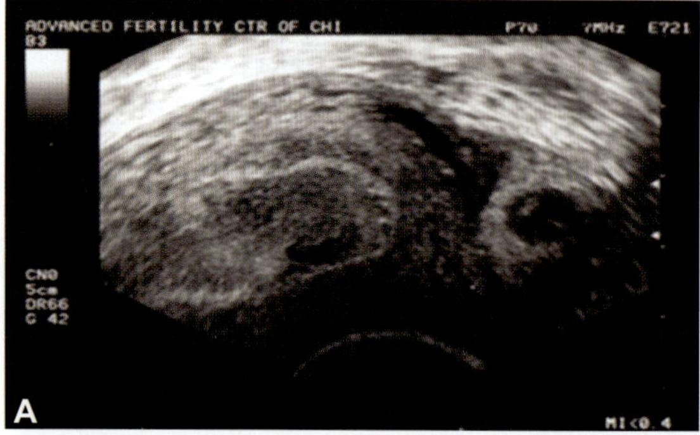

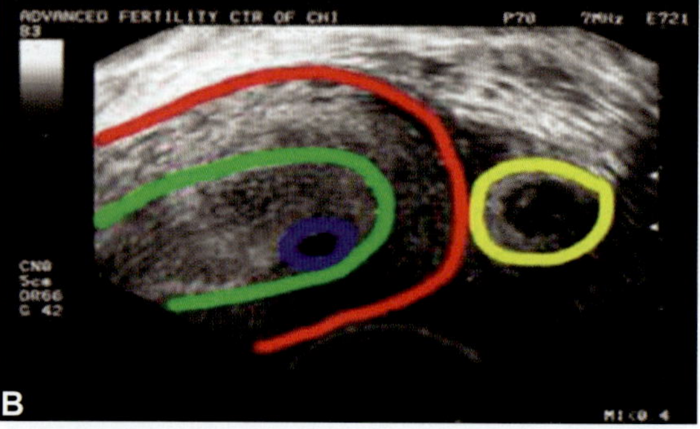

FIGURE 2 Ectopic pregnancy with empty uterine cavity (red outline; green outline is uterine lining) with psudogestational sac (blue outline) and ectopic (yellow outline) seen in the adnexa.

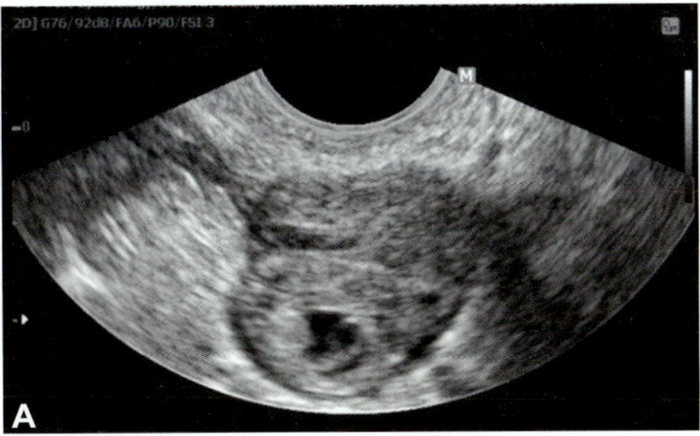

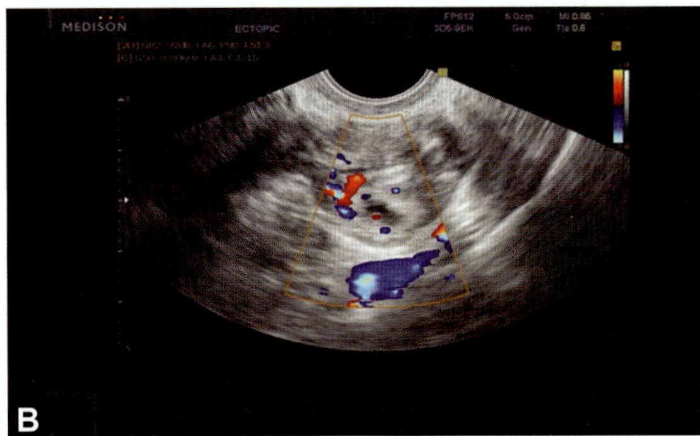

FIGURE 3 **A,** Ectopic gestational sac in the adnexa; **B,** Increased blood flow around the sac.

Extrauterine findings

- Adnexal masses
- Living extrauterine embryo in an unruptured sac
- Extrauterine gestational sac
- Cul de sac fluid.

Negative Signs

Intrauterine pregnancy: living intrauterine embryo with gestational sac and yolk sac - double decidual sign.

False Negative Signs

Intrauterine pseudogestational sac

Indirect Positive Signs

- Empty uterus sign
- Free pelvic and abdominal fluid.

Direct Positive Signs

Adnexal pregnancy

- Living embryo
- Tubal/adnexal ring
- Complex/solid mass
- Abdominal pregnancy.

Tubal Abortion

- The stretching and erosion of the tubal wall result in bleeding into the sac as well as between the tubal wall and the gestational sac
- Once the gestational sac separates from the tubal wall, four events may occur
  - Rupture of the sac into the lumen of the tube
  - Absorption of the gestational sac
  - Abortion into the pelvis
  - A slow blood leak or rupture of the tube leading to pelvic intraperitoneal fluid collection.

Cul de Sac

- The presence of free fluid in an amount larger than normally detected with or without blood clots. The blood clots are depicted as bizarre shaped mass of irregularly echogenic substance. If the probe is gently moved in and out or the patient is asked to tilt her pelvis to the right and left several times, the blood clot may be observed to move. This fluid creates optimal contrast for visualization of the tube improving diagnostic accuracy.
- The absence of free fluid excludes the possibility of active bleeding into the pelvis.

TVS in Diagnosis and Management of Ectopic Pregnancy

The diagnosis or exclusion of an ectopic gestation depends on a combination of two or more of the following features:

- Documentation of intrauterine pregnancy and extraembryonic structures at a very early stage
- Exclusion of intrauterine pregnancy by documentation of the lack of a gestational sac in the uterus
- Sonographic documentation of tubal pregnancy
- Fluid in cul-de-sac.

Beta HCG Correlation

- Failure to locate intra uterine pregnancy sac with beta HCG of 750mIU/mL with missed period, strongly suggests ectopic pregnancy. Even when a beta HCG value does not correlate with the exact period of amenorrhea, suspect ectopic
- A negative beta HCG, ectopic pregnancy can be ruled out
- A subnormal rise of beta HCG less than 66% in 48 hours or plateauing titre of HCG is highly suspicious of ectopic pregnancy
- Discriminatory Zone—the quantitative beta HCG level at which one would expect to be able to identify an intrauterine pregnancy
    - For vaginal sonography— (1000–2000 per ACOG)
    - For abdominal sonography—3000–4000
- If the quantitative β-hCG is at or above the discriminatory zone, and no intrauterine can be identified, the pregnancy may be ectopic

Pseudogestational Sac (Figure 4)

- Seen in 20% of ectopic pregnancies
- Caused by high progesterone levels which lead to thickened endometrium
- No yolk sac

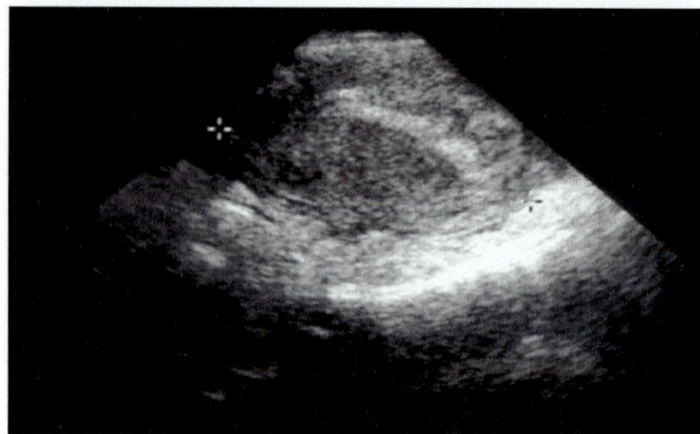

FIGURE 4 Pseudogestational sac.

- No embryo
- ± Double decidual sign
- Doppler will show absent to none peri-trophoblastic flow.

Tubal Ring Sign

Ultrasound appearance

- Cystic mass outside the uterus
- Thick echogenic wall
- Empty uterus with thickened endometrium with or without a pseudogestational sac (Figure 5)
- Embryo may or may not be present (Figure 6).

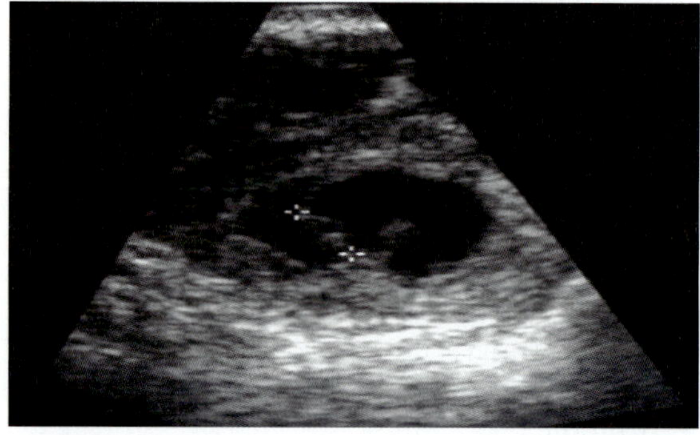

FIGURE 5 Ectopic pregnancy with presence of fetal pole and yolk sac.

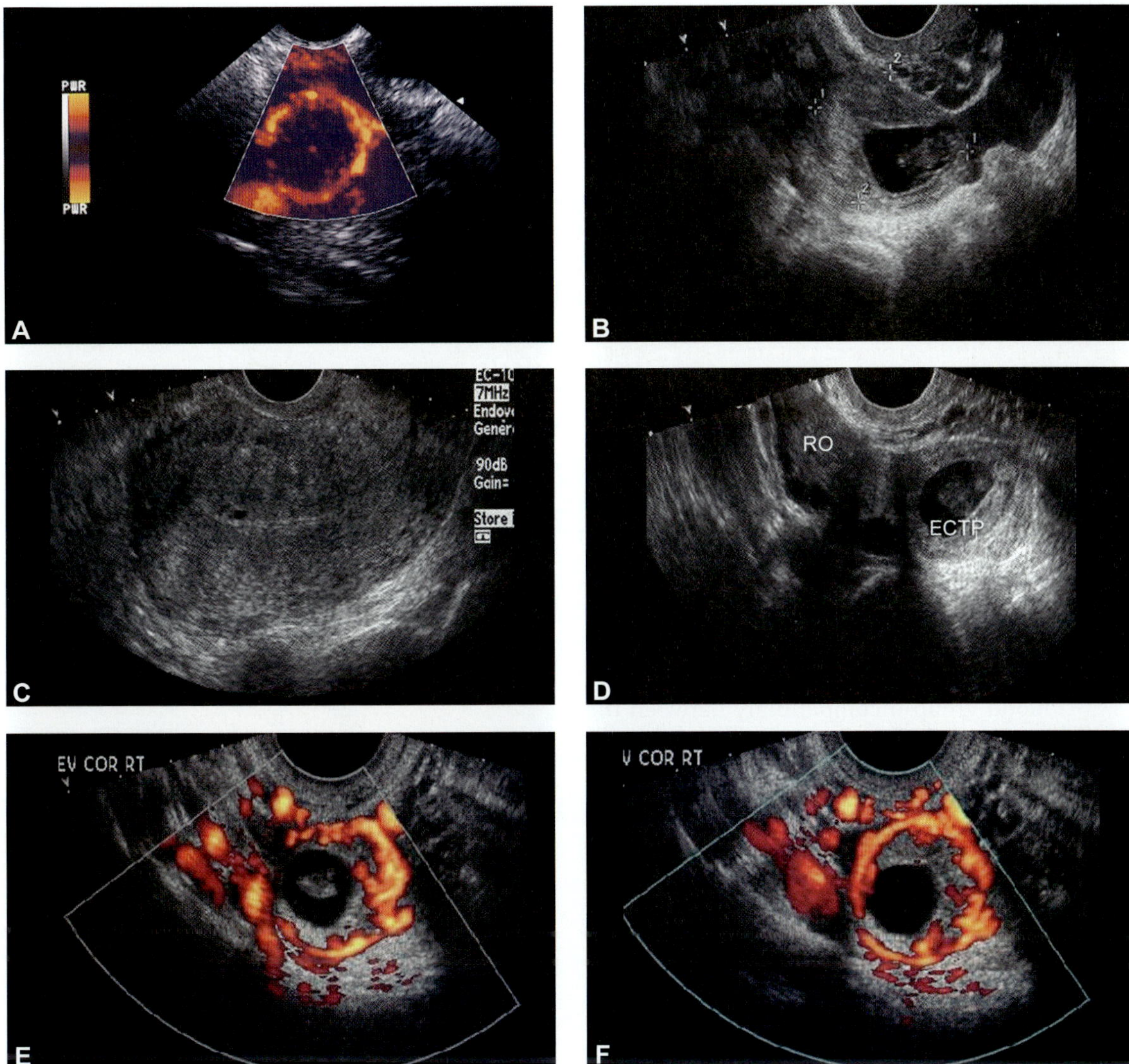

FIGURE 6 **A,** increased blood flow around the ectopic sac; **B,** Shows an ectopic sac with fetal pole; **C,** Pseudogestational sac; **D,** Right tubal ectopic pregnancy; **E,** Ectopic gestational sac with fetal pole with increased blood flow; **F,** Ectopic gestational sac without fetal pole with increased blood flow.

Uncommon Ectopic Sites

- Heterotopic - both intrauterine and extra-uterine; 1/30,000 normal population, as much as 1% with artificial reproductive technology (ART)
- Cervical: 1/2,500–1/18,000 (1%)
- Ovarian: 1/ 2,100–1/60,000 (1–3%)
- Interstitial (1–3%) - swelling adjacent to round ligament. Often misdiagnosed as early, oddly placed intrauterine pregnancy leading to

delay of diagnosis. Associated with uterine rupture
- Abdominal (1.4%) - can go undetected longer resulting in severe hemorrhage, maternal mortality as high as 20%
- Intramural, it occurs within uterine myometrium (It is rare <50 cases reported in literature)
- Cesarean scar pregnancy.

Annexure 13

Fetal Hydrops

It is the pathological accumulation in fluid tissues that leads to
- Ascites
- Pleural effusions
- Pericardial effusions
- Subcutaneous edema.

Two types
- Immune hydrops
  - Blood group incompatibility between the mother and fetus
  - Treatment is intrauterine-fetal blood transfusion
- Non-immune hydrops
  - Prognosis is poor
  - Causes:
    - Cardiac
    - Infections
    - Chromosome abnormalities
    - Twins.

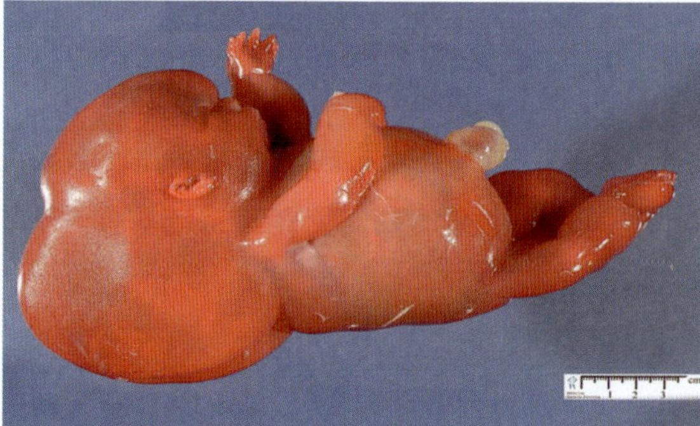

FIGURE 1 Hydropic fetus.

Annexure 14

Nuchal Translucency

Nuchal translucency (NT) is a collection of fluid under the skin behind the neck of fetuses at 11-13+6 weeks that can be measured by ultrasound examination (Figure 1).
- The term translucency is used irrespective of whether it is septated or not, confined to the neck, or envelopes the whole fetus
- NT is increased in fetuses with chromosomal abnormalities, cardiac defects, certain genetic syndromes
- During the second trimester, the translucency usually resolves or it evolves into nuchal edema or cystic hygromas with or without generalized hydrops

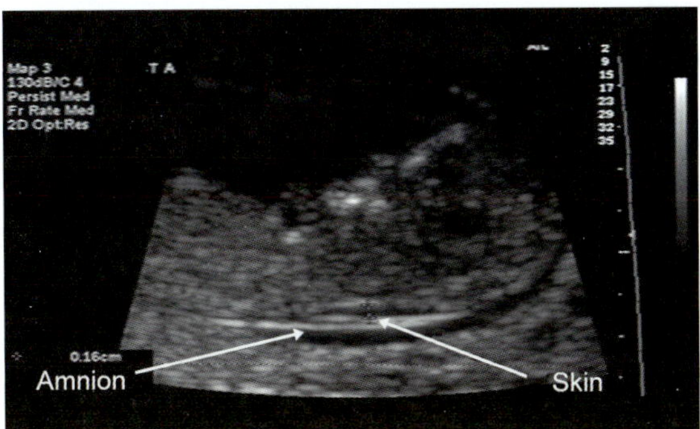

FIGURE 1 Ultrasound (Transvaginal) appearance of nuchal translucency.

- Increased fetal NT thickness at 11–13+6 weeks is a common phenotypic expression of chromosomal defects and a wide range of fetal malformations and genetic syndromes.

First Trimester Nuchal Translucency

- Lymphatic obstruction may be a cystic hygroma or a precursor. It may resolve or persist
- Associated with increased risk of trisomy and cardiac anomalies
- Normal values depend on gestational age
- The wider the translucency, the higher the risk.

Image and Measurement

- The optimal gestational age for measurement of fetal NT is 11 weeks to 13 weeks and 6 days
- The minimum fetal crown-rump length should be 45 mm and the maximum 84 mm
- Transabdominal ultrasound is successful in 95% of cases
- The results from transabdominal and transvaginal scanning are similar
- A mid-sagittal section of the fetus is taken with the fetus is in the neutral position
- Only the fetal head and upper thorax should be included in the image
- The magnification should be as large as possible.
- Care must be taken to distinguish between fetal skin and amnion. This is achieved by
  - Spontaneous fetal movement
  - Asking the mother to cough
  - Tapping the maternal abdomen
  - The maximum thickness of the subcutaneous translucency between the skin and the soft tissue overlying the cervical spine should be measured
  - The callipers should be placed on the lines that define the NT thickness (Figure 2)
  - The crossbar of the calliper merges with the white line of the border and not in the nuchal fluid
  - More than one measurement must be taken
  - The maximum one should be recorded
  - It is good practice to retain at least one image for your patient records.
- In normal fetuses, NT thickness increases with fetal crown-rump length (CRL)
- Increased NT refers to a measurement above the 95th centile
- The median and 95th centile of NT at:
  - CRL of 45 mm are 1.2 and 2.1 mm,
  - CRL of 84 mm are 1.9 and 2.7 mm
- The 99th centile does not change with CRL and it is 3.5 mm (Snijders et al 1998)*
  - NT should be measured with the fetus in the neutral position.
  - When the fetal neck is hyperextended, the measurement can be increased by 0.6 mm.
  - When the neck is flexed, the measurement can be decreased by 0.4 mm.

---

*Snijders RJ, Noble P, Sebine N, Souka A, Nicolaides KH. UK multicentre project on assessment of risk of trisomy 21 by maternal age and fetal nuchal translucency thickness at 10–14 weeks of gestation. Fetal Medicine Foundation First Trimester Screening Group. Lancet. 1998;352 (9125):343–346.

TABLE 1: Screening of chromosomal defects by nuchal translucency

Nuchal translucency	*Chromodomal defects*	*Normal karyotype*		*Alive and well*
		Fetal death	*Major fetal abnormalities*	
<95th centile	0.2%	1.3%	1.6%	97%
95th–99th centiles	3.7%	1.3%	2.5%	93%
3.5–4.4 mm	21.1%	2.7%	10.0%	70%
4.5–5.4 mm	33.3%	3.4%	18.5%	50%
5.5–6.4 mm	50.5%	10.1%	24.2%	30%
≥6.5 mm	64.5%	19.0%	46.2%	15%

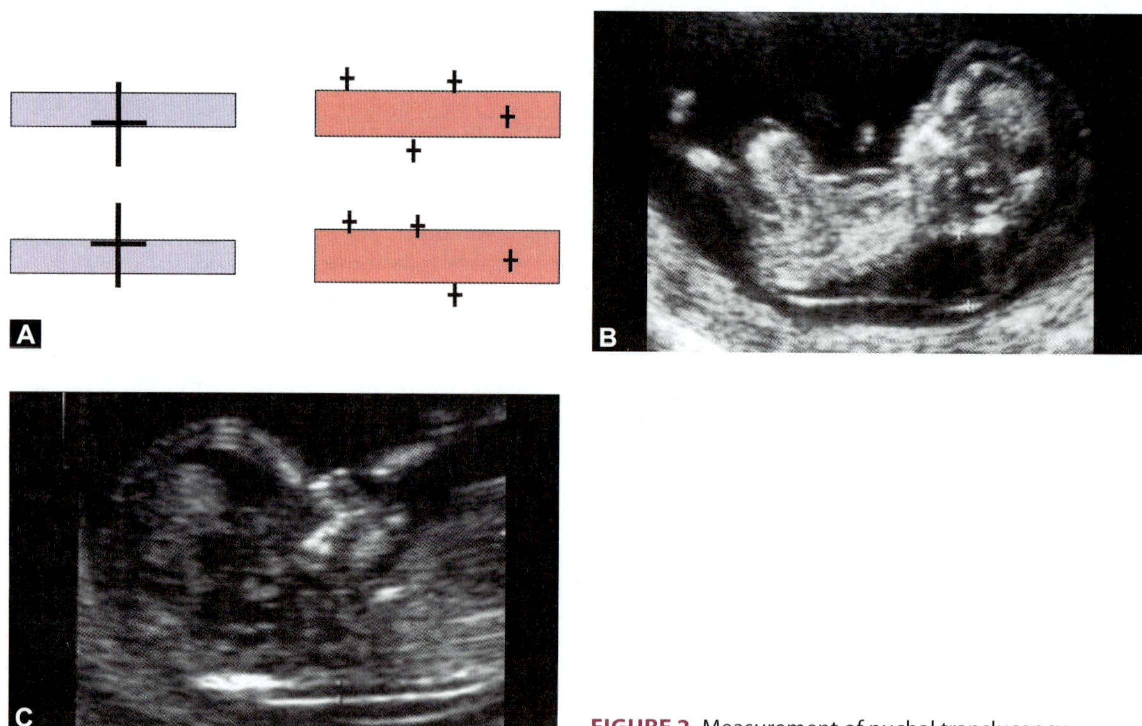

FIGURE 2 Measurement of nuchal translucency.

Screening for chromosomal defects in the first, rather than the second trimester, has the advantage of (Table 1):

- Earlier prenatal diagnosis
- Less traumatic termination of pregnancy
- Disadvantage of earlier screening is that identifies chromosomally abnormal pregnancies that are destined to miscarry spontaneously.

Pathophysiology of Increased Fetal NT

The heterogeneity of conditions associated with increased NT suggests that there may not be a single underlying mechanism for the collection of fluid under the skin of the fetal neck.

The incidence of chromosomal and other abnormalities is related to the size, rather than the appearance of NT

- The correlation between NT and fetal anomalies and perinatal risk is one of the single most important breakthroughs in birth defect screening
- Pathophysiology of increased NT
  - Cardiac dysfunction
  - Venous congestion in the head and neck
  - Altered composition of the extracellular matrix
  - Failure of lymphatic drainage
  - Fetal anemia
  - Fetal hypoproteinemia
  - Fetal infection.

Major Cardiac Defects

In chromosomally normal fetuses, the prevalence of major cardiac defects increases exponentially with NT thickness

- 1.6 per 1,000 for NT below the 95th centile
- 1% for NT of 2.5–3.4 mm
- 3% for NT of 3.5–4.4 mm
- 7% for NT of 4.5–5.4 mm
- 20% for NT of 5.5–6.4 mm
- 30% for NT of 6.5 mm or more
- Increased NT constitutes an indication for specialist fetal echocardiography
- The overall prevalence of major cardiac defects in such a group of fetuses (1–2%) is similar to that found in pregnancies affected by maternal diabetes mellitus or with a history of a previously affected off spring, which are well accepted indications for fetal echocardiography
- Increased NT 99th centile constitutes an indication for specialist fetal echocardiography
- In this population the prevalence of major cardiac defects would be very high
- The best strategy of screening for major cardiac abnormalities is to carry out specialist fetal echocardiography in patients with increased NT at 11-13+6 weeks and in those with an abnormal four-chamber view in the routine mid-trimester scan.

Body Stalk Anomalies

- It is found in about 1 in 10,000 at 10–13+6 weeks
- NT is increased in about 85% of the cases
- The karyotype is usually normal
- The ultrasonographic features are major abdominal wall defect, severe kyphoscoliosis, and short umbilical cord with a single artery.

Diaphragmatic Hernia

Increased NT in

- 40% of fetuses
- 80% of neonatal death due to pulmonary hypoplasia
- 20% of the survivors

Exomphalos

NT Increased in

- 85% of chromosomally abnormal
- 40% of chromosomally normal fetuses
- At 11–13+6 weeks the incidence of exomphalos is 1 in 1,000
- The incidence of chromosomal defects, mainly trisomy 18, is about 60%.

Megacystis

NT increased in

- 75% in chromosomal abnormalities mainly trisomy 13
- 30% normal karyotype.

Annexure 15

Screening for Aneuploidy

- Every woman has a risk that her fetus may have a chromosomal defect
- Background or apriori risk depend on maternal age and gestation
- Individual patient-specific risk is calculated by multiplying apriori risk with a series of likelihood ratios, which depend on results of a series of screening tests carried out during the course of pregnancy
- Women require comprehensive counselling about their access to appropriate diagnostic testing for positive screens including chorionic villous sampling.
- Methods of screening are discussed in table 1. The common chromosomal defects and their prevalence are listed in tables 2 and 3.

TABLE 1: Methods of screening

Method of screening	*DR%*
Maternal age (MA)	30
MA and maternal serum biochemistry at 15–18 wks	50–70
MA and fetal nuchal translucency (NT) at 11–13 +6 wks	70–80
MA and fetal NT and maternal serum free B-hCG and PAPP-A at 11–13+6 wks	85–90
MA and fetal NT and fetal nasal bone (NB) at 11–13 +6 wks	90
MA and fetal NT and NB and maternal serum free B-hCG and PAPP-A at 11–13 +6 wks	95

TABLE 2: Common chromosomal defects in fetuses with sonographic abnormalities

	Trisomy 21	*Trisomy 18*	*Trisomy 13*	*Triploidy*	*Turner*
Nuchal edema	+	+	+		
Cystic hygromas					+
Diaphragmatic hernia		+	+		
Cardiac defect	+	+	+	+	+
Exomphalos		+	+		
Duodenal atresia	+				
Esophageal atresia	+	+			
Renal defects	+	+	+	+	+
Short limbs	+	+		+	+
Clinodactyly	+				
Overlapping fingers		+			
Polydactyly			+		
Syndactyly				+	
Talipes		+	+	+	
Fetal growth restriction		+		+	+

TABLE 3: Prevalence of fetal chromosomal defects in fetuses with isolated and multiple abnormalities

Ventriculomegaly	2%	17%
Holoprosencephaly	4%	39%
Choroid plexus cysts	<1%	48%
Posterior fossa cyst	0%	52%
Facial cleft	0%	51%
Micrognathia	-	62%
Cystic hygroma	52%	71%
Nuchal oedema	19%	45%
Diphragmatic hernia	2%	49%
Heart defects	16%	66%
Duodenal atresia	38%	64%
Exomphalos	8%	46%
Talipes	0%	33%
Growth retardation	4%	38%

Advantages to 1st Trimester Screening

Earlier diagnosis

- Pregnancy is less obvious, more private
  - May be less maternal bonding to pregnancy
- Pregnancy termination easier and safer

CAVEAT: Test needs to have high sensitivity and low false positives

Disadvantages to 1st Trimester Screening

- Patients must present early
- Does not assess neural tube defects
- Chorionic villous sampling is slightly at higher risk, and is not as accurate as amniocentesis
- Difficulties with multiple gestations
- First trimester screening may identify fetuses destined to abort spontaneously.

Approaches to Screening

- Nuchal translucency (NT) alone (Figure 1)
- First trimester biochemistry alone
- Combined: NT and first trimester biochemistry
- Integrated first and second trimester
  - No result until both tests done
- Sequential first and second trimester
  - Results known after first test
- Second trimester screening alone.

Trisomy 18

- 2nd most common chromosomal abnormality (Figure 2)
- 1 : 3000 births
- Ultrasound identified abnormalities:
  - Congenital heart disease

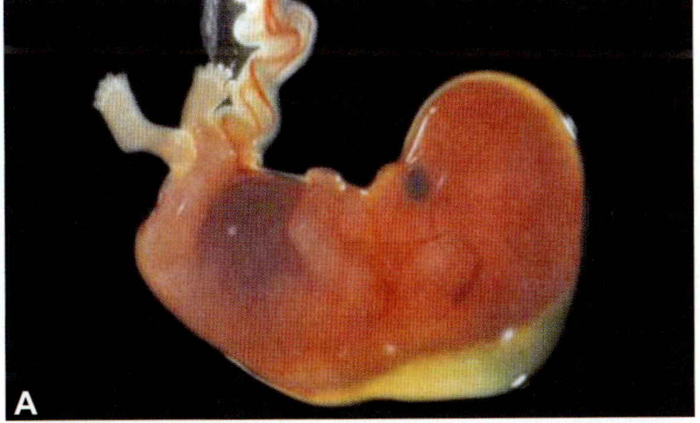

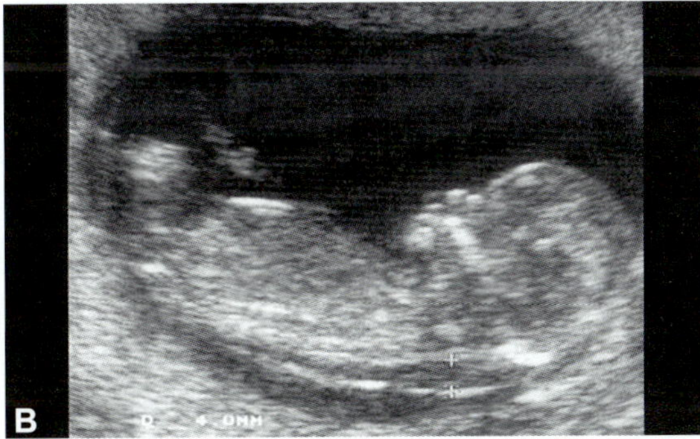

FIGURE 1 Endoscopic image showing increased nuchal transluscency.

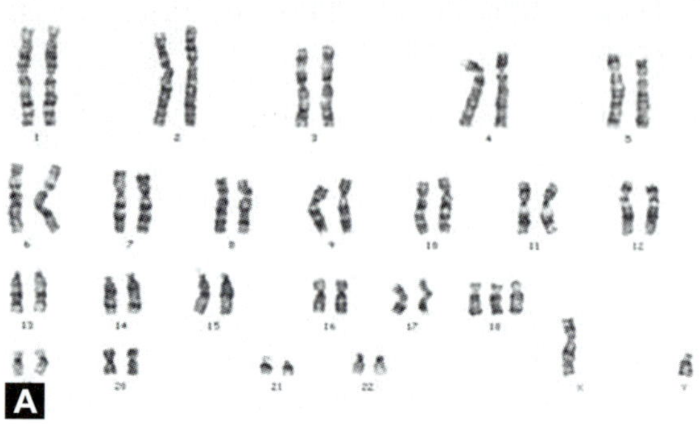
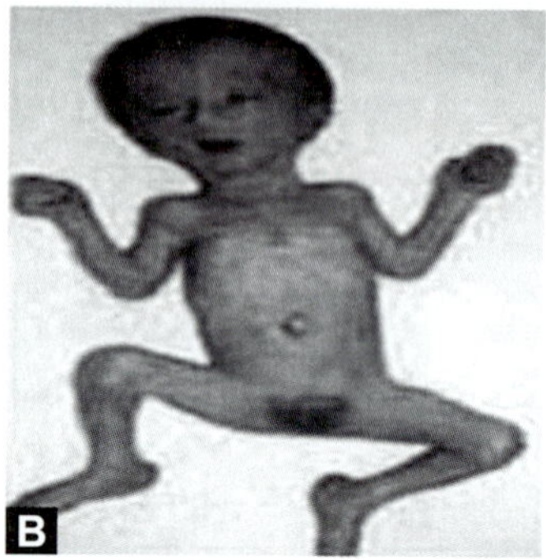
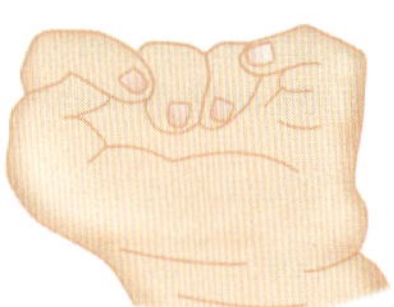

FIGURE 2 **A,** Karyotype of Trisomy 18; **B,** Trisomy 18 (Inset shows clenched hands).

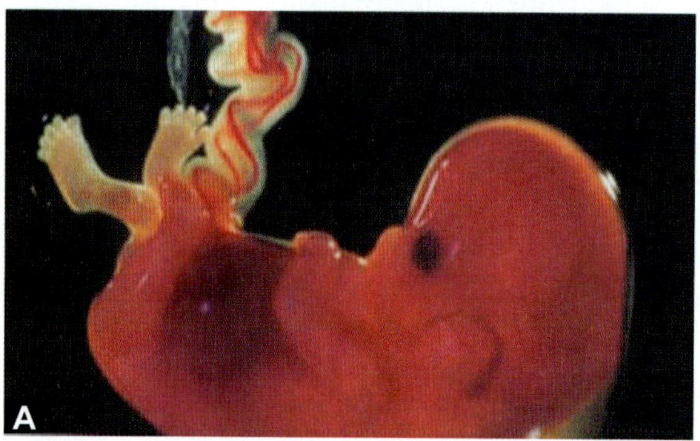
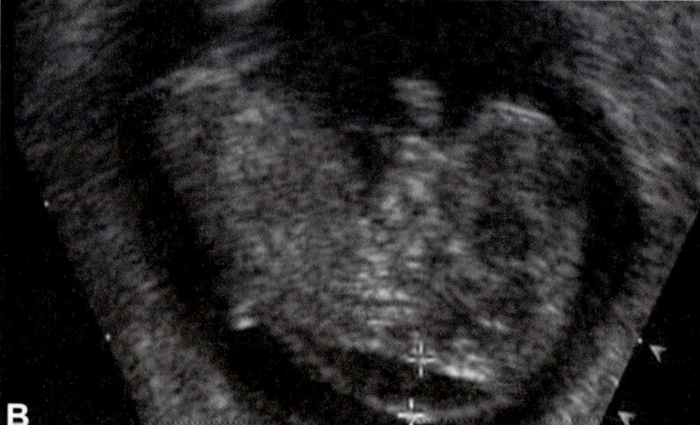

FIGURE 3 Increased nuchal translucency in Trisomy 21 (Down syndrome).

- Congenital diaphragmatic hernia
- Omphalocele
- Neural tube defects
- Dandy-Walker abnormality
- Clenched hands
- Single umbilical artery.

Trisomy 21

First trimester screening for Trisomy 21 (Figure 3) by ultrasound and age is described in table 4.

TABLE 4: First trimester screening for Trisomy 21 by ultrasound and age

Test	Performance
NT	T21 70–80%
NT + Nasal bone	T21 85–90%
Abnormal ductus venosus waveform	T21 78% (at a SP rate of 1.7% in a high risk population)
NT + Nasal bone + abnormal ductus venosus waveform	T21 > 90% at a lower SP rate of 2–3%

NT, nuchal translucency; SP, screen positive.

Annexure 16

Nasal Bone

Examination of Nasal Bone

- The gestation should be 11 to 3 + 6 weeks and fetal crown-rump length (CRL) should be 45–84 mm
- Image should be magnified so that head and upper thorax only are included in screen
- A mid-sagittal view of fetal profile should be obtained with ultrasound transducer held in parallel to direction of nose
- In image of nose there should be 3 distinct lines. The top line represents skin and bottom one, which is thicker and more echogenic than overlying skin, represents nasal bone. A 3rd line, almost in continuity with skin, but a higher level, represents tip of nose
- At 11 to 13 + 6 weeks, fetal profile can be successfully examined in more than 95% of cases (Figure 1)
- In chromosomally normal fetuses, incidence of absent nasal bone is less than 1% in Caucasian populations and about 10% in Afro-Caribbeans.

Nasal Bone Sonography: Criteria

- Magnify until only head and upper thorax visible
- Mid-sagittal plane
- Angle insonation 45^0 to facial plane (Figure 2)
- Tilt probe side-to-side
- 3 lines visible at nose:
  - Top line is nasal skin
  - Bottom line, more echogenic is nasal bone
  - Front line above nasal skin is tip of nose
- Nasal bone absent if not visible or less echogenic than skin (Figure 3).

Nasal Bone –Aneuploidy

- The nasal bone is absent
  - in 60–70% of trisomy 21 fetuses (Figure 4)
  - in about 50% of trisomy 18 fetuses and
  - in 30% of trisomy 13 fetuses.
- For a false positive rate of 5%, screening by a combination of sonography for fetal nuchal translucency, nasal bone, and maternal serum

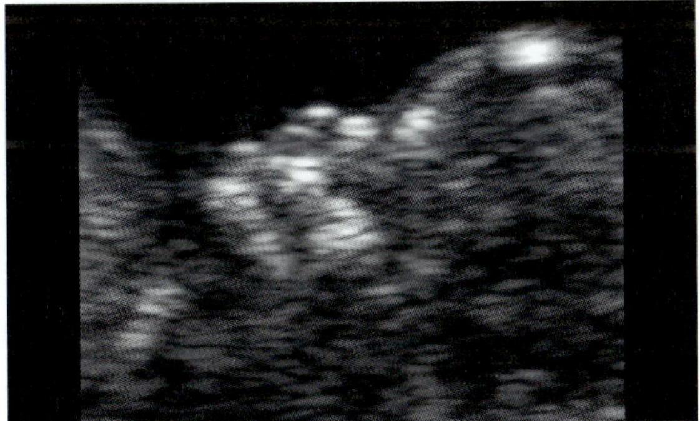

FIGURE 1 Presence of nasal bone in a euploid fetus in first trimester.

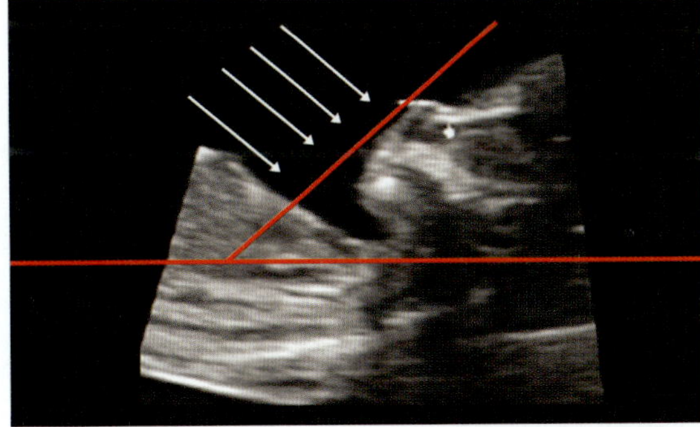

FIGURE 2 Nasal bone sonography: 45^0 angle insonation.

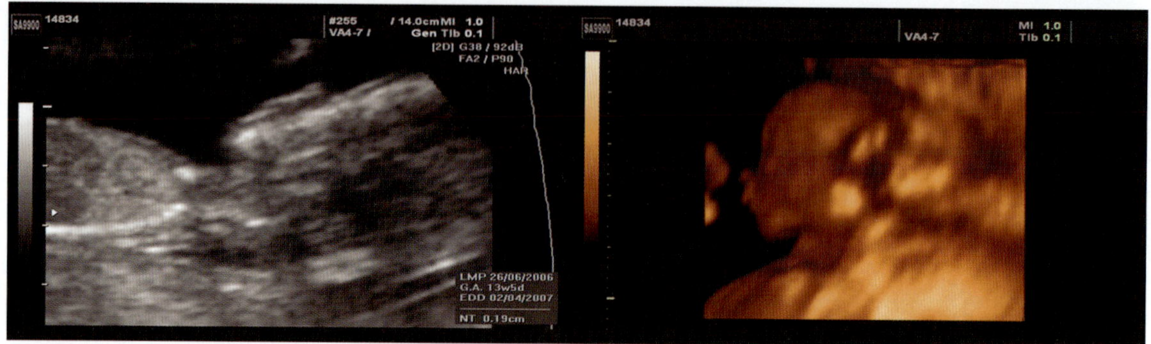

FIGURE 3 Absent nasal bone.

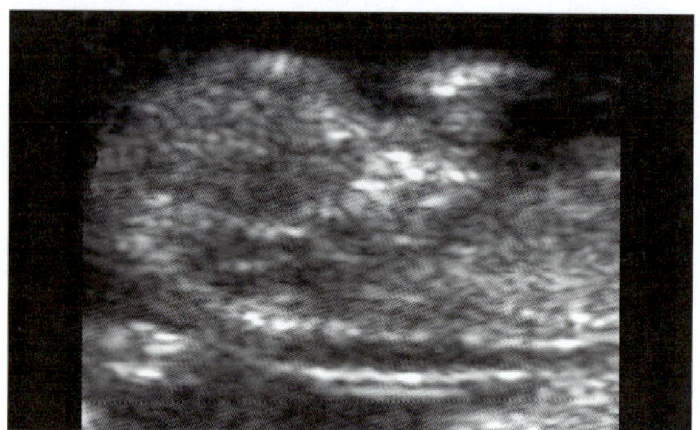

FIGURE 4 Absent nasal bone in a fetus with Trisomy 21 in first trimester.

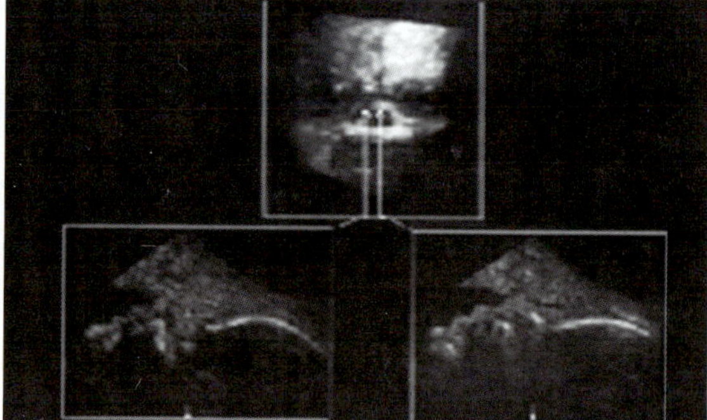

FIGURE 5 Use of 3D ultrasound for detection of absent nasal bone.

free beta human chorionic gonadotropin (B-hCG) and pregnancy associated plasma protein-A (PAPP-A) can potentially identify more than 95% of trisomy 21 pregnancies.

- A 3D and 4D ultrasound improves the detection of absent nasal bone (Figure 5).\

Annexure 17

Maxillary Triangle

Fetal Facial Angle

- Facial angle is quantification of flat facial profile seen in fetuses with trisomy 21. This is also known as frontomaxillary facial angle (FMF angle). Since maxilla is small and set back in these fetuses, angle becomes wider.
- Facial angle is increased (> 95 percentile) in
  - 5% of euploid fetuses
  - 45% of fetuses with trisomy 21
  - 55% of fetuses with trisomy 18
  - 45% of fetuses with trisomy 13.
- Facial angle decreases with an increase in crown rump length (CRL) and the software must therefore include CRL. The angle is measured in same image as nuchal translucency (NT) and nasal bone (NB). Angle is measured between a line along the superior surface of palate and a line drawn from anterosuperior corner of maxilla to anterior surface of frontal bones (Figure 1)
- Assessment of facial angle, in addition to NT, increases detection rate of trisomy 21 from 90 to 94% and decreases false positive rate from 3 to 2.5 %.

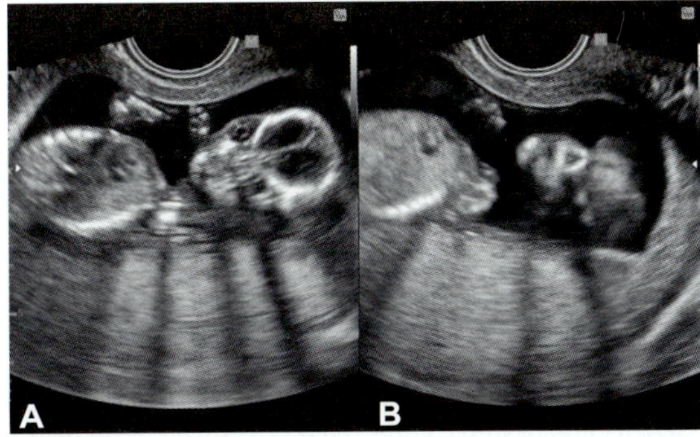

FIGURE 1 **A,** Fetal face; **B,** Maxillary triangle.

Annexure 18

Intracranial Translucency

- Assessment of intracranial translucency (IT) at 11–14 weeks in screening for open spina bifida
- The findings demonstrate that at 11–13 weeks' gestation, the fourth cerebral ventricle is easily recognizable as an intracranial translucency in standard mid-sagittal view of face used routinely in screening for chromosomal abnormalities
- Examination of mid-sagittal view of fetal face is performed routinely for assessment of fetal nuchal translucency (NT) and nasal bone in screening for aneuploidies
- If in this same view, the fourth ventricle is not visible sonographer should be alerted to possibility of an underlying open spina bifida and undertake detailed examination of fetal spine
- Professor Rabi Chaoui presented a "new sign" as possible screen for open spina bifida at 11–14 weeks (absent IT)

- Mid-sagittal view of fetal face is of same view as used for measurement of NT + assessment of nasal bone
- Brain stem and fourth cerebral ventricle are easily visible:
  - The fourth ventricle presents as an IT
  - Parallel to NT and is delineated by 2 echogenic borders
- Between fourth ventricle and occiput there is:
  - Another thinner translucency generated by developing cisterna cerebellomedullaris (Chaoui et al)*.

Absent Intracranial translucency and open spina bifida

- In some cases of open spina bifida, the fourth ventricle is not visible (absent IT)
- This is as a result of leakage of cerebrospinal fluid into amniotic cavity, causing hypotension in subarachnoid spaces leading to downward displacement of brain (Figure 1)
  - The "banana" and "lemon" signs are seen at 16–24 weeks
- The downward displacement of fetal brain is visible as absent IT in first trimester (Chaoui et al.)*.

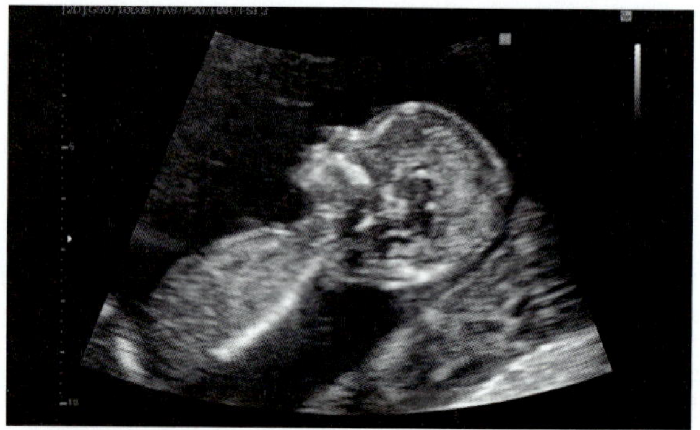

FIGURE 1 Ultrasound showing intracranial translucency.

*Chaoui R, Benoit B, Mitkowaska-Wozniak H, Heling KS, Nicolaides KH. Assessment of intracranial translucency (IT) in the detection of spina bifida at the 11–13-week scan. *Ultrasound Obstet Gynecol.* 2009;34:249–252.

Annexure 19

Ductus Venosus

Abnormal Flow in Ductus Venosus and Chromosomal Defects

- At 11 to 13 + 6 weeks, abnormal ductal flow is observed in 5% of chromosomally normal fetuses and in about 80% of fetuses with trisomy 21
- Assessment of ductus venosus (DV) can be combined with measurement of fetal nuchal translucency (NT) to improve effectiveness of early sonographic screening for trisomy 21.
- Examination of ductal flow is time-consuming and requires highly skilled operators (Figures 1–4). It is therefore unlikely to be used in routine screening, but it could be used in specialist centres to re-evaluate risk in patients with borderline results after screening by fetal NT and maternal serum biochemistry.

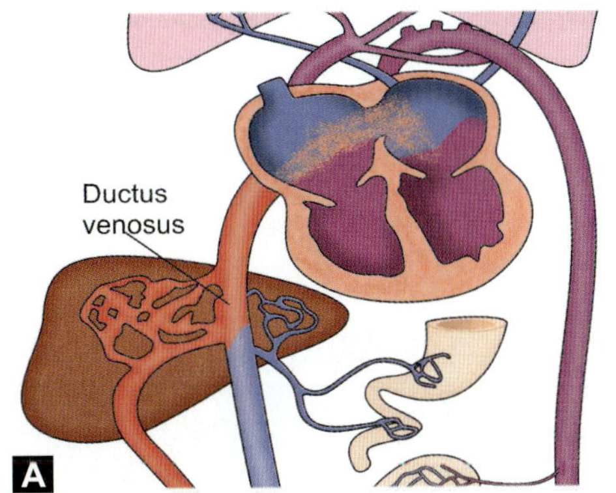

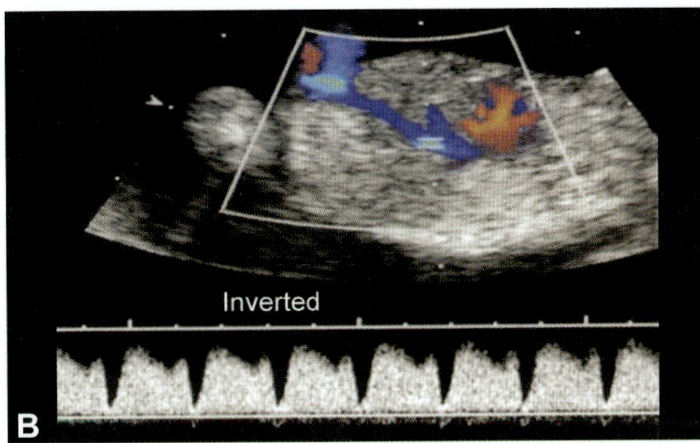

FIGURE 1 **A,** Anatomy of ductus venosus; **B,** Ultrasound showing anatomy of ductus venosus.

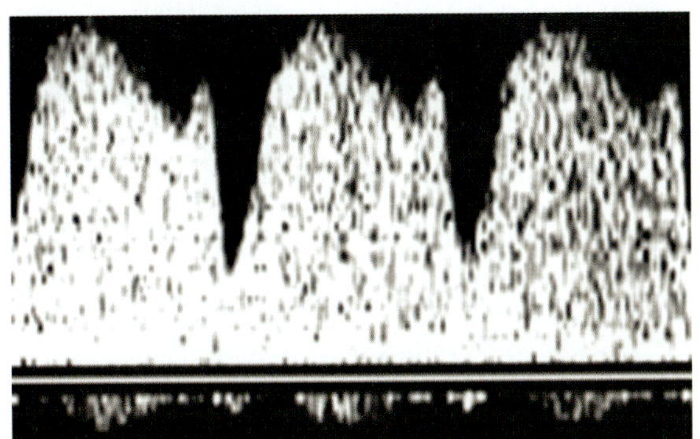

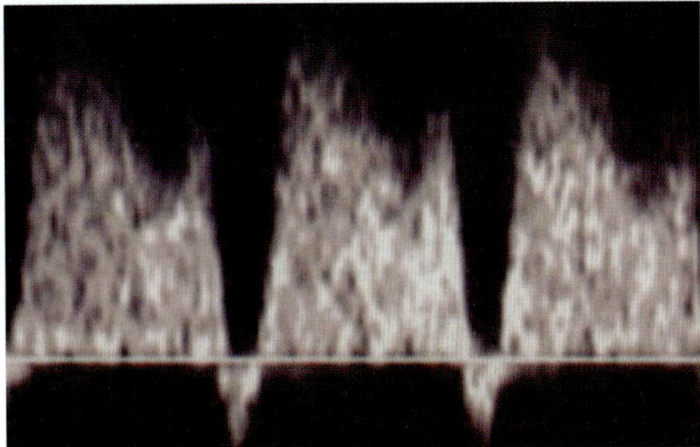

FIGURE 2 Normal ductus venosus waveform.

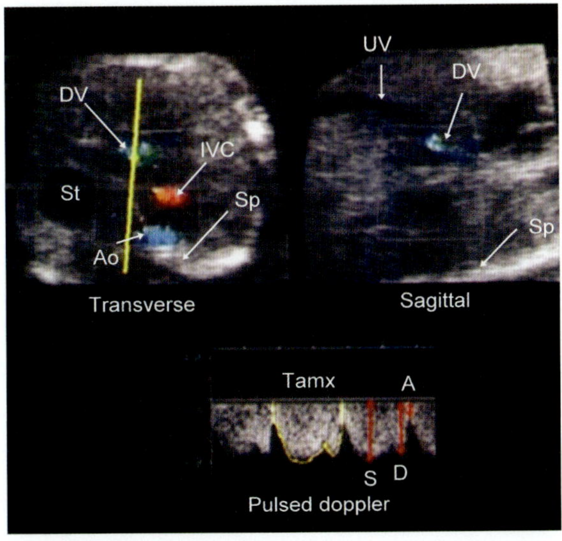

FIGURE 3 Transverse and sagittal section of ductus venosus + Tmax.

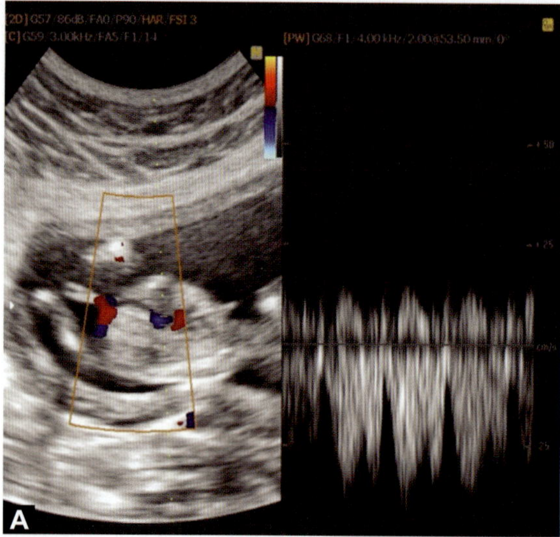

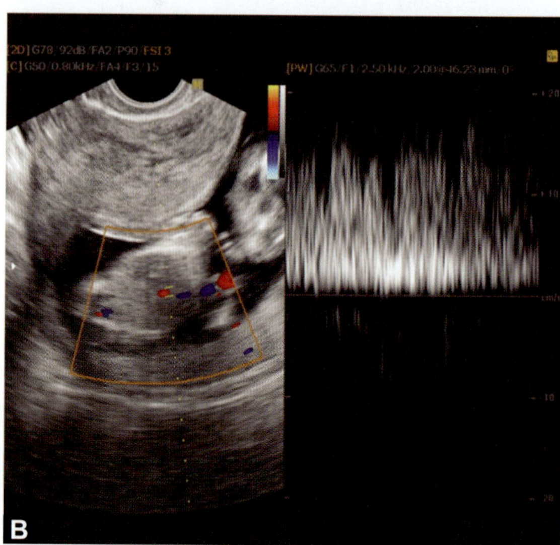

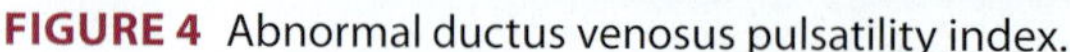

FIGURE 4 Abnormal ductus venosus pulsatility index.

Matias et al 1998* performed ductus venosus Doppler in fetuses with increased NT and observed:

- Abnormal ductus in 57 of 63 (90.5%) chromosomally abnormal fetuses
- Abnormal ductus in 13 of 423 (3.1%) chromosomally normal fetuses
- 7 of 13 with absent or reversed flow had major cardiac defect demonstrated 14–16 weeks.

*Matias A, Gomes C, Flack N, Montenegro N, Nicolaides KH. Screening for chromosomal abnormalities at 10-14 weeks: The role of ductus venosus blood flow. *Ultrasound Obstet Gynecol.* 1998;12:380-4.

Annexure 20

Tricuspid Regurgitation

- The documentation of tricuspid regurgitation (TR) increases the risk for trisomy 21 as well as for cardiac defects
- Fetus should not be moving. An apical 4 chamber view is obtained and magnified so that entire screen is occupied by thorax. Color flow mapping is not used. The insonation angle should not exceed 30 degrees
- The sample volume is positioned across tricuspid valve. The gate should be 2 to 3 mm wide. The sweep speed should be high: 2–3 cm/sec.

- TR is diagnosed if it is found during at least half of duration of systole and with a velocity greater than 60 cm/sec (Figure 1)
- In 1,557 high-risk pregnancies studied* at 11–13 weeks, TR >60/sec was seen in
  - 58/1323 (4%) of normal fetuses
  - 77/114 (68%) of fetuses with Trisomy 21.

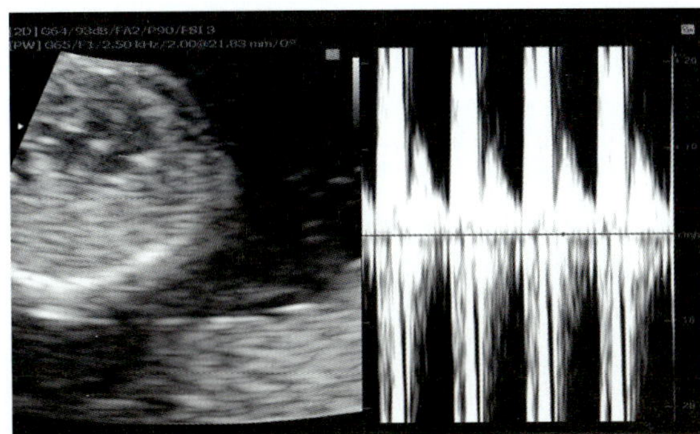

FIGURE 1 Tricuspid regurgitation.

*Falcon et al. Screening for trisomy 21 by fetal tricuspid regurgitation, nuchal translucency and maternal serum free beta-hCG and PAPP-A at 11 + 0 to 13 + 6 weeks. *Ultrasound Obstet Gynecol.* 2006;27(2):151-5.

Annexure 21

Uterine Anomaly and Adnexal Masses

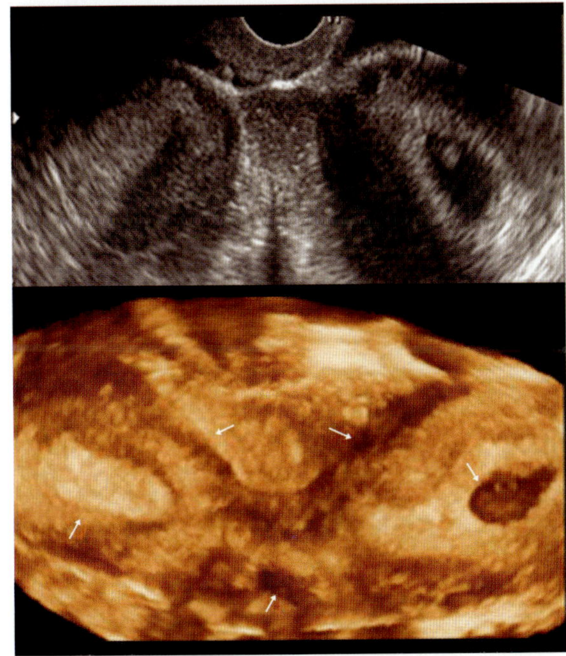

FIGURE 1 2D and 3D appearance of a bicornuate uterus with gestational sac in right horn.

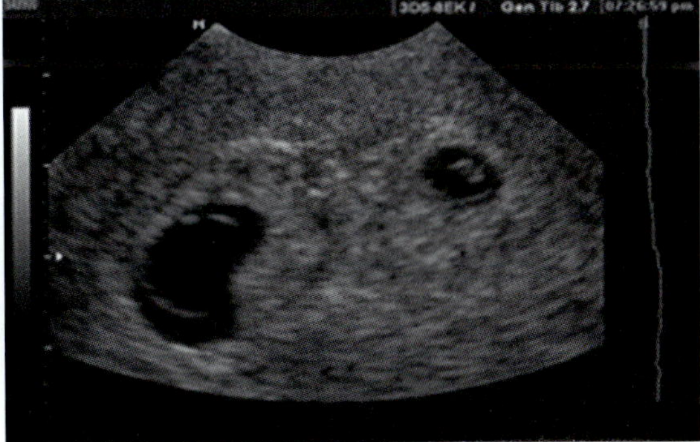

FIGURE 2 2D appearance of a bicornuate uterus with gestational sac in both horns.

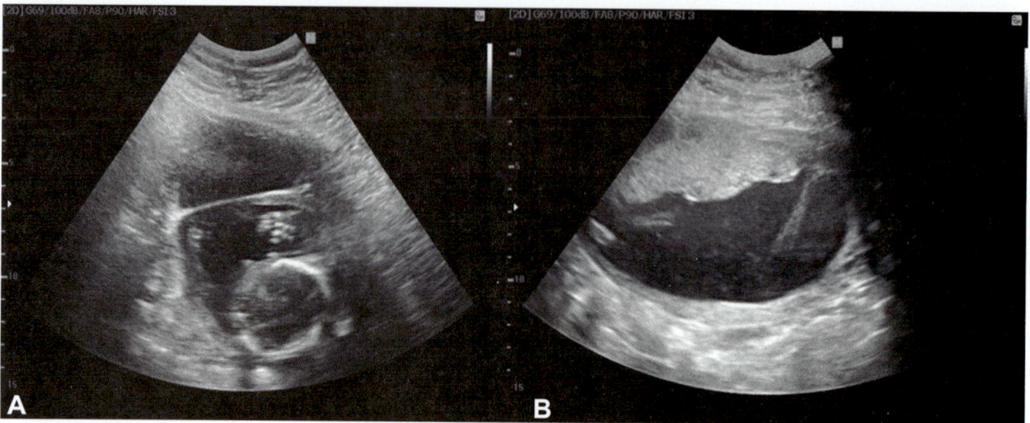

FIGURE 3 Ultrasound showing amniotic band.

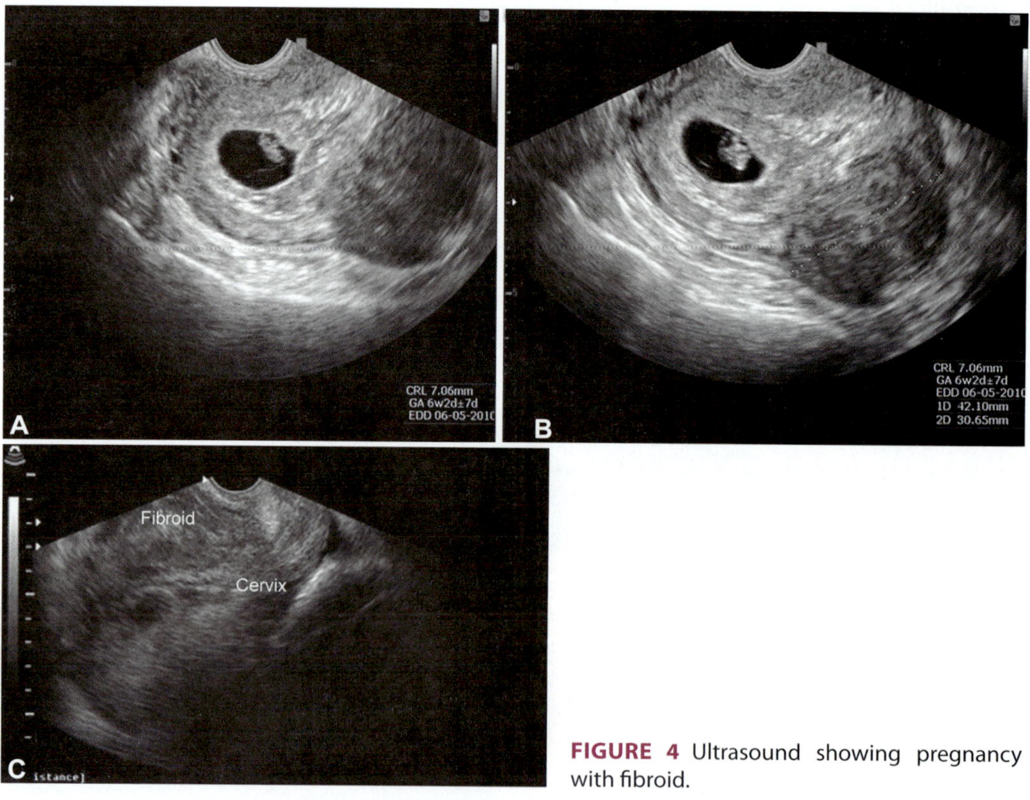

FIGURE 4 Ultrasound showing pregnancy with fibroid.

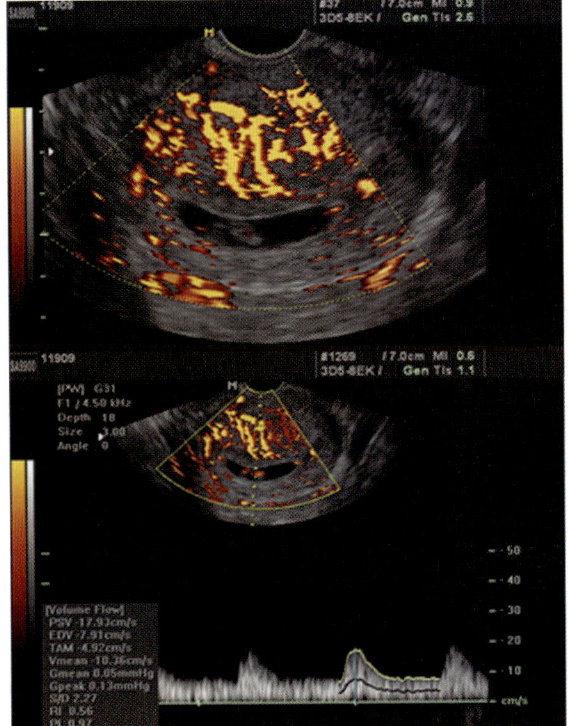

FIGURE 5 Ultrasound showing pregnancy with adenomyosis.

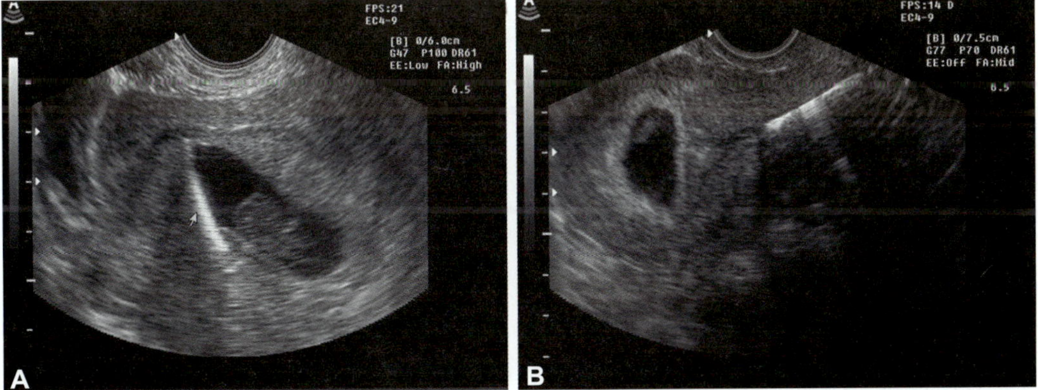

FIGURE 6 Ultrasound showing pregnancy with an intrauterine contraceptive device (IUCD).

Annexure 22

Documentation of First Trimester Ultrasound

1. Intrauterine/extrauterine pregnancy
2. Chorionic plate/placental localization – echogenicity
3. Cervix
4. Biometry – GS/ CRL/BPD/FL
5. Spine
6. Stomach bubble, abdominal wall
7. Extremities – all 4 limbs
8. Face
   - Nasal bone
   - Premaxillary triangle
   - FMF angle
   - Nuchal thickness
   - Intracranial translucency
9. Heart
   - Situs, heart rate, rhythum
   - 4 chamber view
   - 3 vessel view
   - Outflow tract
   - Tricuspid regurgitation
10. Ductus Venosus
11. Uterine masses/adnexal masses/foreign body

GS, gestational sac; CRL, crown rump length; BPD, biparietal diameter; FL, femur length; FMF, frontomaxillary facial angle.

Index

Please note page numbers with *f* and *t* indicate figure and table, respectively.

C

D

E

F

G

H

M

N

O

P

T

U

V

W

X

Y

Z